Nurse Practitioners

The Evolution and Future of Advanced Practice

Fifth Edition

Eileen M. Sullivan-Marx, PhD, CRNP, FAAN, is an associate professor at the University of Pennsylvania School of Nursing and Program Director for the Adult Health and Gerontology Nurse Practitioner Programs. With over 20 years' experience in the nursing field and as a primary care nurse practitioner with a special interest in geriatrics, Dr. Sullivan-Marx has been on the forefront of new trends in nursing practice since 1980. She has established innovative, model practices for nursing in hospital, outpatient, home care, and nursing-home settings. She is a founder, advisor, and consultant with the Gerontological Nursing Consultation Service/PNN Consulting at the University of Pennsylvania School of Nursing. Her trend-setting experience has led to numerous national appointments on policy committees addressing quality of health care and payment issues for nurses. From 1993–2002, she represented nursing in the American Medical Association's Relative Value Update Committee that sets work values for the Medicare Fee Schedule.

Diane O'Neill McGivern, PhD, RN, FAAN, is a professor at the New York University College of Nursing and is currently responsible for teaching professional nursing and health care issues in the baccalaureate and master's programs.

Dr. McGivern has been active in professional nursing and other health organizations and has received honors and awards for her work. She has been a Robert Wood Johnson Health Policy Fellow, was elected to the American Academy of Nursing, and served on the board of the Nurses' Educational Fund. She has produced numerous articles, book chapters, speeches, and presentations during her prolific career, focusing on professional practice preparation, particularly advanced practice nursing.

Julie A. Fairman, PhD, RN, FAAN, is a professor at the University of Pennsylvania School of Nursing and is an internationally renowned nurse historian. She is the director of the Barbara Bates Center for the Study of the History of Nursing. Dr. Fairman is the author of two critically acclaimed books, *Critical Care Nursing: A History* (University of Penn Press, 1998), authored with her mentor, Dr. Joan Lynaugh, and *Making Room in the Clinic: Nurse Practitioners and the Evolution of Modern Health Care* (Rutgers University Press, 2008), an analysis of the American nurse practitioner movement. Both books received distinguished awards from the American Association for the History of Nursing.

Sherry A. Greenberg, MSN, GNP-BC, received both her Bachelor of Science in Nursing and Master of Science in Nursing from the University of Pennsylvania School of Nursing. Ms. Greenberg has worked as a gerontological nurse practitioner in a variety of clinical settings, including a skilled nursing facility, an inpatient acute care for elders unit, and outpatient geriatric primary care practices. Ms. Greenberg was the Coordinator of the Advanced Practice Nursing: Geriatrics Program at New York University College of Nursing from 1997 to 2001. Since then, Ms. Greenberg has worked as a consultant at the Hartford Institute for Geriatric Nursing at New York University College of Nursing. Ms. Greenberg is the Series Co-Editor of the *Try This®* series on Best Practices in Nursing Care for Older Adults and the Resources Manager of the Hartford Institute's clinical Web site, http://www.ConsultGeriRN.org.

Nurse Practitioners

The Evolution and Future of Advanced Practice

Fifth Edition

Editors

EILEEN M. SULLIVAN-MARX, PhD, CRNP, FAAN
DIANE O. McGIVERN, PhD, RN, FAAN
JULIE A. FAIRMAN, PhD, RN, FAAN
SHERRY A. GREENBERG, MSN, GNP-BC

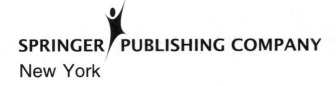

SPRINGER PUBLISHING COMPANY
New York

Springer Publishing Company, LLC
11 West 42nd Street
New York, NY 10036
www.springerpub.com

Acquisitions Editor: Allan Graubard
Production Editor: Pamela Lankas
Cover design: Steve Pisano
Composition: International Graphic Services

E-book ISBN: 978-0-8261-1822-6

10 11 12 13 / 5 4 3 2

The author and the publisher of this Work have made every effort to use sources believed to be reliable to provide information that is accurate and compatible with the standards generally accepted at the time of publication. Because medical science is continually advancing, our knowledge base continues to expand. Therefore, as new information becomes available, changes in procedures become necessary. We recommend that the reader always consult current research and speci?c institutional policies before performing any clinical procedure. The author and publisher shall not be liable for any special, consequential, or exemplary damages resulting, in whole or in part, from the readers' use of, or reliance on, the information contained in this book.

The publisher has no responsibility for the persistence or accuracy of URLs for external or third-party Internet Web sites referred to in this publication and does not guarantee that any content on such Web sites is, or will remain, accurate or appropriate.

Library of Congress Cataloging-in-Publication Data

Nurse practitioners : the evolution and future of advanced practice / Eileen M. Sullivan-Marx ... [et al.], editors.—5th ed.
    p. ; cm.
Includes bibliographical references and index.
ISBN 978-0-8261-1821-9 (alk. paper)
    1. Nurse practitioners. 2. Primary care (Medicine) I. Sullivan-Marx, Eileen. [DNLM: 1. Nurse Practitioners. 2. Primary Health Care. WY 128 N9738 2010]
    RT82.8.N884 2010
    610.7306'92—dc22

                                    2010008764

Printed in the United States of America by Bang Printing

We dedicate this book to our families and to Dr. Mathy Mezey and all the nurse practitioner pioneers who blazed the trails ahead of us

Contents

Contributors   *xi*
Foreword   *xvii*
  Loretta C. Ford, EdD, RN, PNP, FAAN, FAANP
Preface   *xix*
Acknowledgments   *xxi*

PART I: HISTORICAL AND CURRENT SOCIAL CONTEXT   1

1   Historic and Historical Opportunities: Nurse Practitioners and
    the Opportunities of Health Reform   3
    Julie A. Fairman

2   Evolution of Advanced Practice: "Coming to Terms" With Nurse
    Practitioner Definitions and Descriptions   15
    Diane O. McGivern

3   Current Status of Advanced-Practice Nurses in the United States
    and Throughout the Globe   31
    Eileen M. Sullivan-Marx

4   Consumer Role for Nurse Practitioner Care: Center to Champion
    Nursing in America   43
    Brenda L. Cleary, Susan C. Reinhard, Eileen M. Sullivan-Marx, and
    Diane O. McGivern

5   Public Relations Strategies for Nurse Practitioners   49
    Joy McIntyre

**PART II: RESEARCH SUPPORTING NURSE PRACTITIONERS AND
THEIR PRACTICE   63**

6   Research in Support of Nurse Practitioners   65
    Frances Hughes, Sean Clarke, Deborah A. Sampson, Julie A. Fairman,
    and Eileen M. Sullivan-Marx

7 Long-Term Outcomes of Advanced-Practice Nursing   93
Susan W. Groth, Lisa Norsen, and Harriet J. Kitzman

PART III: REGULATORY AND POLICY ENVIRONMENTS   111

8 State Health Care Reform: The Role of Nurse Practitioners
in Massachusetts   113
Nancy O'Rourke

9 Consensus Model for Advanced-Practice Nurse Regulation:
A New Approach   125
Jean Johnson, Ellen Dawson, and Andrea Brassard

10 Politics of Organized Opposition: A Case Example   143
Thomas A. Mackey and Lynda Freed Woolbert

11 The Idiosyncratic Politics of Prescriptive Authority:
Comparing Two States' Legislative Negotiations   149
Deborah A. Sampson

**PART IV: INTEGRATION OF NURSE PRACTITIONERS IN THE HEALTH CARE
ENVIRONMENT   159**

12 Environmental Factors Shaping Advanced Practice   161
Diane O. McGivern

13 Nurse-Managed Health Centers   183
Eunice S. King and Tine Hansen-Turton

14 The Pediatric Nurse Practitioner and the Child With Type 1
Diabetes: Partnership and Collaboration   199
Terri H. Lipman

15 Adult Health and Gerontology Nurse Practitioner Care   205
Melissa A. Taylor and Christine Bradway

16 Nurse Practitioner Contributions to HIV Care   213
Carl Kirton

17 Roles of Nurse Practitioners in the U.S. Department
of Veterans Affairs   223
Karen R. Robinson

18   Ethical Issues in Advanced-Practice Nursing   239
Connie M. Ulrich and Mindy B. Zeitzer

**PART V: BUSINESS AND PAYMENT STRUCTURES
FOR NURSE PRACTITIONERS   255**

19   Business, Policy, and Politics: Success Factors for Nurse
Practitioner Practice   257
Eileen M. Sullivan-Marx

20   Systems of Payment for Advanced-Practice Nurses   271
Eileen M. Sullivan-Marx and David M. Keepnews

21   Nurse Practitioners Navigating Managed Care   295
Elizabeth Miller

22   Community-Based Health Centers:
Nurse Practitioners Contributing to Access   305
Ann Ritter

23   Quality and Safety: Critical Components of a Nurse
Practitioner Business Model   317
Kathryn Fiandt and Joanne M. Pohl

PART VI: GLOBAL HEALTH AND FUTURE CHALLENGES   335

24   Global Health and Future Challenges   337
Helen Ward

25   The Evolution and Future of Nurse Practitioners
in New Zealand   345
Tine Hansen-Turton and Frances Hughes

26   Advanced-Practice Nursing in Ireland   363
Kathleen MacLellan

27   One Look at the Future   375
Diane O. McGivern, Eileen M. Sullivan-Marx, and Julie A. Fairman

28   Online Resources   379
Sherry A. Greenberg

Index   389

Contributors

Christine Bradway, PhD, CRNP
Assistant Professor of Gerontological Nursing
Program Director, Gerontology Nurse Practitioner Program
University of Pennsylvania School of Nursing
Philadelphia, PA

Andrea Brassard, DNSc, MPH, APRN, ANP
ANP Program Coordinator
The George Washington University, Department of Nursing Education
Washington, DC

Sean Clarke, PhD, RN, FAAN
Associate Professor, RBC Chair in Cardiovascular Nursing Research
Lawrence S. Bloomberg Faculty of Nursing
University of Toronto and Peter Munk Cardiac Centre, University
   Health Network
Toronto, ON
Canada

Brenda L. Cleary, PhD, RN, FAAN
Director, Center to Champion Nursing in America
Washington, DC

Ellen Dawson, PhD, APRN, ANP
Chair, Department of Nursing Education
The George Washington University, Department of Nursing Education
Washington, DC

Kathryn Fiandt, DNS, FAANP
Professor and Associate Dean for Graduate Programs and Clinical Affairs
The Finke Distinguished Chair of Nursing Arts
UTMB School of Nursing
Center for Nursing Practice Development
Galveston, TX

Loretta C. Ford, EdD, RN, PNP, FAAN, FAANP
Cofounder, Pediatric Nurse Practitioner Role (1965)
Professor and Dean Emeritus
University of Rochester
School of Nursing
Rochester, New York

Lynda Freed Woolbert, MSN, RN, CPNP-PC
Executive Director
Coalition for Nurses in Advanced Practice (CNAP)
West Columbia, TX

Susan W. Groth, PhD, RN, WHNP-BC
Assistant Professor
University of Rochester, School of Nursing
Rochester, NY

Tine Hansen-Turton, MGA, JD
CEO, National Nursing Centers Consortium
Vice President, Public Health Management Corporation
Philadelphia, PA

Frances Hughes, ONZM, DNurs, FACOMH, FNZCOMH
Adjunct Professor
AUT Auckland and UTS Sydney
WHO PIMHnet Facilitator
Auckland, New Zealand

Jean Johnson, PhD, RN, FAAN
Senior Associate Dean for Health Sciences Programs, School of Medicine
and Health Sciences
The George Washington University, Department of Nursing Education
Washington, DC

David M. Keepnews, PhD, JD, RN, FAAN
Associate Professor
Hunter-Bellevue School of Nursing
New York, NY

Eunice S. King, PhD, RN
Director, Research and Evaluation
Senior Program Officer
Independence Foundation
Philadelphia, PA

Carl Kirton, DNP, RN, ANP-BC, ACRN
Vice President, Nursing & Nurse Practitioner
North General Hospital
Clinical Associate Professor of Nursing
New York University
New York, NY

Harriet J. Kitzman, PhD, RN, FAAN
Professor
University of Rochester, School of Nursing
Rochester, NY

Terri H. Lipman, PhD, CRNP, FAAN
Professor of Nursing of Children
Miriam Stirl Endowed Term Professor in Nutrition
Program Director, Pediatric Acute/Chronic and Pediatric Oncology
　Nurse Practitioner Programs
University of Pennsylvania, School of Nursing
Philadelphia, PA

Thomas A. Mackey, PhD, FNP-BC, FAAN, FAANP
Professor of Clinical Nursing
Associate Dean for Practice
University of Texas School of Nursing at Houston
Houston, TX

Kathleen MacLellan, RGN, MBA, MSc, PhD
Head of Professional Development
National Council for the Professional Development of Nursing and
　Midwifery
Dublin, Ireland

Joy McIntyre
Director of Communications and Marketing
University of Pennsylvania, School of Nursing
Philadelphia, PA

Elizabeth Miller, RN, CRNP, MBA
Genesis HealthCare
Kennett Square, PA

Lisa Norsen, PhD, RN, ACNP
Associate Professor of Clinical Nursing
Director, Masters Nurse Practitioner Programs
University of Rochester, School of Nursing
Rochester, NY

Nancy O'Rourke, MSN, ACNP, ANP, RNC
President, Massachusetts Coalition of Nurse Practitioners
Massachusetts State Representative for American Academy of Nurse
   Practitioners
Hollis, NH

Joanne M. Pohl, PhD, ANP-BC, FAAN
Professor, The University of Michigan School of Nursing
Institute for Nursing Centers
Ann Arbor, MI

Susan C. Reinhard, PhD, RN, FAAN
Senior Vice President, AARP Public Policy Institute and Chief Strategist
Center to Champion Nursing In America
Washington, DC

Ann Ritter, JD
Director, Health Center Development and Policy
National Nursing Centers Consortium
Philadelphia, PA

Karen R. Robinson, PhD, RN, DPNAP, FAAN
Associate Director for Patient Care
Department of Veterans Affairs Medical Center
Fargo, ND

Deborah A. Sampson, PhD, APRN, FNP-BC
Assistant Professor
The University of Michigan
Coordinator, Adult Nurse Practitioner Program
Interim Deputy Director, Occupational Health Nursing Program
The University of Michigan, School of Nursing
Ann Arbor, MI

Melissa A. Taylor, MSN, CRNP
Lecturer
University of Pennsylvania, School of Nursing
Philadelphia, PA

Connie M. Ulrich, PhD, RN, FAAN
Associate Professor of Bioethics and Nursing
Senior Fellow, Center for Bioethics, Department of Medical Ethics
Senior Fellow, Leonard Davis Institute of Economics
University of Pennsylvania, School of Nursing
Philadelphia, PA

Helen Ward, MSc, PGCEA, PG CERT, BSc(Hons), RCN NP Diploma, RGN
Principal Lecturer, Non-Medical Prescribing Programmes
Deputy Course Director, MSc Nurse Practitioner Programme
Faculty of Health and Social Care
London South Bank University
London, UK

Mindy B. Zeitzer, PhD, MBE, CRNP
University of Pennsylvania, School of Nursing
Philadelphia, PA

Foreword

Few of us whose ideas come to fruition in their lifetime survive the journey from innovation to institutionalization. I feel both lucky and blessed to be among the few. The chaotic, uncertain social/political environment was enabling and ripe for change. Still, who would have believed that the first nurse practitioner (NP) educational demonstration project that I and pediatrician Henry K. Silver launched in 1965 would produce almost 150,000 master's-prepared NPs 44 years later? Or that they would be indigenous to every health care delivery service, from ambulatory to acute care facilities, schools and industries, military and veteran services, and even in retail stores? Indeed, at the time, there were many nursing pundits who predicted otherwise.

Not only has the NP movement survived, but it has thrived and transformed the profession of nursing, and affected health care delivery services and the public's perception of nurses. Its progress, potential, and problems have extended beyond the profession and gained the attention of health policymakers and politicians, due in part, to the earlier evidence-based and scholarly publications such as this and earlier editions on the evolvement of the NP.

This journey has been beautifully chronicled in the past four editions of this publication, and is advanced now into the fifth edition. The list of authors in this edition reads like a "Who's Who" in the ranks of scholarly historians, veteran researchers, expert practitioners in specialty services, new organizational initiatives, successful political and health policy leaders, astute business and financial advisors, and futurists with worldly views.

Although this is not a "how-to" book, there are plenty of lessons to be learned, not only from the experiences and insights of these authors, but also from the principles and practices that they have found to be patient-centered, effective, efficient, and economical. Each author's work offers a rich, thoughtful, and realistic account of her/his contribution to *Nurse Practitioners: The Evolution and Future of Advanced Practice, Fifth Edition*. The global view is presented, with the spread of the NP to different countries of the globe. (The ICN Advanced Practice Network has over 1,000 members in 54 countries, so it is apropos to note that this edition will be reaching far beyond our own national borders.)

Today, once again, we have an enabling environment. The public's chaotic, uncertain, and strident demands for social and political changes, including health care reform, offer all advanced-practice nurses and their organizations untold opportunities. These include opportunities to gain increasing respect, recognition, and rewards as they assume the responsibilities of delivering accessible, affordable, accountable, and acceptable affable health care for all. This edition will help all nurses and other health professionals, businesses and corporations, policymakers, and the public toward this goal.

LORETTA C. FORD, EdD, RN, PNP, FAAN, FAANP

This fifth edition of *Nurse Practitioners: The Evolution and Future of Advanced Practice* is fortuitously timed, with the heightened focus on national health care reform. Nurse practitioners (NPs) are situated to play a major role from participation in states' efforts to initiate smaller scale reforms, to broader population-based health promotion and disease management at the primary and acute care levels. The intensive efforts by advanced-practice nurses and their professional organizations to demonstrate their unique contributions and to standardize preparation and scope of practice make this the ideal moment to consider the history, current developments, and future possibilities. Indeed, nursing's organizational efforts to advance health care reform and take its rightful place in the policy debate and implementation of reform was recognized by President Barack Obama in his July 15, 2009, remarks thanking nurse leaders for their role in the debate and support of change.

Not only do these developments define this period for NPs, additional changes are accelerating practitioners' movement to the next level of operation—the pan shortage of health professionals, the limited capacity of health professional programs to meet demand, the rapid spread of disease from country to country, and the diminished economic and infrastructure capacity of many countries to meet their citizens' needs for care and health care personnel.

The potential of NPs in this country and globally to address these challenges and improve health care are documented here, as are the obstacles to full realization of advanced-practice nursing's ability to meet the needs of health system reform.

This edition, which features contributors recognized as foremost in their understanding and analyses of the developmental history, research base, regulatory reform, and innovations in clinical practice, will serve the readers with both a frame of reference and a current and future estimation of NP role development and use. Students in NP programs, seasoned providers, policy makers, and other invested health professionals will gain a totally new perspective on the history of NPs, the mechanics of regulatory and financial recognition of NPs, the effects of managed care, and the opportunities for more democratic sources of care, such as community nursing centers and retail clinics, and the globalization of advanced-practice models.

This rich content is divided into sections highlighting history and research-based support for current and future practice, policy and regulation, first-person accounts of practice innovation, adaptation of the NP model to the requirements of other countries, and last, the distillation of the important policy and political questions to be considered and answered over the next few years. Several bellwether issues are presented here with clarity not found in other discussions: the effects of managed care and reimbursement systems, the creation of a regulatory model, and the future configuration of research questions that could advance practice.

The editors and contributors look forward to your comments, observations, and experiences that will additionally inform the topics presented here. There is no better time for students, providers, policy makers, and consumers to understand the past developments, their shaping of the current status of NP practice, and to use that knowledge to influence the position of practitioners in the restructuring of a more successful and effective health care delivery system.

DIANE O. MCGIVERN, PhD, RN, FAAN
EILEEN M. SULLIVAN-MARX, PhD, CRNP, FAAN
JULIE A. FAIRMAN, PhD, RN, FAAN

Acknowledgments

In every social and professional movement, there are highly visible leaders and many other less well-known participants who effectively create innovation and help sustain these changes over time. Four such leaders inspired the nurse practitioner (NP) role development, institutionalized education and clinical practice advancements by virtue of their academic and organizational positions, and finally, have been central to the editions of this book. Loretta Ford, Claire Fagin, Joan Lynaugh, and Mathy Mezey have, over the last several decades, propelled the NP role in ways unique and powerful, marshalling personal qualities of derring-do, sociability, farsightedness, and plain speaking.

Loretta C. Ford, EdD, RN, PNP, FAAN, FAANP, is, of course, the one who envisioned, with Henry Silver, a community health nurse with expanded skills to provide community-based care for children. Although elements of the expanded role were evident decades earlier, the articulation of the role, drive for organized educational preparation, and advocacy within professional organizations were the essential differences that Dr. Ford's leadership made.

Claire Fagin, PhD, RN, FAAN, influenced the NP movement on multiple levels. Her expositions on the centrality of nursing to health care, on primary care, nursing's disciplinary grounding, and the rightful place of NPs' contribution to national health care create an extraordinary bibliography. Dr. Fagin's academic program influence spans baccalaureate and graduate curricula. Perhaps less heralded, but extraordinarily important, was the early introduction of primary care skills into a baccalaureate program, seeding baccalaureate preparation with the skills now integral to all undergraduate education and expectations for beginning practice.

An early practitioner, faculty member responsible for master's program development, preparation of adult NPs, and arbiter of the skills relevant to advanced practice, Joan Lynaugh, PhD, RN, FAAN, and colleagues developed an adult primary care practitioner program and primary care teams and clinical sites for student experiences. Dr. Lynaugh established and directed NP programs before and after completion of a doctorate focused on health care history. Her collaboration with Barbara Bates, MD, resulted in texts that guided generations of students and faculty in assessment and clinical decision making. A pioneer of master's preparatory programs, and with the eye of an historian, she has helped underscore and explain the legitimacy of the vital links in practitioner role development, particularly in relation to nurse work and with historical research mentorship of her students.

The need for geriatric nursing expertise among baccalaureate and graduate program students and practicing nurses of all preparatory levels was recognized very early by Mathy Mezey, EdD, RN, FAAN. Dr. Mezey's experience in clinical teaching, academic program development, and policy direction through important organizations and foundations has created a momentum that is currently supporting the amalgam of adult and geriatric practitioner expertise, in order to prepare a sufficient number of NPs with knowledge and skills to meet the needs of the majority of the population.

Each of these nurse leaders has provided an authoritative voice through personal style, institutional prominence, multiple organizational leadership positions, academic recognition, clinical credibility, and sustained participation in the evolutionary effort. Lastly, each of them has been a conspicuously unique contributor to this series of books, as well as hundreds of other publications. Few books have the distinction of participation by transformational leaders. Their contributions and authoritative weight have charted the development of the NP role from 1965 through 2010. We gratefully acknowledge their signature leadership and their contribution to the body of literature that supports, explores, and expands the possibilities of NP practice.

Nurse Practitioners

The Evolution and Future of Advanced Practice

Fifth Edition

Historical and Current Social Context

The 4 decades of literature documenting the development of the nurse practitioner (NP) role has included some exciting personal and professional achievements, but has also promulgated some shorthand language that limits the ability of students and new practitioners to fully appreciate this pivotal development in health care. Understanding the historical developments and contemporary context is fundamental to the individual practitioner's ability to articulate the role, advocate for policies that advance autonomy, and confidently interact with patients and other health professionals.

History is powerful, and when the recounting is accurate and nuanced, the reader becomes more engaged and, consequently, a more fluent interpreter of aspects of the current NP role development. Fairman supplies this historical context, McGivern summarizes the semantic and descriptive evolution, and Sullivan-Marx brings us up to the moment with a concise description of the current status of NPs in the broader health care scene. Taken together, the first three chapters serve as a solid and scholarly base from which the reader can delve into many other areas of the book.

Increasingly, nurses and NPs are concerned with how to successfully communicate with the public and, in particular, segments of potential consumer populations and payers. Cleary and Reinhard, speaking with

Sullivan-Marx and McGivern, describe one well-organized campaign with broad network support designed to create sustained messages to professionals, policymakers, and consumers about the importance of nurses and NPs. Several state teams in the Champion Nursing in America initiative describe their efforts, communication services, and products to promote nursing and advanced practice. While Cleary and Reinhard lead an effort to ultimately deliver messages to consumers, how do NPs successfully craft their messages to appeal to their own potential consumers? McIntyre gives us the answer. McIntyre, a media and communication professional experienced in shaping the nursing message for the public, describes how individual and practitioner groups can most effectively explain their services, target potential consumers, and tailor messages to most effectively educate different populations. The chapter is an interesting, concise, and effective guide to useful strategies.

Very often, when questioned about reasons for selecting NP programs or what they anticipate doing upon beginning practice, many students describe future practice as everything antithetical to their current generalist practice. This section will promote an understanding of the nursing component that is foundational to the practitioner role, how the role evolved, its current status and strength, and the scope of responsibilities and possibilities beyond the clinical encounter that will refine and focus new practitioners' contributions.

1

Historic and Historical Opportunities: Nurse Practitioners and the Opportunities of Health Reform

JULIE A. FAIRMAN

At the end of the first decade of the 21st century, the nursing profession is at a critical juncture. It sits at the intersection of its own transformation and its ability to shape health care reform. Nursing is central to the key policy issues, such as the primary care workforce, health care costs, and the functioning of the health care delivery system. How the profession situates itself and clearly develops a descriptive and strategic narrative that engages the public will create the foundation for its future.

Health care reform under the Barack Obama presidency is a main legislative focus of this time period, and policy strategists, professional organizations, and industry representatives have floated numerous tactical initiatives both familiar and innovative. Policy analysts and strategists evoke the historical view at almost every turn, from comparisons with the Clinton-era attempts at reform to references to the Flexner Report on the state of medical education in the early 20th century, as lessons for our current reform efforts (Flexner, 1910). We should do likewise and take time to think about the history of nurse practitioners, how that history positioned them and created opportunities for their role in our modern health policy debates.

One of the most pressing health care issues facing the American public is also one that has been historically persistent—the difficulty certain populations and groups have accessing quality health care services, particularly primary care and the management of chronic illness. These are very variable and historically contingent issues that also shaped the foundation of the development of the nurse practitioner movement in the 1960s. They also persistently and continuously justify and substantiate the role. Of course, people suffering from acute illnesses or emergent health issues can obtain care. But when the "well and well but worried" (Bates, 1971), especially those in rural or poor urban areas or those without health insurance, have basic health needs, seek answers to questions, or need support, they have difficulty finding qualified practitioners.

In spring 2009, The Institute of Medicine (IOM) empanelled the Robert Wood Johnson Foundation Initiative on the Future of Nursing Committee. This group of individuals, constituted from a wide array of stakeholders, including academics, practicing nurses and physicians, corporate representatives, and innovators of health care models, has been tasked with developing a "transformational" report that establishes a "blueprint for action" articulating the future role that nurses can and should play in the design and delivery of high-value care in a reformed health care system. The Committee, and the report it will produce, is propitious, and is positioned to be a watershed for the nursing profession in standing with other noteworthy reports such as the Goldmark Report, the Brown Report, the Report of the Surgeon General Consultant Group on Nursing, and the National Commission for the Study of Nursing and Nursing Education, among others (Brown, 1948; Goldmark, 1923; National Commission for the Study of Nursing and Nursing Education, 1970; U.S. Department of Health, Education, and Welfare. Surgeon General's Consultant Group on Nursing, 1963). These historically significant reports have been forgotten by most policy makers and strategists, but they were extremely important. When considered in the broad context of the time in which they were situated, the reports stimulated a host of policy strategies that shaped the nursing profession, including federal and private funding for nursing education and development of expanded practice roles for nurses. The reports also provided evidence for enlarging the nursing workforce and set standards for the education faculty needed to train the next generation of nurses for clinical practice. This new report is well-positioned to be the next step—an innovative vision of how the nursing workforce should be employed in evidence-based, outcome-focused care to meet the health care needs of the American public (Robert Wood Johnson Foundation, 2008). Nurse practitioners are at the forefront of these deliberations.

Several historical factors make nursing and nurse practitioners salient participants in reform. Nursing, as a female-gendered profession with social and cultural mandates to provide a broadly defined array of care services, is situated at the fulcrum where health disparities and social justice movements are balanced. Its history illustrates this nexus through its long tradition of focusing on the issues of equity, and interceding between the dominant power of local and national governments and medical men and women, and disenfranchised groups and populations. We see this in examples such as the settlement house movement and Lillian Wald's work with others to establish the Children's Bureau in the early 20th century, midwife Mary Breckinridge and the Frontier Nursing midwifery service and school, the clinics and nurse midwifery programs of the Maternity Center Association in New York City, and the later school nurse movement (Buhler-Wilkerson, 2001; Connolly, 2008; Dawley, 2001; Keeling, 2007). Equity, to be sure, is a noble aim, but it is not a driving force of the modern health reform debates. Even so, nurse practitioners' advocacy and supporting roles position them in the tangential discussions about health care equity that will, in the long term, remain a factor shaping new programs and services.

In this current environment, much of the policy debates revolve directly and indirectly around the cost of, and payment for, health coverage. Although these issues are important, they cause us to lose sight of the systematic problems in the design of the health care delivery system that are highly amenable to strategies that involve nurses. The health care reforms undertaken by the state of Massachusetts are one example of this conflicting focus. Although the state has now achieved near-universal coverage through more inclusive eligibility benefits for Medicaid, it is struggling with increased demand for services, particularly for primary care providers (PCPs), and subsequently, increased program costs. Advanced-practice nurses as PCPs can help meet demands for services, in addition to developing, testing, and demonstrating models that promote patient inclusion into the health care system at all levels. But similar to trends in the past, there may not be sufficient numbers of nurse practitioners to fulfill the public's primary care needs, even when combined with the numbers of practicing primary care physicians. In a greater proportion than physicians, nurses are attracted to generalist, PCP roles for practice independence and satisfaction from relationships with families and patients (U.S. Department of Health and Human Services, 2004, 2006). But, similar to physicians, nurse practitioners have always and will continue to specialize along clinical, procedural, and age-based areas.

From the history of the nurse practitioner movement, we can see how the development of the role and the support earned from patients positioned nurse practitioners for this historical time and place. In my book, *Making Room in the Clinic* (Fairman, 2008a), I describe in detail the social, political, and health care environment that supported nurses' response to patient need and to practice opportunities in the mid-1960s to the 1980s. Some of the problems patients and practitioners faced are familiar. For example, health care costs were sharply rising, especially after the passage of Medicare and Medicaid in the mid-1960s. A shortage of PCPs (due to low status and pay) and the medical specialization trend created severe access-to-care issues for many Americans in rural and poor urban areas, as well as for middle-class families. Some of the same population groups, women, children, and young adults, accessed the health care system only with great difficulty. The chronically ill and the elderly found continuity of care to be illusive, and constituted some of the fastest growing and most expensive population groups in the health care arena.

In turn, nurses were looking for opportunities to practice their skills to the fullest extent whenever and wherever possible, both stimulating and building on the new educational programs that were emerging in colleges and universities in the 1960s and 1970s. Physicians on the ground were looking for help to better serve their patients, and negotiated and collaborated in good faith to form new models and partnerships with nurses. On the other hand, both medical and nursing organizations (The American Medical Association and the American Nurses Association) pursued strategies that were, at times, incompatible with practitioner efforts and too slow to make a marked difference. They perhaps inadvertently stimulated a fragmented conglomeration of specialty organizations that were difficult to harness to generate policy consensus (Fairman, 2008a).

The nurse practitioner movement was also fed by the social movements of the time, including the women's and civil rights movements. Many women working in the free women's health clinics of the 1960s and 1970s labored side by side with nurses, and found their gendered practice paradigm a comforting alternative to the paternalism they found in medicine. Many of these women later made their way into nursing and nurse practitioner education programs (Candib, 1995). Women of various racial and ethnic groups gained greater entry into nursing education programs after the Nurse Training Acts of 1975 and 1980, and through the progressive health care management structure of the United States Military and its generous support of higher education for nurses (Sarnecky, 2000).

Powerful, smart, and wise women, such as Loretta Ford, Barbara Resnick, Joan Lynaugh, and Harriet Kitzman, among many others, also ensured that innovative nursing models emerged from their synergy and collaboration with enlightened physician colleagues. Loretta Ford, with pediatrician Henry Silver, developed the earliest certificate training program for nurse practitioners at the University of Colorado (Ford & Silver, 1967). Barbara Resnick and Charles Lewis, in response to the low level of interest from medical fellows and residents in ambulatory care at the University of Kansas, implemented a medical clinic model that provided patients with a nurse-run practice (Lewis & Resnick, 1967). Joan Lynaugh and Barbara Bates set up a series of training modules—that later became the physical diagnosis text used in many nurse practitioner training programs—to educate nurses in the hospital clinics and community to work collaboratively as partners in physician practices in Rochester, New York (Bates & Lynaugh, 1973). Harriet Kitzman developed a similar model in the Rochester-area pediatric clinics, and she later went on to help shape the nurse–family partnership with David Olds (Charney & Kitzman, 1971; Olds & Kitzman, 1990). Nurse practitioners (until the early 1960s, all nurses were labeled nurse practitioners) emerged out of this contextual milieu, building a new role upon their already substantial and growing clinical care skills, honed in public health and community nursing. Working with physician colleagues and patients who understood nurses' promise and potential, they carved out enlarged nursing territory, and education followed. Federal funding for nursing education and practice demonstration models supported this trajectory, starting with the special projects embedded in the 1964 Nurse Training Act, as did support from private foundations such as Robert Wood Johnson for programs like the Clinical Nurse Scholars, and Commonwealth Foundation (Newbergh, 2005).

These nurses were the pioneers—they practiced independently or in collaboration with physician colleagues who were available for support on site, but many times only by phone or occasional visits. From these practitioners and the media, the public learned of nursing's capabilities and value. Nurse practitioners received broad coverage in popular newspapers and magazines of the 1970s and 1980s, as well. *Look* magazine published one of the earliest stories in the popular press in 1966 (Berg, 1966). The *Wall Street Journal* and *Today's Health* referred to nurse practitioners as "super nurses," expressing perhaps surprise at their competence, as well as recognition of their ability to provide high-quality services. By 1985, The *New York Times, Washington Post,* and The *Wall Street Journal* reported on nurse practitioners in the main or health sections, and printed letters to the editor over 150 times. *McCall's* magazine, a leading popular women's magazine at the time, ran articles about nurse practitioners starting in 1975 (e.g., Clift, 1975; Lublin, 1974; Safran, 1975).

As nurse practitioners negotiated and experimented with their physician colleagues, they created new types of practice models, both in and out of hospitals, for providing increased access to care for populations across the board. They also showed typical entrepreneurial spirit, long associated with the nursing profession, by seeking out practice areas without the constraint of institutional oversight. In public health and hospital clinics, nurse practitioners demonstrated that they could provide a different type of care and much-needed continuity, advocacy, and education to patients long ago abandoned by much of mainstream medicine for the more complex and highly acute cases. In this way, nurse practitioners became essential to a system of care fragmented by medical specialization.

Although they became crucial providers in particular places for certain populations, nurse practitioners still faced legal and political obstacles that limited patient access to services. Political action by organized medical groups at the state and national levels to restrict nurse practitioners' practice, resources, and adequate payment kept attention on legislative battles. Physicians' traditional normative status, their gender, higher class, and their cultural authority as scientific clinicians ensured nurse practitioners a prolonged battle to engage policy makers. As attention of the organizations was focused on territorial and contextual disputes, nurse practitioners were emboldened to develop new modes of care—nurse-managed centers, Program of All-Inclusive Care for Elders (PACE) programs, and independent practices emerged. Except in public health and home care, in which nurses have long been recognized as essential providers, nurse practitioners fought against traditional conceptualizations of the physician as the normative authority on the public's recovery from illness.

And, it is here—in the difference between health care and medical care—that nurse practitioners found their voice and their strategy to position themselves in the last 3 decades as essential to health care reform. Although the dichotomy that nurses care and physicians cure is not a useful way of showing nursing's capabilities and value, embedded in this old trope is the nurses' claim to expertise in prevention and promotion of the public's health. Of course, nurse practitioners do diagnose and treat illnesses in the traditional medical model, but they do so from a paradigm that is flexible enough to move back and forth from medical care to a much broader nursing perspective to meet the fluid needs of patients.

As they positioned themselves from the 1960s on across multiple settings, their ingenuity and flexibility served them well and provided a standpoint for the current policy debate surrounding the primary care work force, health insurance, and emerging care models. Numerous studies have shown the high quality of care nurse practitioners provided to particular populations across time. There is little need to document efficacy and efficiency of care, except as a strategy to build on current clinical issues. This does not mean that we no longer need to test new models with different populations, but that the role in general, and the competency of nurse practitioners, already has proven salience and value. Nurse practitioners do need to be included on health maintenance organization (HMO) panels and receive equitable payment for rendering services that are comparable to physician services. Their exclusion is a legacy of the politics of health care reimbursement, our complicated payment systems, and the politics of practice. Because a service or skill has been traditionally rendered by physicians does not justify less payment to other health professionals for the same work, particularly when the quality indicators for nurse practitioners are the same or better than traditional physician-only care. Our system has become accustomed to privileging payment to physicians over any other form; discussions surrounding equitable pay for particular services (rather than by who provides the services) become a political tempest.

One argument against equitable payment is its cost—it raises the cost of health care in general by adding to, rather than decreasing, costs. Another argument against equitable payment is physicians' traditional explanations of expertise based on their more detailed science education. Only recently, as explored and supported by the Institute of Medicine study *Crossing the Quality Chasm,* has this traditional approach been challenged. This is a shift in the traditional paradigm of privileging professional medicine and its legislative allies to categorize ownership of skill sets. For example, clinical decision making, diagnosis, and prescription are now the domains of several different health professionals, and should no longer be considered solely in the medical domain. This is becoming increasingly true as developing nations train nurses and community health workers in assessment, diagnostic, and treatment skills (see chapters 24 and 25 in this book; Sheer & Wong, 2008).

Strategies focusing on advanced-practice nursing cannot be part of health reform without the insight, information, and guidance provided by an examination of basic nursing, which is the foundation for the nurse practitioner role. A key example of this connection is the lack of resolution in American nursing regarding entry level into general practice, with both the associate and baccalaureate entry points recognized by state licensing boards. In many ways, education level has become the proxy for power in the discussions surrounding nursing's participation in health care reform and debates about professional status across professions. We see this in the general discussions about how much education nurses need, and how educational preparation helps define role and practice boundaries, again a discussion that shows great historic stamina. The general entry-level inconsistency intrinsically influences graduate education for advanced-practice nurses, because it means there can be no expectations for a student's consistent knowledge and skill level on admission or after program completion. Also relevant to this discussion will be how the Doctor of Nursing Practice requirement for advanced-practice nurses, as well as the Clinical Nurse Leader role, will be integrated into health care systems and health policy debates. These models are untested and have engendered intense scrutiny from medical professional organizations, as well as nurses themselves. But again, changes in nursing education have always gained support from nursing in general with great difficulty. Across nursing's history, the fight for nurse registration and graduate preparation in general at both the master's and doctoral levels (PhD) has always been highly contentious.

We tend to get into difficulties in these debates when the profession locates its source of power in its education models, rather than its practice capabilities. Although these are, indeed, linked concepts, the profession has, over time, more heavily relied on the education strategies to boost its legitimacy, rather than practice. However, conflict should not deter us from developing and testing new models of nursing education. We have done this in the past with more or less success, as nursing education entered into higher education institutions that were not always welcoming, or into programs that channeled nurses into advanced programs in the basic and social sciences and the humanities (Fairman, 2008b). As in the past, strategies for redesigning the education system to ensure an adequate supply of nurses prepared to meet health care demands, for more diverse nurse recruitment, and for retention of nurses, in general, will also have a great impact on advanced-practice nursing.

The historical roots of nurse practitioners should provide much-needed perspective to the debates over health reform now and in the future. From their history, the issues of cost containment, access to care, and work force issues seem, perhaps, less intractable. Despite practice, reimbursement, and political barriers, nurse practitioners have created new models of care that provide relief for patients of all types and in all locations. These are important lessons. Nurse practitioners are central to the functioning of the health care system, and their history shows their great adaptability and flexibility to meet the health care needs of the nation.

REFERENCES

Bates, B. (1971, February). *Can a screening unit do it?* Rough draft of paper presented at the 165th Annual Convention, Medical Society of the State of New York, New York, NY, 7, Barbara Bates Collection, Barbara Bates Center for the Study of the History of Nursing, University of Pennsylvania, School of Nursing, Philadelphia, PA.

Bates, B., & Lynaugh, J. (1973). Laying the foundations for medical nursing practice. *American Journal of Nursing, 73*(8), 1375–1379.

Berg, R. B. (1966, 6 September). More than a nurse, less than a doctor. *Look,* pp. 59–61.

Brown, E. L. (1948). *Nursing for the future: A report prepared for the National Nursing Council.* New York: Russell Sage Foundation.

Buhler-Wilkerson, K. (2001). *No place like home: A history of nursing and home care in the United States.* Baltimore: Johns Hopkins University Press.

Candib, L. C. (1995). *Medicine and the family: A feminist perspective.* New York: Basic Books.

Charney, E., & Kitzman, H. (1971). The child-health nurse (pediatric nurse practitioner) in private practice. *New England Journal of Medicine, 285*(24), 1352–1357.

Clift, E. (1975). The new family doctor is a nurse. *McCall's, 103*, 35.

Connolly, C. (2008). *Saving sickly children: The tuberculosis preventorium in American life, 1909–1970.* New Brunswick, NJ: Rutgers University Press.

Dawley, K. L. (2001). *Leaving the nest: Nurse-midwifery in the United States, 1940–1980.* Unpublished doctoral dissertation, University of Pennsylvania, Philadelphia.

Fairman, J. (2008a). *Making room in the clinic: Nurse practitioners and the evolution of modern health care.* New Brunswick, NJ: Rutgers University Press.

Fairman, J. (2008b). Context and contingency: The post World War II history of nursing scholarship. *Journal of Nursing Scholarship, 40*(1), 4–11.

Flexner, A. (1910). *Medical education in the United States and Canada.* New York: Carnegie Foundation for the Advancement of Teaching.

Ford, L. C., & Silver, H. K. (1967). The expanded role of the nurse in child care. *Nursing Outlook, 15*, 43–45.

Goldmark, J. (1923). *Nursing and nursing education in the United States, Report of the committee for the study of nursing education.* New York: Macmillan.

Keeling, A. W. (2007). *Nursing and the privilege of prescription, 1893–2000.* Columbus, OH: Ohio State University Press.

Lewis, C. E., & Resnick, B. A. (1967). Nurse clinics and progressive ambulatory patient care. *New England Journal of Medicine, 277*, 1236–1239.

Lublin, J. S. (1974, July 3). Filling the gap: 'Supernurses' provide care for thousands. *Wall Street Journal.* Retrieved July 29, 2008, from ProQuest Historical Newspapers, *Wall Street Journal* (1889–1991) database. Document ID: 72274513.

National Commission for the Study of Nursing and Nursing Education. (1970). *Abstract for action.* New York: McGraw Hill.

Newbergh, C. (2005). The Robert Wood Johnson foundation commitment to nursing. In S. L. Isaacs & J. R. Knickman (Eds.), *To improve health and health care* (Vol. VIII, The Robert Wood Johnson Foundation anthology). San Francisco: Jossey-Bass.

Olds, D., & Kitzman, H. (1990). Can home visitation improve the health of women and children at environmental risk? *Pediatrics, 86*, 108–116.

Robert Wood Johnson Foundation, Commission on Investing in the Future of Nursing at the Institute of Medicine. (2008). *Background.* Retrieved September 18, 2009, from http://www.iom.edu/CMS/28312/64233/64236.aspx

Safran, C. (1975, July–August). Their patients call them supernurses. *Today's Health Care, 21*, 23, 51.

Sarnecky, M. T. (2000). *A history of the U.S. Army Nurse Corps.* Philadelphia: University of Pennsylvania Press.

Sheer B., & Wong, F. K. Y. (2008). The development of advanced nursing practice globally. *Journal of Nursing Scholarship, 40*(3), 204–211.

U.S. Department of Health, Education, and Welfare. Surgeon General's Consultant Group on Nursing. (1963). *Toward quality in nursing: Needs and goals* (PHS publication 992). Washington, DC: U.S. Government Printing Office.

U.S. Department of Health and Human Services, Health Resources and Services Administration. (2004). *The registered nurse population: Findings from the 2004 national sample survey of registered nurses.* Retrieved September 19, 2009, from http://bhpr.hrsa.gov/healthworkforce/rnsurvey04/appendixa.htm

U.S. Department of Health and Human Services, Health Resources and Services Administration. (2006). *Physician supply and demand: Projections to 2020.* Retrieved September 19, 2009, from http://bhpr.hrsa.gov/healthworkforce/reports/physiciansupply-demand/currentphysicianworkforce.htm

2

Evolution of Advanced Practice: "Coming to Terms" With Nurse Practitioner Definitions and Descriptions

DIANE O. McGIVERN

INTRODUCTION

There are advantages to codifying the advanced-practice definitions and descriptions, including that of the nurse practitioner (NP), in order to communicate more clearly with the public, payers, and health professionals. An examination of the linear development of terms over time is difficult to describe, except in the most general chronological way, appreciating that research, case studies, position papers, regulations, and policy statements of professional and special interest groups may begin at one temporal point and not be available for dissemination, analysis, adoption, or refutation until a much later time.

The descriptions of the NP role are determined on multiple levels that have defied consensus for some time. Descriptions/definitions are proposed by national professional organizations, state statutes, institutional policies and procedures, and unique role requirements that are determined by the service or populations and nuanced by the individual's role interpretation and implementation.

The evolution of terms defining and describing the NP is informative, reflecting a preoccupation with different aspects of the role and the goals of organized nursing to firmly establish desired parameters of practice. These sequential definitions advanced by various sectors invariably lagged behind actual practice, and reflected an attempt to bring official recognition to already established clinical practices.

Three elements have characterized the definitional and descriptive changes over time: type of preparation, growing list of knowledge and skills, and degree of emphasis on professional role attributes. The first element is the transition of preparation from certificate, continuing education, or baccalaureate education to completion of graduate education, followed by certification. The second began rather simply with the focus on health promotion and maintenance, physical assessment and clinical decision making, and later followed by emphasis on the three Ps: physical assessment, pharmacology, and pathophysiology. Currently, we have an increasingly detailed listing of clinical knowledge and skills that supports expert practice. Last, the role attributes that occupied a significant part of the early dialogue included autonomy, change-agent skills, leadership, collaboration, and the characteristics associated with primary care (McGivern, Mezey, & Baer, 1976). Autonomy and accountability have become the shortened version of the necessary internalized qualities (Johnson, Dawson, & Brassard, 2010; National Organization of Nurse Practitioner Faculties, 1995).

The intensive work to arrive at a more uniform, inclusive, and coherent construction of advanced practice and the place of the NP is coming to fruition. This will be an important milestone in the short history of a concept that flourished and diversified with each clinical, academic, and jurisdictional modification.

The original NP model that expanded the public health nurse's role in the community-based care of adults (Lewis & Resnick, 1967) and children (Ford, 1982) morphed into a variety of roles and population foci as funding, educational preparation, and competing controlling interests, including hospitals, physicians, and community agencies tailored practitioner programs to suit their mission and goals. Consequently, the definition/description of NP took on different emphasis from decade to decade. The 4-decade shift from primary care to primary and acute care and introduction of specialties and subspecialties is currently culminating in delimitations of six population foci: family/individual, adult–gerontology, primary and acute care, neonatal, pediatrics primary and acute care, women's health, and psychiatric–mental health (APRN Consensus, 2008). This latest description of advanced practice, including NP practice, is an attempt to make the definition consistent, transparent, and understandable to the public and payers (see chapter 9, this volume).

IN THE BEGINNING

The initial conceptualization of the NP role is formally linked with the mid-1960s, when Loretta Ford and Henry Silver launched a program to provide nurses with skills to meet the primary care needs of children in the community. The original conceptualization was a nursing model upon which additional skills were grafted (Ford, 1982). However, this formal point on the timeline was preceded by many decades during which nurses, by virtue of patient need, military necessity, isolation from other providers, or specialization in anesthesia or midwifery, developed the diagnostic and treatment skills currently associated with NP practice (Fairman, 2008; Keeling & Bigbee, 2005; Lewis, 1982; Lewis & Resnick, 1967; Lynaugh & Fairman, 1992). The advent of the NP role was spurred by the recognition by nurses and others (Lewis, 1982) that nurses could be used more effectively, and that nurses wanted to expand their professional skills and improve care outcomes. Ford's assessment of the times as providing the *opportunity* to take advantage of nursing's potential and create new roles was based on an assessment of the larger social context—a period of conflict, demand for services, and an environment in which new and humanistic values were being embraced, driving a demand for rights, including civil, health, and gender (1982).

Ford's original conceptualization was a community health nurse prepared with additional clinical expertise to care for children in an ambulatory setting. The new provider was a *pediatric public health nurse practitioner* (Ford, 1982). The elements of the role were advanced clinical content that stressed physical and psychosocial assessments, leading to clinical judgments and plans of intervention. Because the focus was on the child, the health history had a strong developmental and family component (Ford, 1986). The health focus rested on knowledge of growth and development, family dynamics, and effective use of family and community strengths. To meet the health goals, the pediatric NP also focused on health teaching and supportive counseling. As important and explicit as these clinical functions were, there were also strong emphases on professional role attributes and professional development that supported the internalization of the role change while maintaining collegial relations with other health professionals.

Early writers defined the NP as a nurse who had completed a course of study, had responsibility for health care, and used knowledge and skills formerly identified as medical. The identified behaviors stressed health histories and performance of physical examination, managing health and selected deviations from health, and interventions that were agreed upon by nursing and medicine (Browne, 1970; McGivern, 1974; Mussallem, 1969).

The primary care origins of the NP role continued to be the dominant theme of advanced practice with emphasis on wellness, assessing and supporting clients/patients, ability to pursue health promotion, and maintenance. The meaning of health promotion and health maintenance activities also produced much discussion; in particular, how were screenings and management of stable chronic illnesses part of the scope of primary care (McGivern, 1986)? The concept of primary care, a reiteration of the definition of comprehensive care, was characterized as ambulatory, interdisciplinary, and family-centered, and then broadened to indicate first contact care, longitudinal responsibility, and integration of all other aspects of care, including health promotion and management of acute and chronic problems (McGivern, 1986).

Ultimately, primary care took four definitional routes: as a method of delivery of services, the content and type of services rendered, which health professional provided the care, and as nursing's academic discipline and scope of practice (Fagin, 1986; McGivern; 1986) with continued emphasis on health, accountability, and continuity. Considerable debate ensued about which primary care definition should dominate, though some, anticipating that NPs would provide care beyond the ambulatory setting, suggested that the primary care/NP link would be too limited, given other populations and settings in need (Lewis, 1982; Mezey, 1986a). But the concept of primary care became the *sine qua non* of the NP role and focus in the United States.

The difficulty with definitions was discussed by the 1974 American Nurses Association (ANA) Congress of Nursing Practice, which noted that the various descriptions, rather than clarifying, were confusing nurses and other health professionals. Confusion abounded because individual state agencies defined terminology differently, individual nurses had title preferences, and education and employment organizations defined terms to meet curricular or job goals. The ANA Congress noted the need for a process that would produce uniformity of definition while allowing for updating. The ANA Congress of Nursing Practice advanced its own definition: an a NP had skills acquired through formal continuing education or baccalaureate preparation. The advanced skills were physical and psychological assessment of individuals, families, and groups through health history taking and physical examination (ANA, 1974).

In 1976, approximately 10 years after the establishment of the first practitioner program, the Division of Nursing, U. S. Department of Health, Education and Welfare undertook a longitudinal study to determine the effects of federal funding of NP programs and to identify the roles, functions, and practice experiences of nurses. The study was predicated on the definition of a NP as a "nurse whose education extends beyond the basic requirements for licensure as a registered nurse. NP education is formally planned to prepare students for expanded function in diagnostic and treatment needs of patients" (Sultz, Zeilezny & Kinyon, 1976, p. 1).

The survey included 87 institutionally sponsored certificate programs and 46 master's degree programs that indicated that their programs prepared students for ambulatory care, and focused on the "primary care skills of history taking, physical examinations, ordering of laboratory tests and assessing the medical management of uncomplicated care" (p. 5). The second and third phases of the survey (Sultz, Zielezny, Gentry, & Kinyon 1978,1980) found the majority of NPs were providing pediatric and family primary care, and the dominant function was direct care, including health history, physical assessment, routine tests, teaching, coordination, and referral. Consultative and teaching functions were undertaken primarily by practitioners with academic program preparation (Sultz et al., 1978, pp. 83, 114).

The early conceptualizations were discussed and challenged within and outside nursing. According to Fagin (1976), the NP was a primary care provider, community based and responsible for accessible, affordable, and continuous care. The more basic of the newly identified skills moved from certificate programs and were rapidly integrated into baccalaureate and master's degree programs (McGivern, Mezey, & Baer, 1976). During the resulting turmoil in academic and clinically based nursing regarding what constituted "appropriate" knowledge and skills, supporters cited earlier examples of the evolution of practice; nurses using equipment and procedures previously designated as medical, and the belief that nurses were being prepared for practice beyond what they "were allowed" to do. Early certificate and academic programs focused on primary care skills, and how primary care skills could be taught in clinical preparatory programs that still relied on secondary and tertiary clinical settings. The role attributes were also prominent; discussion of leadership, change-agent skills, and decision-making skills were part of the rhetoric, if not the clinical practice (Fagin, 1986; Health Professions Education Extension Amendments, 1992; McGivern, Mezey, & Baer, 1976).

The primary care focus, first in pediatrics, then in other community-based populations, continues to dominate NP specialization. Approximately 80% of NP students and graduates identify primary care as their focus of preparation and practice (Fang, Tracy, & Bednash, 2009). Primary care, as the basis of the preparatory programs and clinical practice, is consistent with the Institute of Medicine's (1996) definition of primary care: "Primary care is the provision of integrated, accessible health-care services by clinicians who are accountable for addressing a large majority of personal health care needs, developing sustained partnership with patients and practicing in the context of family and community" (p. 2).

The usefulness of the primary care–NP linkage was well described by Diers and Molde (1983), "accepting the initial definition of the scope of practice for nurses in primary care—that of well-child, well-adult care—was expedient and probably strategically correct. Indeed, to have specified anything greater would have been so provocative as to ensure failure" (p. 474). Eventually, it was outweighed by the desirability of implementing broader roles across settings and populations, and adding more specific functions and activities to the definition. The essential link between well-child care, primary care, and NP practice slowly gave way to definitions that incorporated a stronger emphasis on medical management, and populations including family, adult, geriatric, and obstetric/gynecology (Ford, 1982; McGivern, 1986).

A NURSE FOR ALL SETTINGS

Despite the continued focus on primary care, NPs had begun to provide services in acute care settings, learning "on the job" through the 1970s–1980s (Becker & Richmond, 2003; Jarvis, 2003). On the one hand, competencies and domains were seen to be common to both primary care and acute care (National Organization of Nurse Practitioner Faculties, 1990, 1995, 2000). However, unlike the primary care NP description that is embedded in the definition of primary care, the description of acute care practice reflected greater variability created by institutional and clinical services, practitioner skills, and agreements among providers in specific settings. The central competency was and is direct clinical practice, including diagnosis and management of rapidly changing problems, but also includes health promotion and disease prevention. Emphasis on the six core competencies of teaching/coaching, consultation, research use/participation, leadership, collaboration, and ethical decision making vary; their relative weights fluctuating with the specialty population and the setting (Cajulis & Fitzpatrick, 2007; Hravnak, Kleinpell, Magdic, & Guttendorf, 2005).

Without losing focus on primary care, many anticipated what Ford described, "the NP is a nurse for all settings" (1979, p. 245) noting in particular the opportunities for effective management of the elderly, chronically ill, and the acutely ill. Mezey (1986b) also reflected on the shift from a practitioner based solely in primary care, and predicted the blending of the role to meet the needs in both acute care inpatient and ambulatory settings.

The elaboration of conceptual models and diversification of NP roles proceeded from the 1970s through the 1990s. The expansion of the definition of NP from primary care, including adult/geriatrics, family, and women's health (National Organization of Nurse Practitioner Faculties & American Association of Colleges of Nursing, 2002) to other areas of emphasis was slowly achieved through the 1970s with the creation of the neonatal NP, critical care NP, and other specialty roles.

In 1993, the Association of Academic Health Centers sponsored a workshop on roles of physician assistants and NPs in primary care. However, the participants suggested there should be a "dramatic change" in academic programs' focus, creating primary care programs and specialty and acute care programs (Clawson & Osterweis, 1993, p. 5). Participants acknowledged that this clinical practice trend had already begun, partially modeled on the inpatient specialty practice of clinical nurse specialists (Ryan, 1993).

In fact, academic programs in acute and subspecialty care were being offered in the late 1980s, and by the mid-1990s, two more developments further refined the NP description relative to acute care: the establishment of standards of clinical practice and the development of the certifi-cation examination. The Standards of Clinical Practice and Scope of Practice for the Acute Care Nurse Practitioner developed by the ANA and the American Association of Colleges of Nursing (AACN; 1996) defined the acute care NP as "a provider of advanced nursing care across the continuum of acute care services to patients acutely and critically ill." The certification examination, developed initially by the ANA and AACN, and now offered by the ANA's Credentialing Center, recognized the evolution of the acute care role, specific to patients with acute care needs, but not to setting.

The juxtaposition of NPs defined as primary care providers with acute care NP developments is seen as late as 1995–1996. An early examination of state-by-state legislation determining NP practice (Burns, 1996) was based on recognition that "nurse practitioners are capable of providing primary care services that have long been available only from physicians" (p. 5). The individual state's descriptions varied widely, however, allowing diagnosis and prescriptive measures (Alaska, p. 12) to functioning in a collaborative relationship with other providers and making independent nursing decisions (Texas, p. 120).

The National Council of State Boards of Nursing (NCSBN, 1992) described advanced-practice nursing as based on knowledge and skills required in basic nursing, registered nurse licensure, graduate degree, and experience in a designated area of practice, including advanced nursing theory, substantial knowledge of physical and psychosocial assessment, and appropriate intervention (NCSBN, p. 4). Professional role attributes listed by NCSBN included caring, advocacy, accountabil-ity, accessibility, autonomy, independence, and collaboration.

In 1993–1994, The American College of Nurse Practitioners (ACNP) was established to create a platform for NP participation in health care reform, policy development, and other agenda items im-portant to NPs. The ACNP contributed yet another definition of NPs. This definition stressed two components—the preparation of the NP and the scope of activities. Preparation included registered nurse licensure, completion of master's education, and clinical training. The scope of clinical activities included preventive care, including health promotion and maintenance and acute care including health assessment, diagnosis, and treatment of common acute care problems.

By 1995, The American Nurses Association Social Policy Statement (1995) emphasized that advanced practice included expansion of knowledge and skills, advancement, or building on new knowledge and increasing specialization. There is a cycling feedback loop—nursing has responded to the need for specialization by creating specialty organizations, leading to the creation of more narrowly defined educational programs, and institutionally and community-tailored roles. More narrowly defined specialties and subspecialties required assessments/portfolios or certification examinations (Brown, 1998; Hanson & Hamric, 2003).

At this point in 1995, the NP is defined more broadly as a provider with graduate-level preparation, certification, and equipped to practice in a variety of settings. But descriptions also became extremely more detailed in terms of enumerating knowledge, skills, responsibilities, and competencies (American Association of Colleges of Nursing, American Organization of Nurse Executives, & National Organization of Associate Degree Nursing, 1995; National Organization of Nurse Practitioner Faculty, 1995). A *Model for Differentiated Nursing Practice* (American Association of Colleges of Nursing, American Organization of Nurse Executives, & National Organization of Associate Degree Nursing, 1995) created a workforce blueprint that recognized different education levels and work–environment demands. Whereas the document included some discussion of master's education but not specific roles, it did note that the advanced-practice nurse is master's-degree prepared, provides care across settings, focuses on wellness and illness, is prepared in physiology, pharmacology, and physical assessment, uses protocols and case-management strategies, and integrates and coordinates care with other professionals and payers (p. 27). Although less detailed, it is consistent with the National Organization of Nurse Practitioner Faculies (NONPF; 1995) document that contained extensively detailed functional descriptions.

THE GOAL OF STANDARDIZATION

Pressure for greater standardization and specificity of preparation and practice was brought by nursing's professional organizations, regulatory agencies, and third-party payers. The last 15 years have seen intense efforts to achieve standardization of the definition and description of the NP, and ultimately, agreement among regulatory, accrediting, and reimbursement entities. Others have argued for increasing specificity in the distinctions among advanced-practice professionals that have included not only NPs, clinical nurse specialists, certified nurse anesthetists, and midwives, but also case managers, informaticists, physician assistants, holistic practitioners, and many others, not necessarily direct providers.

The American College of Nurse Practitioners (ACNP; 2001) stated that NPs function independently and collaboratively, but are also active in a broad array of specialties and settings, managing both medical and nursing problems. The ACNP current definition includes the preparation and functional elements. Preparation is based on graduate-level education and clinical training. The functional elements include performing health histories and physical examinations, diagnosing and treating acute and chronic problems, interpreting diagnostic studies, prescribing and managing medications, teaching and counseling, emphasizing health maintenance and disease prevention, and referring to other health professionals (http://www.acnpweb.org).

In 2002, the NONPF and the AACN developed a consensus document to describe entry-level primary care competencies in adult, geriatric, pediatric, family, and women's health for all master's and postmaster's program graduates. The general competencies included health promotion and disease prevention and treatment; practitioner–patient relationship, teaching–coaching function, professional role, managing and negotiating health care delivery systems, monitoring and ensuring the quality of health care practice, and cultural competence (pp. 13–20).

The ANA Scope & Standards of Advanced Practice Registered Nursing (2004) definition is more parallel to others, in that it begins with the preparation of registered nurses in graduate education at the master's or doctoral levels; then lists all the functions included in practice, including health promotion, disease-prevention activities, differential diagnoses, ordering and interpreting tests, prescribing, managing nursing and medical problems in primary care, acute care, and long-term care settings. Like the 1996 definition, it emphasizes autonomous practice and collaboration (pp. 16, 1250).

The definitions of advanced-practice nursing, and NPs in particular, posed by professional organizations and authors/researchers have created a spectrum of complex to more simple descriptive models of the NP role. For example, as recently as 2009, the AACN report (Fang et al., 2009) on enrollment and graduations defined the NP as a "registered nurse, who through a graduate degree program in nursing, functions in an independent health care provider role addressing a full range of patient/client health problems within an area of specialization" (p. xii). This recent description emphasizes academic preparation for an independent provider role without the detailed listing of practice activities (Fang et al., 2009).

There is an argument that stressing the commonalities among the four categories of advanced practice would emphasize the specialized knowledge base gleaned through graduate education, highlight the scope of practice, and clarify role confusion that potential consumers and advanced-practice nurses alike experience (MacDonald, Herbert, & Thibeault, 2006). Supporting this view, Hamric (2005) proposed "core" definitions, criteria, and competencies for advanced practice that stress advanced academic and clinical preparation, certification, and direct clinical practice focused on patients and families (p. 89).

Work began in the early to mid-1990s to attempt to codify the requirements for advanced practice. Representatives of state boards of nursing and many nursing organizations invested in advanced practice labored intensively from 2003 to 2008 to produce a consensus statement on advanced practice (APRN Consensus Work Group, 2008). The definition of NP rests on the description of advanced practice: elements common to advanced practice include preparation in an accredited graduate-level program, national certification, acquisition of advanced knowledge and skills that focus on health promotion and maintenance, assessment, diagnosis, problem management, prescription of pharmacologic/nonpharmacologic agents, and provision of direct care across the wellness–illness spectrum, recognizing accountability and responsibility.

On this foundation, the NP is a direct primary care or acute care provider across settings and points on the health–illness continuum. The knowledge, skills, and functions embedded in advanced practice can be reiterated, with additional emphasis on care that is initial, ongoing, and comprehensive, and includes autonomous and team-based practice, education, and supportive counseling.

These definitions and descriptions are intended to clarify and inform all parties involved in providing and consuming services, and serve as the springboard for regulatory reform. A common definition and standardized credentialing should enhance the acceptance and use of NPs (Stanley, 2009). The 40 years of definitional/descriptive flourishes are now woven together to achieve a more precise standard that will serve as a uniform reference.

CONCLUSIONS

We have come a long way from early attempts to describe to colleagues and the public what an NP was by saying, "think of it as being like a Dr. Welby," the 1969 television series character played by Robert Young who epitomized the primary care physician, employing little more than a stethoscope and kindness in his family practice. The initial descriptions elaborated upon over time by the practice successes of early practitioners, state regulations, positive and negative influences of third-party payers, and efforts by nursing organizations to strengthen and standardize the role preparation and practice have created a story, intense, rich, and exciting in all its possibilities. The currently and widely agreed-upon description of the what and who of advanced practice and the NP sets the stage for the next major era in nursing.

Adherence to one definition or descriptive model may enhance understanding of the role, reassure consumers, regulators, and payers, and provide the consistency necessary to establish an appropriate and central role in health care service delivery. A long and eventful regulatory journey is next.

REFERENCES

APRN Consensus Work Group, & National Council of State Boards of Nursing APRN Advisory Committee. (2008). *Consensus model for APRN regulation: Licensure, accreditation, certification & education.* Retrieved March 23, 2009, from http://www.aacn.nche.edu

American Academy of Nursing. (1976). *Primary care by nurses: Sphere of responsibility and accountability.* Kansas City, MO: American Nurses Association.

American Association of Colleges of Nursing, American Organization of Nurse Executives, & National Organization of Associate Degree Nursing. (1995). *A model for differentiated practice.* Washington, DC: Authors.

American College of Nurse Practitioners. (2001, November). *What is a nurse practitioner?* Retrieved September 16, 2009, from http://www.acnpweb.org/i4a/pages/index.cfm?pageid=3479

American Nurses Association Congress for Nursing Practice. (1974). *ANA definitions: Nurse practitioner, nurse clinician, clinical nurse specialist.* Kansas City, MO: American Nurses Association.

American Nurses Association. (1996). *Scope and standards of practice. Scope and standards of advanced practice registered nursing.* Washington, DC: Nursebooks.org.

American Nurses Association. (2004). *Scope and standards of practice. Scope and standards of advanced practice registered nursing* .Washington, DC: Nursebooks.org.

American Nurses Association. (1995). *Nursing's social policy statement.* Silver Springs, MD: Author.

American Nurses Association and American Association of Colleges of Nursing. (1996). *The standards of clinical practice and scope of practice for the acute care nurse practitioner.* Washington, DC: American Nurses Association.

Becker, D. E., & Richmond, T. S. (2003). Advanced practice nurses in acute care services. In M. D. Mezey, D. O. McGivern, & E. Sullivan-Marx (Eds.), *Nurse practitioners: Evolution of advanced practice* (4th ed., pp. 135–149). New York: Springer Publishing Company.

Brown, S. J. (1998). A framework for advanced practice nursing. *Journal of Professional Nursing, 14,* 157–164.

Browne, H. (1970). Family nurse practitioner project. *Frontier Nursing Service Bulletin, 46,* 23.

Burns, P. A. (1996). *National directory of nurse practitioner legislation.* Buffalo, NY: Rural Health Research Center.

Cajulis, C. B., & Fitzpatrick, J. J. (2007). Levels of autonomy of nurse practitioners in an acute care setting. *Journal of American Academy of Nurse Practitioners, 19,* 500–507.

Clawson, D. K., & Osterweis, M. (Eds.). (1993). *The roles of physician assistants and nurse practitioners in primary care.* Washington, DC: Association of Academic Health Centers.

Diers, D., & Molde, S. (1983). Nurses in primary care: The new gatekeepers? *American Journal of Nursing, 83*(5), 742–745.

Fagin, C. M. (1976). Nature and scope of nursing practice in meeting primary health care needs. In *American Academy of Nursing: Primary care by nurses: Sphere of responsibility and accountability.* Kansas City, MO: American Nurses Association.

Fagin, C. M. (1986). Primary care as an academic discipline. In M. D. Mezey & D. O. McGivern (Eds,), *Nurses, nurse practitioners: The evolution of primary care* (pp. 29–36). Boston: Little, Brown.

Fairman, J. (2008). Making room in the clinic: Nurse practitioners and the evolution of modern health care. New Brunswick, NJ: Rutgers University Press.

Fang, D., Tracy, C., & Bednash, G. (2009). *Enrollment and graduations in baccalaureate and graduate programs in nursing.* Washington, DC: American Association of Colleges of Nursing.

Ford, L. (1979). A nurse for all settings: The nurse practitioner. *Nursing Outlook, 27*(8), 516.

Ford, L. (1982). Nurse practitioner: History of a new idea and predictions for the future. In L. Aiken & S. Gortner (Eds.), *Nursing in the 1980s: Crises, opportunities, challenges.* Philadelphia: J. B. Lippincott.

Ford, L. (1986). Nurse, nurse practitioners: The evolution of primary care. Review. *Image: Journal of Nursing Scholarship, 18,* 177–178.

Hamric, A. B. (2005). A definition of advanced practice nursing. In A. Hamric, J. Spross, & C. M. Hanson (Eds.), *Advanced practice nursing: An integrative approach.* (3rd ed., pp. 85–105). St. Louis, MO: Elsevier/Saunders.

Hanson, C. M., & Hamric, A. B. (2003). Reflections on the continuing education of advanced practice nursing. *Nursing Outlook, 51*, 203–211.

Health Professions Education Extension Amendments of 1992. (PL 102-408, Section 204). *Nurse practitioner and nurse midwife programs*, 102nd Congress, 2nd session, p. 87. Retrieved June 17, 2009, from www.eric.ed.gov

Hravnak, M., Kleinpell, R. M., Magdic, K. S., & Guttendorf, J. (2005). The acute care nurse practitioner. In A. Hamric, J. Spross, & C. M. Hanson (Eds.), *Advanced practice nursing: An integrated approach* (pp. 475–514). St. Louis, MO: Elsevier/Saunders.

Institute of Medicine. (1996). *Primary care: America's health in a new era*. Washington, DC: National Academy Press.

Jarvis, S. D. (2003). Surgical intensive care unit nurse practitioner. In M. D. Mezey, D. O. McGivern, & E. M. Sullivan-Marx (Eds.), *Nurse practitioners: Evolution of advanced practice* (4th ed., pp. 347–354). New York: Springer Publishing Company.

Johnson, J., Dawson, E., & Brassard, A. (2010). Consensus model for advanced practice registered nurse regulation: A new approach. In E. Sullivan-Marx, D. O. McGivern, J. A. Fairman, & S. A. Greenberg (Eds.), *Nurse practitioners: The evolution and future of advanced practice* (5th ed., pp. 125–142). New York: Springer Publishing Company.

Keeling, A. W., & Bigbee, J. L. (2005). The history of advanced practice nursing. In A. Hamric, J. Spross, & C. M. Hanson (Eds.), *Advanced practice nursing* (pp. 3–45). St. Louis, MO: Elsevier/Saunders.

Lewis, C. E. (1982). Nurse practitioners and the physician surplus. In L. Aiken & S. Gortner (Eds.), *Nursing in the 1980s: Crisis, opportunities, challenges* (pp. 249–289). Philadelphia: J. B. Lippincott Company.

Lewis, C. E., & Resnick, B. (1967). Nurse clinics and progressive ambulatory patient care. *New England Journal of Medicine, 277*, 1236–1241.

Lynaugh, J., & Fairman, J. (1992). New nurses, new spaces: A preview of the AACN history study. *American Journal of Critical Nursing, 1*(1), 19–24.

MacDonald, J., Herbert, R., & Thibeault, C. (2006). Advanced practice nursing: Unification through a common identity. *Journal of Professional Nursing, 22*(3), 172–179.

McGivern, D. O. (1974). Baccalaureate preparation of the nurse practitioner. *Nursing Outlook, 22*, 94.

McGivern, D. O. (1986). The evolution of primary care nursing. In M. D. Mezey & D. O. McGivern (Eds.), *Nurses, nurse practitioners: The evolution of primary care* (pp. 3–14). Boston: Little, Brown.

McGivern, D., Mezey, M., & Baer, E. (1976). Teaching primary care in a baccalaureate program. *Nursing Outlook, 24*, 7–10.

Mezey, M. D. (1986a). The future of primary care and nurse practitioners. In M. D. Mezey & D. O. McGivern (Eds.), *Nurses, nurse practitioners: The evolution of primary care* (pp. 37–51). Boston: Little, Brown.

Mezey, M. D. (1986b). Issues in graduate education. In M. D. Mezey & D. O. McGivern (Eds.), *Nurses, nurse practitioners: The evolution of primary care* (pp. 101–119). Boston: Little, Brown.

Mussallem, H. (1969). The changing role of the nurse. *American Journal of Nursing, 69*, 514.

National Council of State Boards of Nursing. (1992). *Position paper on the licensure of advanced practice nursing*. Unpublished manuscript.

National Organization of Nurse Practitioner Faculties. (1990). *Advanced nursing practice: Curriculum guidelines and program standards for nurse practitioner education.* Washington, DC: Author.

National Organization of Nurse Practitioner Faculties. (1995). *Advanced nursing practice: Curriculum guideline and program standards for nurse practitioner education.* Washington, DC.

National Organization of Nurse Practitioner Faculties. (2000). *Advanced nursing practice: Curriculum guideline and program standards for nurse practitioner education.* Washington, DC.

National Organization of Nurse Practitioner Faculties, & American Association of Colleges of Nursing. (2002). *Nurse practitioner primary care competencies in specialty areas.* Rockville, MD: Department of Health and Human Services, Health Resources and Services Administration.

Ryan, S. (1993). Nurse practitioners: Educational issues, practice styles, and service barriers. In K. Clawson & M. Osterweis (Eds.), *The roles of physician assistants and nurse practitioners in primary care.* Washington, DC: Association of Academic Health Centers.

Stanley, J. (2009). Reaching consensus on a regulatory model: What does this mean for APRNs? *The Journal for Nurse Practitioners, 2,* 99–104.

Sultz, H. A., Zielezny, M., & Kinyon, L. (1976). *Longitudinal study of nurse practitioners, phase I.* Bethesda, MD: U.S. Department of Health, Education, and Welfare.

Sultz, H. A., Zielezny, M., Gentry, J., & Kinyon, L. (1978). *Longitudinal study of nurse practitioners, phase II.* Bethesda, MD: U.S. Department of Health, Education, and Welfare.

Sultz, H. A., Zielezny, M., Gentry, J., & Kinyon, L. (1980). *Longitudinal study of nurse practiioners, phase III.* Bethesda, MD: U.S. Department of Health, Education, and Welfare.

United States Department of Health, Education, and Welfare, Secretary's Committee to Study Extended Roles for Nurses. (1972). Extending the scope of nursing practice: A report of the secretary's committee. *Nursing Outlook, 20,* 46.

3

Current Status of Advanced-Practice Nurses in the United States and Throughout the Globe

EILEEN M. SULLIVAN-MARX

Since 1965, nurse practitioners (NPs) have evolved from a unique provider type to a mainstream profession potentially capable of meeting the United States' needs in primary care, acute care, and a number of specialty care areas. Richard Cooper and colleagues noted in 1998 that the health care workforce would be dominated by a pluralistic workforce, rather than a medical monopoly, citing that by 2010, there would be a growth of approximately 130,000 NPs (Cooper, Laud, & Dietrich, 1998). The 2004 Department of Health and Human Services' Registered Nurse (RN) Sample Survey exceeded Cooper's predictions by reporting that there were 141,209 NPs in the workforce, and that RNs with master's or doctoral degrees rose to 376,901, an increase of 37% from 2000 (U.S. Department of Health and Human Services [USDHHS], 2004). This growth in the NP workforce has occurred during a time that the physician workforce has declined in the United States (Association of American Medical Colleges [AAMC], 2006). A current estimate of the number of NPs in the United States is 147,295; 44 years in the making (Pearson, 2009).

For the most part, NPs in the United States are Caucasian/Northern European (89.4%), 3.0% are Hispanic, 2.7% are African American, and 2.6% are of Asian/Pacific Islander ethnicity. In contrast, the U.S. minority RN population is 1.7% Hispanic, 4.2% African American, and 3.1% Asian (Sipe, Fullerton, & Schuiling, 2009; USDHHS, 2004). None of these figures are representative of the national minority ethnic profile in the United States. Moreover, the U.S. nurse and NP population has remained a female-gender-dominated profession; men represent only 5% of NPs and 5.8% of RNs (USDHHS, 2004). Of note, 44.5% of certified RN anesthetists are men. Most NPs have a master's degree (84.8%) as their highest earned degree, and the average national salary ranges between $70,000–$85,000, compared with the average RN salary of $57,784 and physician salary of $150,000 (Kung & Porterfield, 2009; Sipe, Fullerton, & Schuiling, 2009; USDHHS, 2004).

The two top employment settings for NPs in the United States are physician-owned practices and hospitals, although the exact arrangements of employment relationships are not known. For example, NPs may be employed in a physician group practice and have a high level of autonomy to care for their own patients, or they may be employed to follow all patients in a practice who reside in nursing homes. Acute care NPs, particularly in medical centers, are employed by hospitals, but are increasingly engaged in highly autonomous practices, including managing critical care and postoperative surgical patients. Highly specialized acute care NPs, such as those in organ transplant services, provide assessment, treatment, and consultation services, both within academic medical centers and to referring and primary care physicians (National Organization of Nurse Practitioner Faculties, 2004; Barbara Todd, personal communication, September 11, 2009; Sipe, Fullerton, & Schuiling, 2009).

As NPs emerge in nations other than the United States, issues of title and scope of practice are being explored in relation to nursing practice and societal needs in the respective countries (Sheer & Wong, 2008). Nurses and lay health workers in developing countries are known to perform clinical tasks that only NPs or other advanced-practice nurses (APNs) might perform in the United States, out of necessity, access to care, or because some countries prepare nurses to perform functions that are not taught in U.S. basic education, such as management of maternal delivery. However, for the NP role to be recognized in any country as a professionally advanced career, the NP must have the skills, autonomy, and authority to practice and be recompensed directly for his/her services. Hence, both the International Council of Nursing (ICN) and nursing organizations and regulatory agencies throughout the world have been more active in the last 25 years in building advanced nursing careers in their countries (Schober & Affara, 2006; Sheer & Wong, 2008).

The development of NPs, first in the United States and now around the world, follows a development model outlined in Figure 3.1 that describes four spheres of interaction: (a) innovation, (b) policy, (c) meeting needs in services, and (d) nursing careers provide impetus for the growth of NPs. The development of advanced careers for nurses, for example, as NPs, can have starting points in any of the four spheres outlined. For NP roles to fully emerge and mature, all spheres need to be active. In the United States, Ford and Silver (Fairman, 2008) are credited with development of the NP model that grew to address gaps in health promotion and disease prevention for children in rural Colorado in the mid-1960s. Fairman (2008) has pointed out that the Colorado NP model also occurred at a time when professional nursing was ripe to advance nursing careers in many sectors, stemming from intensive care nursing in the 1950s and 1960s. Policy changes in Medicare and Medicaid in the 1960s set the stage for creating access to care for formerly uninsured senior citizens and others with low income, propelling the U.S. Federal Government to provide funding to universities and colleges for NP programs, training of faculty, and student tuition support. Meanwhile, nurses in public health service, private physician offices, and elsewhere, with entrepreneurial spirit and skills, drove the impetus of NP movement in the United States. In this chapter, I will highlight how the NP movement continues in the United States and internationally using the framework of the NP Development Model (Figure 3.1).

GLOBAL CONTEXT

The ICN defines an NP or APN as an RN who has acquired the expert knowledge base, complex decision-making skills, and clinical competencies for expanded practice. A master's degree is required, yet each country has its own particular context and issues for development of an NP role (ICN, 2009). In the United States, APNs are categorized as either NPs, clinical nurse specialists (CNSs), certified nurse midwives (CNMs), or certified RN anesthetists (CRNAs). In some countries, India, for example, RNs are prepared as both midwives and nurses at the basic

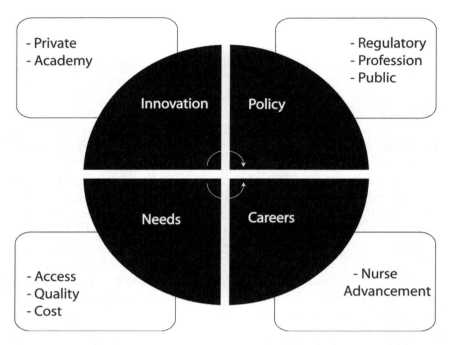

Figure 3.1. Nurse Practitioner Development Model by E. Sullivan-Marx.

level of preparation, and so, to define nurse midwifery as an advanced skill would be different in the United States and India (IKP Centre for Technologies in Public Health [ICTPH], 2009; Patidar, 2009). In many countries, the concept of CNS and NP are blended, as in the United Kingdom. To address the emerging growth of advanced nursing practice throughout the globe, the ICN has developed scope, standards, and competencies of practice to guide development of advanced practice. The International Nurse Practitioner/Advanced Practice Nursing Network (INP/APNN) and the ICN will host biannual conferences to explore how advanced nursing practice can respond to the many demands placed on health care systems in a global environment of constant change (Schober & Affara, 2006; Tropello, 2009).

As McGivern points out, writing on the environmental context for NPs later in this book, context is of paramount importance for the development of NP models. In today's world, there is great demand on the workforce of professionals, technical staff, and direct care workers, yet, the context of economic constraints, ongoing health reform, emerging technologies, and consumer demand influences the global development of NPs, and makes it difficult to focus on simple formulas of supply/demand and training of professionals and workers.

NEEDS IN SERVICES

Health services needs vary based on population and economic differences in regions and nations. For the most part, needs in services are shaped by access, quality, and cost issues. Developing countries have greater needs, due to misdistribution or geographic challenges in service access, than wealthier nations. Health problems from nutrition, infectious and pathogen-borne illnesses to chronic diseases of hypertension and diabetes are increasing in significance in developing countries (World Health Organization [WHO], 2008). Developed countries are faced with a growing aging population who requires a new perspective on integration of social and health services that promotes health and function, regardless of biological age or presence of chronic illness. NPs are well prepared to address these concerns. Addressing gaps and needs in services is often the impetus for developing NP models or new positions for NPs. In New Zealand, primary care needs of the Maori people set in process a movement to develop NPs by the New Zealand health ministry (see chapter 25, this volume). A think tank on the development of NPs in India took place in Chennai, India, in 2009 to address rural health needs (ICTPH, 2009). Gaps in services alone can not propel the development of NPs; consequently, simultaneous activity in policy, evidence from innovation feasibility projects, and career advancement must occur to complete the full development of NP roles.

INNOVATION

Small creative and innovative projects that demonstrate the feasibility and success of the NP role have spurred the initial development and ongoing growth of NPs in the United States. Entrepreneurial nurses who garnered funds or risked their own financial assets emerged in the 1970s to provide advanced nursing services as NPs. They were a driving force in demonstrating that not only could nurses expand their scope, but they were well received by patients and had good outcomes (Dickerson & Nash, 1985; Lang, 1983; Lewis & Resnick, 1962; Sullivan, 1992).

Academic institutions have partnered with communities for many years to provide gaps in services with NP faculty who engage in health promotion, education of students, and role model careers in health (Lang & Evans, 2004). In 2004, Belgian professors established CNS and NP roles at the Catholic University in Louvain to address unmet health needs (Sheer & Wong, 2008). In Vellore, India, the Christian Medical College of Nursing has run a rural nurse-managed clinic for several years, and subsequently developed a family NP program that is recognized as an innovation and potential source of career advancement for nurses in India (Jayakaran, 2009).

Rogers (2003) maintains that innovation is diffused through communication. The innovation of NP models of care must be diffused not only through scholarly publications, but also through visibility in everyday public life and through consumer education. Momentum in NP development in the United States has recently been catalyzed by placement of NPs in retail convenience clinics in shopping centers, in which "customers" can receive care for common, short-term problems, as well as health promotion education (Mehrotra, Wang, Lave, Adams, & McGlynn, 2008; Ryan, 2009). The publicity and front-line exposure of NPs to the public has created opportunity for NPs to be regarded as autonomous providers who meet the public's need in a safe and cost-effective manner (Thygeson, Van Vorst, Maciosek, & Solberg, 2008).

NURSING CAREERS

As advances in nursing practice have emerged throughout the globe, nursing careers have been enhanced. In the mid-20th century, nursing career advancement was tied to careers in administration and education, and supported by graduate degrees for nursing in these areas (Fairman, 2008). Advanced-practice careers in nursing emerged slowly, starting in the 1940s to the 1970s, in Canada, Korea, and the United States (Sheer & Wong, 2008). As educational programs grew and were federally funded and supported with student stipends in the 1970s and 1980s, NP careers became a catalyst for nurses to advance their careers at the graduate level without leaving practice for the relatively limited education and administrative positions. There are 350 higher education institutions that prepare NPs in the United States as of 2009. As the supply of NPs grew, so did demand, thus drawing and attracting people to nursing careers. A fast-growing segment of applicants to nursing schools in the United States is comprised of individuals with bachelor's degrees in other fields who seek accelerated programs for nursing degrees and advanced-practice careers (American Association of Colleges of Nursing [AACN], 2009).

The ICN recommends that education for advanced-practice nursing is at the master's level, and largely, this is the recommendation followed throughout the world. In the last several years in the United States, professional doctorate degrees have become more common among health professions. For NPs, a doctorate in nursing practice (DNP) degree has been implemented in many higher degree institutions to reflect the amount of content and course work needed to prepare NPs, particularly in the areas of evidence-based practice, quality assurance/improvement, and financial preparation in leadership and management (Kung & Porterfield, 2009). The impetus for a doctorate degree in nursing practice, advocated by the AACN was to create a practice-focused doctorate degree, distinct from doctorate or philosophy degrees that focus on research careers (AACN, 2006). DNP programs were created to produce a workforce of doctorate-prepared practitioners who could fill faculty needs, and bring parity to nursing within the health care hierarchy. An NP with a practice doctorate degree would have equivalent status to peer health professions, such as those in medicine, pharmacy, and physical therapy. The AACN promulgated recommendations that specified the DNP as the required degree for advanced-practice nursing by the year 2015. Although work had been done for 2 years prior to gain input from nursing practice and nursing academic stakeholders, nonetheless, the AACN recommendations stirred vigorous debate in professional nursing circles. Critics of a DNP model have identified potential consequences such as discouraging nurses from research careers, marginalizing nurses with DNPs from academic promotion opportunities, and creating confusion at a time when nursing as a profession in the United States and elsewhere must speak with one voice in health care reform discussions, and in meeting the health needs of the world (AACN, 2006: Meleis & Dracup, 2005; O'Sullivan, Carter, Marion, Pohl, & Werner, 2005). Proponents of the DNP degree argue that NPs need programs that reflect the amount of skills and knowledge required to meet basic competencies for practicing, and that NPs who seek such degrees would not have sought a PhD degree (Kung & Porterfield, 2009; Spear, 2005). Nonetheless, the 2015 DNP mandate for advanced practice (described previously) did not seem to be feasible or forthcoming in 2009, given the full range of consequences and implications to be considered. In 2009, according to AACN data, 92 DNP programs in the United States were active, with a similar number of schools planning DNP programs. In the same time period, applications to PhD nursing programs have increased by nearly one-third. Further study to identify trends that impact enrollment in both DNP and PhD programs needs to inform the nursing community about the impact of both degrees on NP workforce capacity and faculty careers.

As United States nurse leaders engage with our global counterparts in nursing, we must continue to be clear about the development of NP models and the potential for the advancement of careers that NP education and roles can provide to professional nursing in any country. As some nations struggle with advancing nursing education and professional nursing, the DNP versus MSN degree issue will need to be clarified and put into context, so that nursing throughout the globe grows to fully realize our potential to address health concerns everywhere.

POLICY

If any lesson is to be learned from over 40 years of NP development in the United States, it is that regulation, credentialing, licensing, and policy of NP practice must be controlled through nursing regulatory bodies in the public/governmental sector, and in nursing professional organizations. The success of NP practice through innovation and urgency to fill gaps in services may stand in contrast to the painstaking and time-consuming work in bureaucratic agencies to recognize and set standards of care for NP work. Yet, without public recognition and nursing professional standards, movements to establish the NP role outside of nursing or regulatory bodies will be short-lived. Feasibility studies, pilot projects, and waivers to allow innovations in NP practice by nursing policy, professional, and regulatory bodies are useful to maintain momentum as NP practice evolves prior to full recognition of standards and scope of practice. In the United States, early recognition by governmental agencies linking NP practice with physician regulatory agency oversight has been problematic both for physician regulating agencies and NPs, because physician regulatory bodies cannot and should not regulate nursing practice (Fairman, 2008).

Consensus bodies of 70 regulatory and professional organizations have been meeting in the United States since 2005 to re-establish the regulatory environment for APNs in the United States (see chapter 9 of this book; Stanley, 2009). As NP and other APN models grew in the United States, different regulations in 50 states, 3 territories, and 1 district, and variations in definitions and scope created difficulties for standardizing practice across state borders or to set federal funding guidelines for education and reimbursement of NPs. The proposed model distinguishes licensure, regulation, credentialing, and education regulation from professional specialization certification, so that consistency across legal entities, particularly at the level of the state boards of nursing, can occur. Professional bodies can then determine specialty certification standards as practice knowledge and opportunities evolve (Stanley, 2009).

In the United Kingdom, Ireland, Europe, Taiwan, Thailand, and New Zealand, efforts to establish regulatory policy for advanced practice are occurring at the national level. Taiwan, for example, formally recognized NPs in 2004, and Thailand established national certification of NPs in 2003 (see chapter 24 in this book; Sheer & Wong, 2008). Such efforts to establish national policies under the control of nursing will continue to drive NP development as long as it is done in concert with meeting societal needs, providing needed service, and promoting nursing careers.

SUMMARY

NPs are the most numerous of the advanced-nursing practice categories in the United States following more than 40 years of development. Global interest and commitment to an NP model follows a framework conceptualized in Figure 3.1. The interplay of nurses to provide needed services, create innovation, develop nursing careers, and establish nursing policy to support NP practice catalyzes and propels the NP model across the globe. Although it is a challenge to maintain this interplay for the profession of nursing, it is crucial to adhere to these dynamics, so that advances in health can be met in any region or country.

REFERENCES

American Association of Colleges of Nursing. (2009). *Fact sheet: Accelerated baccalaureate and master's degrees in nursing.* Retrieved September 24, 2009, from http://www.aacn.nche.edu/Media/FactSheets/AcceleratedProg.htm

American Association of Colleges of Nursing. (2006, October 20). *DNP roadmap task force report.* Washington, DC: Author.

Association of American Medical Colleges. (2006). *Help wanted: More U.S. doctors.* Washington, DC: Author.

Cooper, R. A., Laud, P., & Dietrich, C. L. (1998). Current and projected workforce of nonphysician clinicians. *Journal of the American Medical Association, 280,* 788–794.

Dickerson, P. S., & Nash, B. A. (1985). The business of nursing: Development of a private practice. *Nursing and Health Care, 6,* 327–329.

Fairman, J. (2008). *Making room in the clinic: Nurse practitioners and the evolution of modern health care.* New Brunswick, NJ: Rutgers University Press.

IKP Centre for Technologies in Public Health (ICTPH). (2009, August 22). *Equitable healthcare through alternate human resources.* ICTPH press release.

International Council of Nursing. (2009). *Definition and characteristics of the role.* Retrieved September 24, 2009, from http://66.219.50.180/inp%20apn%20network/practice%20issues/role%2 0definitions.asp

Jayakaran, R. (2009, August). *The NP programme in CMC Vellore.* Paper presented at the IKP Centre for Technologies in Public Health conference on "Alternative human resources for health in India: Innovative models for improving primary healthcare," Chennai, India.

Kung, Y. M., & Porterfield, S. (2009). The DNP: A need for standardized educational policies. *American Journal for Nurse Practitioners, 13*(5), 34–46.

Lang, N. M. (1983). Nurse managed centers: Will they survive? *American Journal of Nursing, 83,* 1290–1291.

Lang, N. M., & Evans, L. K. (2004). A vision and a plan for academic nursing practice. In L. K. Evans & N. M. Lang (Eds.), *Academic nursing practice: Helping to shape the future of health care* (pp. 3–19). New York: Springer Publishing Company.

Lewis, C. E., & Resnick, B. A. (1962). Nurse clinics and progressive ambulatory patient care. *New England Journal of Medicine, 277,* 1236–1241.

Mehrotra, A., Wang, M. C., Lave, J. R., Adams, J. L., & McGlynn, E. A. (2008). Retail clinics, primary care physicians, and emergency departments: A comparison of patients' visits. *Health Affairs, 27,* 1272–1282.

Meleis, A., & Dracup, K. (2005). The case against the DNP: History, timing, substance, and marginalization. *Online Journal of Issues in Nursing, 10*(3), manuscript 2. Retrieved on January 27, 2010, from http://www.nursingworld.org/MainMenuCategories/ANAMarketplace/ANAPeriodicals/OJIN/TableofContents/Volume102005/No3Sept05/tpc28_216 026.aspx

National Organization of Nurse Practitioner Faculties. (2004). *Acute care nurse practitioner competencies.* Washington, DC: Author.

O'Sullivan, A. L., Carter, M., Marion, L., Pohl, J. M., & Werner, K. E. (2005). Moving forward together: The practice doctorate in nursing. *Online Journal of Issues in Nursing, 10*(3), manuscript 4. Retrieved January 27, 2010, from http://www.nursing world.org/MainMenuCategories/ANAMarketplace/ANAPeriodicals/OJIN/Tableof Contents/Volume102005/No3Sept05/tpc28_416 028.aspx

Patidar, J. S. (2009, August). *Launch of an NP model in Gujarat.* Paper presented at the IKP Centre for Technologies in Public Health conference on "Alternative human resources for health in India: Innovative models for improving primary healthcare," Chennai, India.

Pearson, L. J. (2009). The Pearson report. *American Journal for Nurse Practitioners, 13*(2), 8–71.

Rogers, E. M. (2003). *Diffusion of innovations* (5th ed.). New York: Free Press.

Ryan, S. F. (2009). Providing the right level of care. *Nurse Practitioner Journal, 34,* 6–7.

Schober, M., & Affara, F. (2006). *International Council of Nurses: Advanced nursing practice.* Malden, MA: Blackwell.

Sheer, B., & Wong, F. (2008). The development of advanced nursing practice globally. *Journal of Nursing Scholarship, 40,* 204–211.

Sipe, T. A., Fullerton, J. T., & Schuiling, K. D. (2009). Demographic profiles of certified nurse-midwives, certified registered nurse anesthetists, and nurse practitioners: Reflections on implications for uniform education and regulation. *Journal of Professional Nursing, 25,* 178–185.

Spear, H. J. (2005, September 30). Letter to the editor on "Doctor of nursing practice..." [Letter to the editor]. *Online Journal of Issues in Nursing.* Retrieved January 27, 2010, from http://www.nursingworld.org/MainMenuCategories/ANAMarketplace/ANA Periodicals/OJIN/LetterstotheEditor/HilaJSpearLetter.aspx

Stanley, J. (2009). Reaching consensus on a regulatory model: What does this mean for APRNs? *Journal for Nurse Practitioners, 5,* 99–104.

Sullivan, E. (1992). Nurse practitioners & reimbursement: Case analyses. *Nursing & Health Care, 13*(5), 236–241.

Thygeson, M., Van Vorst, K. A., Maciosek, M. V., & Solberg, L. (2008). Use and costs of care in retail clinics versus traditional care sites. *Health Affairs, 27,* 1283–1292.

Tropello, P. D. (2009). International Council of Nurses Meeting. *Nurse Practitioner World News, 14*(11/12), 21–22.

U.S. Department of Health and Human Services, Health Resources and Service Administration. (2004). *The registered nurse population: Findings from the 2004 national sample survey of registered nurses.* Retrieved September 24, 2009, from http://bhpr.hrsa.gov/ healthworkforce/rnsurvey04/

World Health Organization (WHO). (2008). *The world health report 2008: Primary health care: Now more than ever.* Geneva: WHO Press.

Consumer Role for Nurse Practitioner Care: Center to Champion Nursing in America

4

BRENDA L. CLEARY, SUSAN C. REINHARD,
EILEEN M. SULLIVAN-MARX, AND DIANE O. McGIVERN

The *Center to Champion Nursing in America* is a joint initiative of the AARP Foundation and the Robert Wood Johnson Foundation, with a mission to ensure that every American has access to a highly skilled nurse, when and where they need one. We spoke with Susan Reinhard (**SR**), PhD, RN, FAAN, Senior Vice President, AARP Public Policy Institute and Chief Strategist, Center to Champion Nursing in America, and Brenda Cleary (**BC**), PhD, RN, FAAN, and Director of the Center. Conducted by Eileen Sullivan-Marx (**ESM**), the interview focused on partnerships with consumer organizations to promote advanced-practice nursing and how advanced-practice nurses can address consumer concerns.

ESM: Nurses and nurse practitioners (NPs) have had strong partnerships with consumers throughout their history. How can nurse practitioners today, and in the future, strengthen these partnerships?

BC: To the consumer, nurse practitioners are a viable alternative to current care. At the Center, we want every consumer to have access to a highly skilled nurse. Consumers should also have a choice of primary care providers, such as nurse practitioners. It is clear that people who receive services from a nurse practitioner have a good experience with high satisfaction, but if you have never had that kind of experience with an NP, it is not in your repertoire of choices. It is hard to believe in the 21st century that everybody does not know about nurse practitioners, what NPs do, and that they give really good care and can handle a great deal of people's basic health care needs.

SR: Nurse practitioners need to be able to define what they do, so consumers can better understand the nurse practitioner's role and value. I call it "thinking out loud." For example, as the nurse is assessing the patient, she or he says, "What I am doing now is listening to your lungs so I can tell whether there is any fluid; this is one way I can tell whether your medication is working or whether I can offer more advice on how you can manage your heart problem." Nurses are so good at demystifying what they do. That is one of our major gifts to society. But consumers do need to understand that what nurse practitioners are doing is very complex.

ESM: Tell us more about the mission of the Center to Champion Nursing in America, "to ensure that every American has access to a highly skilled nurse, when and where they need one."

BC: At the Center, we are trying to partner nurses with consumer organizations to raise awareness about nursing, and ensure that consumers have a choice for basic care when and where they need it. We have more work to do to keep consumers informed about the range of nursing care and services. Although it is surprising that there is still much to do to inform consumers, it is important to recognize the deficit in their understanding and make a plan to deal with it. Through AARP and Susan Reinhard's leadership in public policy at AARP, the Center is embedded in AARP, which provides opportunities for mutual strategies to meet the mission of ensuring every American has access to a highly skilled nurse when and where they need one. Champions are voices of nurses at high-level meetings and grass-roots community meetings who raise awareness of what nurse practitioners really do. Operationalizing the voice of nursing through our campaigns and board membership is a key and critical activity.

SR: The mission is evolving. When I started the Center in 2007, I articulated the mission as ensuring that, "Americans have the nurses they need, now and in the future." But in 2008, the AARP Public Policy Institute initiated research on consumer and family experiences in chronic care, and it become evident that they need health care professionals who have the knowledge and skills to manage chronic conditions and transitions between health care settings. And we need nurses who can help individuals and families discuss advanced illness management, including end-of-life and palliative care. So, we need more nurses, but even more important, we need a highly skilled nursing workforce. And we need those highly skilled nurses in all settings—especially in the community (in which so many nurse practitioners practice). So we changed our mission to emphasize ACCESS and SKILLS—in all settings.

ESM: In addition to boardrooms or policy tables, how can NPs or NP students in local communities increase this awareness to the consumer and make these same alliances?

BC: It is hard to have impact when you are just one person in a community, so I suggest that NPs and nurses link with community organizations that would be good alliances with AARP, such as Rotary International or Better Business Bureaus. An NP can present messages from the Center to Champion Nursing in America to local meetings and present what he or she does in his or her practice every day. In addition, NPs can connect with local AARP chapters. AARP has volunteers in every community in the United States. It is helpful for the local chapters to hear messages from the national organization and spread the word. If all "sing with one chorus," it is quite stirring and can reach a tipping point.

Questions about NPs and what they do can be added to polls and focus groups by AARP. NPs can send local stories about NP care to the Center or AARP at the national level. The AARP infrastructure for dissemination and reaching out to the nation is quite strong. We already know from polls that overwhelming numbers of Americans do say that nurses have a huge role in health care reform, as far as primary care and chronic care are concerned, and that nurses are held in high regard. So, NPs could use this good will for nurses, in general, both nationally and regionally to spread the word about what they have to offer. NPs could then present the barriers that they face as a need for consumers to work with them to improve access to NPs, and also remove barriers that prevent NPs from practicing to the level of their education and abilities. For example, helping consumers understand that NPs can be full primary care providers and refer directly to specialists for serious problems.

ESM: I think that one of the messages that gets jumbled for nurse practitioners is finding their own voices and identities in the physician-centered health reform conversation. This leads to invisibility for NPs and other advanced-practice nurses in health reform discussions. Consumers are often surprised to learn that NPs have their own distinct education, licensure, and regulatory standards. How can NPs' contributions to health care reform get to the American public?

BC: In relation to health care reform, we need the workforce so that the American consumer should have access to a highly skilled nurse when and where they need one, and to have a nursing workforce that has a skill set that people will need in the 21st century. To achieve this, some of the Center's strategic priorities are to focus on expanding both nursing education capacity and nurse leadership development and retention. For advanced-practice nurses, there should be a strong interface between their practice and these strategies. We need a dramatic increase in the advanced-practice nurse workforce. Along with increasing the numbers of advanced-practice nurses, we need to make sure at state levels that NPs can practice to their full capacity without limits. Some AARP state offices, in partnership with state nursing health reform groups, have a primary focus on expanding capacity in nursing education. State NP organizations can partner with the state AARP groups to get technical assistance and inform the consumers in the state about NP issues. Standardization for advanced-practice nurses is a significant issue for both increasing the supply of NPs, and deploying them to their fullest capacity, and at the national level, AARP is keeping abreast of these issues. This is keeping with the Center's mission, for consumers to have access to nurses with these advanced skills; they need to be able to provide the care that they were prepared to give.

ESM: One of your goals is to increase the number of nurses remaining in the workforce past traditional retirement age. How can nurse practitioners fit into this goal?

BC: We are concerned that the bottleneck in nursing education is only emphasized at the front end of education. No matter what we do on the front end of nursing education to increase the supply, there is still going to be a number of years when we are probably not going to have enough nurses. In 2010, we are going to roll out a project on older nurses in the workforce. This project will go beyond the basic foundation of improving ergonomics and assistance in physical care, to a focus on what environments would look like in primary care, home care, or hospitals for the older nurses to make them want to stay in the workforce, if that is their career choice. Right now, the economy is a factor to keep older nurses working, but to take a long view for nurse practitioners, perhaps a seasoned NP would like a reduced case load, but would be really interested in being a mentor for a nurse practitioner in a residency program. We think that use of the older workforce is going to be important to get over the hump of the nursing shortage. Interventions to keep the baby boomers engaged in the nursing workforce are going to be very important.

ESM: I see what you mean about the importance of helping NPs be able to continue to contribute their strengths and experience. We also need NPs to stay sharp and skilled in their competencies in clinical expertise; this can create a tension between "winding down" and staying highly skilled.

BC: We want NPs to stay engaged, but perhaps reduce the physically demanding aspects of their practice, and transfer their knowledge. We want to use this golden opportunity of a large retirement-age nurse workforce with knowledge and experience to help transfer knowledge. Older workers can provide younger nurses with insights into their thinking about certain aspects of practice that work best in a given situation. The older nurse workforce project is a natural opportunity for AARP to work with nurses and NPs, because of its infrastructure to support older workers. The message to AARP members is that everybody deserves to retire, but if you are not ready, maybe there is something in your work life that could be a little more interesting and manageable, for you to stay in the workforce. This would be good for consumers and for nurses.

ESM: It seems that one of the solutions to the shortage of nurses and nurse practitioners lies in reaching out to men and diverse groups who are underrepresented in the American nurse workforce. What efforts are you undertaking toward diversity of the nursing workforce?

BC: One of the dilemmas we face is the shortage of faculty, and schools that have had to turn away students due to a lack of capacity, at the same time that we are trying to recruit a broader range of people to nursing. The Center is supporting federal policies to increase diversity in the nurse workforce. A more diverse nurse workforce would be a stronger workforce, and also fit with the population at large. Diversity at the advanced-practice level would be essential to fostering leadership roles for all nurses.

We also consider that second-degree entrance students are a diverse group of people to enter nursing, because they bring a range of backgrounds that are very exciting. We are planning to add models to our Web site that work for recruitment and workforce as an interactive feature for consumers and others to learn about the wide variety of care that nurses and advanced-practice nurses provide. As it relates to nurse practitioners, we want to emphasize for our consumers that NPs, as primary care providers, are experts focusing on health promotion and disease prevention (a major area of interest to consumers), coordinating care, and providing transitional care and chronic care management.

SUMMARY

The goal of the AARP, the AARP Foundation, and the Robert Wood Johnson Foundation Campaign to Champion Nursing in America is to ensure a sufficient number of generalists and advanced-practice nurses to meet American's health care needs. In particular, the mission of the Center, and the goal for nurses and consumers, is "access and skills in all settings," including highly skilled nurses such as community-based nurse practitioners (www.championnursing.org).

The overall collaboration is underway, with state teams framing messages to policymakers, nurses, and the general public. Although state teams are at different levels of organization and message development, their common goal is to produce effective communications tailored to various constituent groups. Supported by their broad organizational coalition and extremely experienced state team members, the developing campaign is producing a variety of interesting and potentially important information networks.

Two examples of the Center to Champion Nursing in America campaign efforts include the Colorado Center for Nursing Excellence and the Washington Center for Nursing's contributions to consumer information. The Colorado Center for Nursing Excellence (www.colora donursingcenter.org) produces a lengthy, data-rich weekly communication regarding health care and nursing sent to its advisory committee and board members. The Washington Center for Nursing's (www.wa centerfornursing.org) online publications include the "Be A Nurse" brochure, which describes generalist and advanced-practice nursing career options.

As additional state teams' messages and communication products mature, their messages will become more targeted to the full range of constituent groups the Center plans to reach. Reinhard and Cleary's goal and emphasis is on a highly organized and orchestrated effort that will reach into states and locales. The Center's strength rests on a broad organization of teams such as these, working at the state level.

5 Public Relations Strategies for Nurse Practitioners

JOY McINTYRE

Nurse practitioners (NPs) are practically considered invisible in the media (Edmunds, 2002; Norwood, 2001). Despite the many contributions made by nurses, the respect that the American public holds for them (Morales, 2008), and their significant numbers in the workforce (Health Resources and Services Administration, 2007), nurses and NPs are rarely seen in television and print ads as health care providers, nor are they quoted in the media as experts in health care delivery or policy.

This apparent dichotomy has been the message of a bumper crop of journal articles, books, and blogs. The former Center for Nursing Advocacy cataloged many major news stories in the interest of assessing coverage of nurses, and found only a few involving NPs, usually staffing "quick clinics" (Center for Nursing Advocacy, 2004). As such, the coverage seems to question whether nursing care is equal to a physician's, while showing the NP, in a retro image, waving a hypodermic needle. The state of affairs is so dire that Peter Buerhaus and colleagues (Buerhaus, Donelan, Ulrich, Norman, & Dittus, 2006) and other well-known nursing researchers have investigated whether the current portrayal of nurses has contributed to the projected nursing shortage. Logically, this may affect NPs as well as a much smaller group: future NPs. It's hard for teenagers to decide on a career they've never heard of.

This can be changed. This chapter aims to demonstrate some of the strategies that can be employed to help NPs polish their individual reputations and practices, while also raising the visibility of the profession.

CHANGING PERCEPTIONS TO CHANGE BEHAVIOR

Public Relations is the art of persuasion based on a relatively simple cause-and-effect equation: our perceptions form our attitudes, which, in turn, shape our behaviors. In order to change behaviors, then, you must first change the perception that leads to taking that action (Bernays, 1945). It's simple, yet frustratingly difficult to achieve.

To illustrate: If NPs are invisible, or if they are seen in only minor roles, the logical belief is they have no independent body of knowledge, no real science, and therefore are not "qualified" to take care of the nation's families. The predictable behavior that follows is that an NP may not be chosen as a health care provider, and may be seen as "second best" to a physician, may be devalued in the workplace, and might even have difficulty achieving parity in pay or reimbursements with physicians. Changing these behaviors requires changing the public perception of what the NP knows and can do. Change perceptions to change behaviors.

The nation's marketing gurus have known this for decades. We take for granted that teeth need to be white, wrinkles nonexistent, washed clothes smelling "fresh;" however, these values have been created through advertising that has, over time and with millions of dollars, altered our perceptions. A generation ago, yellowed teeth were considered a normal part of aging, and the attitude was acceptance, leading to marketers learning that brushing once a day with ordinary toothpaste was not good for sales.

So advertising created the "need" for an ever-growing abundance of products that changed the mind-set, and thus, the behavior, of the American public, made easier by linking the desired behavior to other habits. For instance, using a moisturizer is linked to the morning wash-up ritual or going to bed so as to foster moisturizer use, even though it works perfectly well at other times of day.

These same principles can be applied to health care. Take the spread of disease in underdeveloped nations. The *New York Times* reported that "A few years ago, a self-described 'militant liberal' named Val Curtis decided that it was time to save millions of children from death and disease. So Dr. Curtis, an anthropologist then living in the African nation of Burkina Faso, contacted some of the largest multinational corporations and asked them, in effect, to teach her how to manipulate consumer habits worldwide" (Duhigg, 2008, p. 1).

What did she want to do? She wanted people in developing nations to wash their hands with soap to halt the spread of diseases that kill a child almost every 15 seconds.

Partnering with consumer-product companies, she formed the Global Public–Private Partnership for Handwashing with Soap in Ghana, a country in which soap was readily available, but rarely used after toileting. Why was this happening when soap was both plentiful and cheap?

The aid workers set out to find out why. Questioning local people in information-gathering sessions, they found that a modern toilet was *not perceived to be dirty*. In fact, compared to the latrines of their youth, Ghanaians believed the toilet was a clean place, rendering hand-washing with soap simply unnecessary. Critical to their success, the health care workers knew what the perception was they were trying to change—that the bathroom was clean. They communicated new information about germs, linking them to feelings of disgust. Ads were developed showing mothers' and children's hands dripping with purple slime after toileting, which changed the perception that a modern toilet was clean. That changed behavior, leading to a 13% increase in handwashing in the bathroom, and a 41% increase in using soap before eating (Duhigg, 2008).

So how do we craft a similar equation to change the public perception of NPs without massive advertising budgets? It helps to know what current perceptions of NPs are. Not enough is known. And what is known is rather a mixed bag.

CURRENT PERCEPTIONS OF NURSING

"In the past, nurses have not been a public voice for either themselves or their patients. Consequently, this silence has led to misunderstanding and lack of awareness of the nature, scope, and contributions of NPs. This can be seen in the perceptions of NPs by health care consumers and the medical community, and even among nurses themselves," according to Counts (2005, p. 292).

Susan Norwood's 2001 review of 96 health-related articles and 100 advertisements in popular magazines found that the media continues to portray physicians as the source of health care advice, leading readers "to assume [NPs] have little influence, standing, and authority" (Norwood, 2001, p. 129).

Despite our physician-focused media coverage, the American public trusts nurses, even if they're not exactly sure what it is that nurses *do*. In their annual "Honesty and Ethics of Professions" poll, the Gallup Organization has found that nurses have consistently topped the list every year, except in 2001, when firefighters took first place after the events of September 11. However, perhaps providing further proof that nursing is an "invisible profession," nurses have only been included in the poll since 1999 (Saad, 2008). And NPs have yet to be included on the list.

Sigma Theta Tau International, the international nursing honor society, collected survey data more than a decade ago indicating that the image of nursing in the public mind was out of date, not matching what nurses know and can do. The longstanding image of nurses as "caring angels" is the stuff of legend, but does not reflect the emphasis of the current nursing curriculum, which is grounded in principles of critical thinking, theories of nursing practice, anatomy, pharmacology, and pathophysiology, and prepares students to employ ethical decision making, use increasingly high-tech equipment, and gain competence in independent assessment and action in today's managed care environment (Sigma Theta Tau International, 1997).

Perhaps it is this complex organizational health environment that accounts for some of the differences in perception between nurses and the general public. In their 2006 study, Buerhaus, Donelan, Ulrich, Norman, and Dittus compared the attitudes of nurses to those of the general public in order to shed light on the projected shortage of nurses. These findings show that discrepancies in perception may extend beyond the media to the profession itself. Nurses were more likely to think of nursing as "caring" (20%) than the general public (16%); nurses were less likely to consider nurses highly knowledgeable, qualified, and skilled (6%) than the general public (17%); and nurses were less likely (4%) to think of themselves as "smart or highly educated" than the public (7%). However, somewhat shockingly, only 8% of the public considered nurses to be "professionals," compared with 23% of nurses. How can this be when there are 2.9 million professional nurses in the United States alone (Health Resources and Services Administration [HRSA], 2007)? It might just be because no one knows who the nurse is. A bus conductor wearing a uniform, a minister wearing a collar, and a chef in an apron and toque are all highly visible and identifiable.

Although discarding the "starched whites" long associated with nursing may have been desirable for many reasons, it also deprived nurses of their visual identity. Learning a valuable lesson from this, NPs who wear a white lab coat with a visual identifier can help buck the trend toward invisibility in the workplace. But clothes alone do not make the NP.

As Suzanne Gordon (2005) notes in her seminal book, *Nursing Against the Odds*, sociologist Erving Goffman researched how people present themselves by making "definitional claims." "The patient for whom a nurse cares is both an actor, someone acted upon, and a spectator in the broader health care drama. Along with lessons on how to take their medication or change their diet, the patients are absorbing messages about status and legitimacy as they observe the intricate choreograph of hierarchy that takes place around them. When subtle messages of deference conflict with the nurses' definitional claims, patients usually take notice, as do their families and friends" (p. 215).

What Gordon goes on to suggest is that nurses must stake their claim, identify themselves firmly as Nurse Smith, announce their work with authority, and not fall victim to the idea that nursing work needs to be shrouded in "a jargon of theoretical functions and abstractions" in order to be seen as important. "This understandable attempt to give status to nursing work ends up concealing it from those who have a need to know" (Gordon, 2005, pp. 218–219), particularly journalists.

What do we know? Although nurses are the most trusted professionals, nurses are not quoted as health care authorities in the popular press. NPs have not always spoken with a public voice, which has led to a public misunderstanding of the scope and breadth of the role of NPs as independent health care providers who can prescribe and treat (Counts, 2005). And there is ample evidence that nurses are still seen primarily as "caring" in the hospital or health care setting, instead of as the highly educated, knowledgeable, and skilled providers that they are.

If NPs want the public to view them as health care authorities, they need to alter perceptions by sharing knowledge; identifying themselves as those who can diagnose, prescribe, and treat; identifying themselves professionally by title; and conveying a specialized body of knowledge. And it is important to do this in a way that is memorable.

MESSAGING

A catchy or memorable phrase helps to create what public relations professionals think of as a clear message. A quick review of the *New York Times* "Quote of the Day" reveals what journalists value and what others are willing to say to get their point across. Brief, concise, and understandable, such comments confer power and authority on the speaker.

"We have in our hands the power to reduce the risk of heart disease by a lot," said David Waters, Professor of Medicine at the University of California, San Francisco, in a front page story in the *New York Times* (Kolata, 2004). By contrast, the actual study lasted 2 years, involved 4,162 patients hospitalized for sudden heart pain, and investigated whether reducing cholesterol levels beyond 100 milligrams, the current standard, was beneficial by comparing two popular statin drugs (Kolata, 2004). Importantly, even *The New York Times* uses a quote that is simple, short, clear, and jargon-free.

Knowing how to translate the information simply and compellingly does not detract from the status of the "expert;" rather, it adds to it. Think of the Nobel Laureate who determined that the vulnerability of the O-ring to cold was a possible cause of the Challenger disaster by putting a piece of the material in a pitcher of ice water and going to lunch. When he came back, it was brittle. There is power in simplicity, especially when a news story may run no more than 20 seconds on television, or 6 inches of type in a newspaper, a few sentences in a blog post, or just 140 characters on Twitter.

One critical element of public relations is changing, however, and very quickly. Traditional public relations rely upon a third-party endorsement; that is the belief that a story in the newspaper is more believable and changes opinions more readily than an advertisement. But what happens when there are no newspapers? NPs and everyone else now have the ability to self-publish on a website and link interested parties, clients, and what reporters are left, to the website for information. Social media such as Twitter and Facebook are ways to do this.

But if the goal is to change perceptions, crafting a targeted message is critical to the process. Bill Clinton's winning campaign strategy was based upon a few key messages tacked to the campaign wall: for example, "It's the economy, stupid!" More can be learned about the technique by watching Sunday morning talk shows during a political campaign. No matter what question is asked, a masterful politician will provide answers that frame the same message points. Repeating the thought is another way to get it to "stick" in the public mind in order to alter perceptions, to change attitudes about the candidate, and to change behaviors in order to garner support or gather votes. Think of what message you want to get across to frame your practice.

"Stickiness" is literally what sticks in people's minds, and changes them. In *Made to Stick*, Heath and Heath (2007) illustrate this concept through movie popcorn. When the Center for Science in the Public Interest (CSPI) wanted to warn consumers of the fat content of movie popcorn, they did not put out a warning that a standard serving had 37 grams of fat, simply assuming that the media would carry such a dry story or that consumers would understand it and act appropriately. Most lay people don't memorize what nutritional guidelines are, so they might not even realize how much of anything was good for them or bad.

Instead, at their press conference, the CSPI reported: "A medium-sized 'butter' popcorn at a typical neighborhood movie theater contains more artery-clogging fat than a bacon-and-eggs breakfast, a Big Mac and fries for lunch, and a steak dinner with all the trimmings—combined!" In front of reporters, investigators laid out the entire "day's worth of food" on a table for the television cameras (Heath & Heath, 2007, pp. 6–8).

Up to that point, popcorn was probably perceived as a nutritious choice, more nutritious than candy. But this idea "stuck," changing perceptions and behaviors. Consumers stopped buying popcorn at the movies. And some of the nation's largest theater chains announced they would stop adding coconut oil to their popcorn (Heath & Heath, 2007, p. 8).

There are common characteristics of ideas that sell. In *Made to Stick*, the authors describe them as: Simplicity, Unexpectedness, Concreteness, Credibility, Emotions, and Stories. Easily remembered by the acronym S-U-C-C-E-S, there is no room for jargon in that lineup (Heath & Heath, 2007).

In nursing, there are examples of "stickiness." Consider Linda Aiken and her colleagues' study, "Hospital nurse staffing and patient mortality, nurse burnout, and job dissatisfaction," which was published in 2002 (Aiken, Clarke, Sloane, Sochalski, & Silber, 2002). Since publication, the article has been widely cited by researchers, as well as the lay press. The findings, exhibiting the characteristics of "stickiness," were memorable because the results were expressed as Simple in a color-coded bar chart. The findings were Concrete and Credible. The issue of Unexpected patient deaths is as Emotionally charged as it gets. And the public saw the Story of overworked nurses so clearly there were editorial cartoons illustrating the issue.

REACHING THE AUDIENCE

In the case of the CSPI and campaign against unhealthy popcorn, the desired behavior was a change to healthier eating habits. The story was picked up by mass media, making the front pages of major newspapers and television shows.

But for most individual NPs, the stories are local. And thinking of changing behaviors leads us to an important question: Whose?

If the general public's perceptions are to change, then getting the attention of the mass media can be the option. But if the goal is to get more patients into a clinic, or advanced-practice nurses (APNs) on a committee in the hospital, or younger nurses into the profession, the target audience might be vastly different.

Local radio or newspaper outlets might help with clinic attendance. A hospital newsletter could establish nurses as experts within the hospital culture. Web sites or other tech-friendly media might be needed to reach today's high school and college students and encourage them to think of earning a master's degree in nursing.

Knowing which slice of the general public is actually the target audience for the message is central to the process, because demographic information, especially age, changes the means for delivering the information. Older Americans still read newspapers, but younger ones get their information from the Internet, or the rapidly growing social networking sites such as Facebook and Twitter. Even television is being eroded as the source of most Americans' information. What is under-stood about the audience's knowledge, attitudes, and beliefs will dictate the goals of your communications. It is no secret that newspapers are dying: Major cities once had two; now just one in each city is struggling. With circulations dropping and prices, especially newsprint and delivery costs, rising, many pundits are predicting the demise of the American newspaper, at least if it's printed on paper. As of December 2008, 36% of those 18–29 got their information from the Internet, compared with 14% of those 65 and older. When it came to reading the local paper, the percentages were reversed, with 68% of older Americans still reading the paper, and only 22% of the young adult demographic. It's not hard to see where this is heading. Before the Fall 2008 stock market meltdown, the stock values of the cofounders of Google exceeded the value of the entire newspaper industry in the United States (Morales, 2008).

The Gallup Organization polled Americans to find that most use local television as a source for their local news. But the venerable polling organization also found striking trends based on age—only 36% of 18–29-year-olds watch local television news, compared with 63% of those 65 years old and older.

As of December 2009, exactly the same percentage of 18–29-year-olds (36%) was getting information from the Internet. But that percent-age had grown 10% in 2 years, whereas television watching had declined 8% (Morales, 2008).

Clearly, a seachange is taking place in how Americans get their information. Not surprisingly, the Internet has shown the biggest in-crease in popularity as a news source, with 31% of Americans now saying it is now a *daily* news source (Morales, 2008). This marks a nearly 50% increase since 2006, and a more than 100% increase from 2002. Use of the Internet as a news source has increased each time Gallup has asked about it, beginning in 1995 (Morales, 2008).

Some of the most striking trends are by age. Knowing who is getting their news from which medium can begin to direct a public relations campaign. If you want to reach younger people, the better place to speak to them may be through social networking sites on the Internet such as Facebook or Twitter or your own Web site, whereas a geronto-logical NP may want to consider reaching potential clients through the local newspaper.

Looking at the local television news, in 2008, 36% of 18–29-year-olds watched, compared with 63% of those 65 years old and older. So looking at it as a delivery vehicle for messaging, more older people are going to hear it than younger, which is effective only if older people are the target market. Local newspapers are the source for news for only 22% of the younger group, but 59% of the older group. To reach a market of younger consumers, 78% of 18–49-year-olds get their news on the Internet (Morales, 2008).

Looking at this demographic information before developing a program helps determine which media should be used, depending on which population is the target market. If a gerontological NP wants to reach the market, using the local newspaper might find the most potential users. But a young mother looking for a health care provider for her infants might be looking on the Internet for an especially informative website for a practice in her area. Thinking through who the target audience is then helps decide which medium to use.

Summing up, there's a perception to be changed to spark a desired change in behavior. A key message has been developed with a story that can "stick." The target audience has been established that informs us about the medium best used to reach them, whether it's print, television, radio, or an internal communication, such as a hospital newsletter.

WRITING THE PRESS RELEASE

Now it is time to write the press release, right?

Not so fast. Very few press releases match any of the criteria for effective communication discussed previously. What is contained in a news release generally will not change perceptions to change behavior, nor will they sell a message that "sticks," hit a discreet target audience, or tell a compelling story. At best, press releases that announce a grant, award, honor, or even a new practice will only get a slender mention in a column that lists similar honors for a host of others.

A press release is only one of an array of tactics used to inform editors and the public, and unless there is actual "stop-the-presses" news, it is not usually chosen by public relations professionals. NPs can consider establishing themselves as experts through letters to the editor and opinion pieces, becoming an "expert" guest on a radio show, or even cold-calling an editor and "pitching" a story idea. It helps if that story is somewhat broad-based and not only about the virtues of a practice. Editors are likely to think of the latter kind of story as advertising that needs to be purchased, and not a story written for the greater good. Producing publications or a Web site allows for more targeted messaging and more control, but it is harder to know whether anyone is reading it.

CONCLUSIONS

All of the examples given previously can be thought of as adding up to one directive: Tell the story proactively and with conviction—and most importantly, do it often and well.

In *Becoming Influential, A Guide for Nurses*, Eleanor Sullivan (2003) describes five steps for telling the story of nurses:

1. Consciously develop your own belief that nursing is essential to the health care system. Emphasize that conviction to your colleagues.
2. At every opportunity, be willing to tell the public and the media what nurses do and how nursing care affects health and recovery.
3. Collect three anecdotes about your work and be prepared to share them with others.
4. Cultivate a "voice of agency" (authority).
5. Let both internal and external media know that you are willing to speak to health care audiences, public groups, and the media about nursing.

Case Study and Conclusions

Looking through the lens of all that has been discussed, we can take on the case of an APN who may want to draw attention to her practice in gerontology while also working to upgrade the public image of NPs. It is always worthwhile to consider the image of the entire profession because a rising tide floats all boats.

Literally taking a page out of the Buresh and Gordon (2006) book, the NP will develop that "voice of agency" by identifying herself confidently as an NP. The ongoing column written by Tom Bartol, NP, CDE,

"Promoting the NP Profession," which runs regularly in *The American Journal for Nurse Practitioners*, offers tips for building self-confidence and negotiating the role of the NPs in the health care system: in short, showing how to do public relations on a personal level every day. One way is to consistently define the NP in a succinct sound-bite style messaging as someone who can "evaluate, prescribe, and treat." That tells the public the distinct nature of the advanced-practice role without sorting through the list of alphabetic credentials at the end of a title. Television viewers and newspaper readers are not detectives. That "voice" should be paired with a professional appearance, and for that, we might look through the eyes of a child.

Use the "voice of agency," define the visual appearance with a white coat and stethoscope, and define the role of the APN as someone who can "evaluate, prescribe, and treat."

In gerontology, the APN might approach local newspaper editors, offering expert advice on what older people should do in heat waves to protect their health, or guard against falls, showing the APN as an expert. Local newspapers are read by older people, but if the behavior the APN is addressing (such as nursing home placement) is made by a different audience (middle-aged children), then a different venue, such as drive-time radio, could be considered to reach working people. Check the demographics to find *your* audience.

And when messaging, using everyday language helps. Speaking of "old people," the "World War II generation," or "the elderly," instead of "frail elders," resonates with busy family members and can help get a message to stick. Think of a message that is surprising and succinct, such as, "Should Mom take her medication in a heat wave?" while explaining, as an expert, that dehydration can lead to an overdose of maintenance medications and giving exact information. The result is that the right audience will think of the APN as credible, expert, and memorable.

And the profession will begin to move the needle of public opinion, and not just be identified with using one.

REFERENCES

Aiken, L., Clarke, S., Sloane, D., Sochalski, J., & Silber, J. (2002). Hospital nurse staffing and patient mortality, nurse burnout, and job dissatisfaction. *Journal of the American Medical Association, 288*(16), 1987–1993.

Bernays, E. (1945). *Public relations.* Boston: Bellman Publishing Company.

Buerhaus, P. I., Donelan, K., Ulrich, B. T., Norman, L., & Dittus, R. (2006). State of the registered nurse workforce in the United States. *Nursing Economics, 24*(1), 6–12.

Buresch, B., & Gordon, S. (2006). *From silence to voice: What nurses know and must communicate to the public.* Ithaca, NY: Sage.

Center for Nursing Advocacy. (2004). *Quick clinic NPs: Neos in the health care matrix?* Retrieved January 20, 2009, from http://www.nursingadvocacy.org/news/2004jul/18_nyt.html

Counts, M. (2005). Speaking with one voice. *Journal of the American Academy of Nurse Practitioners, 17*(8), 292–294.

Duhigg, C. (2008, July 13). *Warning: Habits may be good for you.* Retrieved January 20, 2009, from http://www.nytimes.com/2008/07/13/business/13habit.html?_r=1& ref= world

Edmunds, M. (2002). Advocacy in practice: Market to the media. *Nurse Practitioner, 27*(3), 72.

Gillin, P. (2008, December 6). *Tale of the tape.* Retrieved February 26, 2010, from http://www.newspaperdeathwatch.com/tale-of-the-tape.html

Gordon, S. (2005). *Nursing against the odds.* Ithaca, NY: Cornell University Press.

Health Resources and Services Administration (HRSA). (2007). *The registered nurse population: Findings from the March 2004 national sample survey of registered nurses.* U.S. Department of Health and Human Services. Retrieved January 20, 2009, from http://bhpr.hrsa.gov/healthworkforce/rnsurvey04/

Heath, D., & Heath, C. (2007). *Made to stick.* New York: Random House.

Kolata, G. (2004, March 9). *Cholesterol targets should be set far lower, study finds.* Retrieved January 13, 2009, from http://www.nytimes.com/2004/03/08/health/08 CND-STAT.html?ex=1394168400&en=fcce26d7310b1cf0&ei=5007&partner= USERLAND

Morales, L. (2008, December 15). *Gallup poll: Cable, internet news sources growing in popularity.* Retrieved May 12, 2009, from http://www.gallup.com/poll/113314/Cable-Internet-News-Sources-Growing-Popularity.aspx

Norwood, S. (2001). The invisibility of advanced practice nurses in popular magazines. *Journal of the American Academy of Nurse Practitioners, 13*(3), 129–133.

Saad, L. (2008, November 24). *Gallup poll: Nurses shine, bankers slump in ethics ratings.* Retrieved February 19, 2009, from http://www.gallup.com/poll/112264/Nurses-Shine-While-Bankers-Slump-Ethics-Ratings.aspx

Sigma Theta Tau International. (1997). *The Woodhull study on nursing in the media– Healthcare's invisible partner.* Retrieved February 19, 2009, from http://www.nursing-society.org/Media/Pages/woodhall.aspx

Sullivan, E. (2003). *Becoming influential: A guide for nurses.* Upper Saddle River, NJ: Prentice Hall.

Research Supporting Nurse Practitioners and Their Practice

Part II provides a fresh look at the rapidly evolving research related to the nurse practitioner (NP) role, as well as the elements and nature of the NP's practice. The Groth, Norsen, and Kitzman chapter on long-term outcomes presents not only examples of the work of NPs to improve care for their patients and families, but also a thorough discussion of the elements of the current methods that NPs must know to conduct and interpret research. Fairman and Sullivan-Marx, as editors, have added an epilogue to the chapter on research in support of NPs, which was originally published in the fourth edition.

The chapter remains an excellent piece that will take the reader through the practice, policy, and scientific work that has undergirded the United States and emerging worldwide development of NPs. In the discussion of four areas of research supporting nurse practitioner practice, the authors synthesize work that was done from the early 1960s to present day. Rather than only highlight the chronology of studies about NP practice, however, the authors demonstrate how clusters of work have evolved from providing the worth of NPs, to demonstrating innovations in quality and cost, focusing on outcomes, and finally embarking on significant questions for the future.

6

Research in Support of Nurse Practitioners

FRANCES HUGHES, SEAN CLARKE, DEBORAH A. SAMPSON, JULIE A. FAIRMAN, AND EILEEN M. SULLIVAN-MARX

Since the 1960s, researchers published numerous studies to describe, explain, and justify the nurse practitioner (NP) role to society; in this chapter, we present a focused review of research examining NPs, and propose new directions that go beyond the traditional approaches of effectiveness, use, and comparison. Although it is not an exhaustive review, our approach takes a broad perspective of NP research and the prevailing themes of the last 3 decades, categorized in three eras. We then categorize the eras and themes: Era I (1960–1979) focuses on the theme of proving the worth of NPs, Era II (1975–1995) describes research of innovations, quality, and cost of NPs, and Era III (1990–present) examines current themes and the status of research. Researchers in this area have successfully chronicled the value and justification for advanced-practice nurses (APNs) in health care. Following our review of the state of advanced-practice nursing research to date, we will discuss strategies to move the research agenda forward and away from traditional themes of justification, efficiency, and comparison, and toward evidence-based practice (also see chapter 7 of this book).

ERA I: PROVING WORTH, 1960–1979

Nurses worked in expanded roles well before the 1960s. The public health nurses of the early 20th century, nurse midwives in the Frontier Nursing Service of the 1920s and 1930s, military nurses during World War II, and the early intensive care nurses of the 1950s all practiced in expanded roles. The NPs of the 1960s were not an exception. The foundational differences, however, between the earlier practitioners and NPs of the 1960s were rooted in more formalized education programs and the rapidity with which the idea of expanded practice disseminated, albeit haphazardly.

The Social Context

The research studies of the 1960s and 1970s reflected the social transition and growth occurring in society and influencing nursing practice. Within the context of the women's movement, the civil rights movement, Lyndon Johnson's Great Society programs, and Vietnam War protests, changes in health care and nursing were not surprising. Enactment of Medicare and Medicaid legislation in 1965, and the commensurate increased demand for primary care providers (PCPs), revealed the inherent deficit of a health system geared for acute care. At the same time, the Division of Nursing of the Department of Health and Human Services and private funding sources, such as The Robert Wood Johnson Foundation, made incredibly innovative and highly political decisions to provide money both for postgraduate nursing education and for demonstration projects to fill the gaps in care, particularly for women and children, and people in rural settings. From this context, the pediatric NP program developed by Loretta Ford and Henry Silver emerged in 1965 at the University of Colorado, and focused on caring for rural families and their children. Arising from a foundation of public health nursing, Ford and Silver designed this program to prepare NPs at the graduate level through a certificate program funded, in part, with federal dollars (Silver, Ford, & Stearly, 1967).

The Research Context

As the 1960s matured, more nurses entered academic collegiate settings, and nursing practice focused on patient-centered clinical problems.

Nursing research slowly and reluctantly followed the changes in education and practice. Small groups of nursing scholars posed new types of research questions and defined new nursing values that redirected knowledge development from functional studies toward clinical research and scholarly inquiry.

Few nurses had the knowledge and education to conduct or participate in research, and of those very few nurses who completed doctoral work, many earned their degrees in schools of education, or departments of anthropology and sociology. Their research focus necessarily was guided by their particular educational framework, rather than clinical practice. Until 1976, more than half of *Nursing Research*'s pages were filled primarily with studies about curriculum, methodological issues, or student concerns (Baer, 1997). Similarly, Sigma Theta Tau did not fund a clinically focused study until 1966 (Sigma Theta Tau International, 1996). Even so, nurse researchers, who were primarily clinicians themselves, were eager to focus on the new NP role. They asked questions and collected data according to the tools and skills they had at hand, via essays, surveys, or polls, implementing basic descriptive quantitative studies using samples of convenience. Early on, they focused their analysis at the very basic level: How many patients did they care for over particular periods of time, what did they actually do, what kinds of skills and knowledge did they add to their nursing repertoire in order to practice in an enlarged role, how did they "get along" with their physician colleagues? Patient-centered studies, other than quantitative analysis of patient satisfaction, came much later. However, when NPs became more commonplace as health care providers and less self-conscious about their place in the health care system, and nurses in general became more nuanced researchers, different types of studies emerged in later decades.

Research Exemplars

The studies conducted during the early 1960s and through to the mid-1970s were primarily descriptive in nature, reflecting the early state of nursing research. Many studies, when read closely, carried a sometimes not-so-subtle subtext reflecting nurses' utter excitement and satisfaction with their enlarged roles, as if they finally had escaped the bonds of traditional practice. The studies also implied, again subtly at first, that nurses provided certain kinds of care, such as the well baby care, and performed certain tasks, such as immunizations or physical examinations, as competently as their physician colleagues (Fairman, 1997; Geolot, 1990).

One of the earliest reported experiments came in 1961, from the Collaborative Study of Prenatal Factors in Cerebral Palsy and Neurological Diseases in Providence, RI. Specially trained public health nurses conducted screenings of infants to detect physical defects, a task previously performed only by physicians. In this study, public health nurses were found to be as highly effective as pediatricians in screening efforts (Solomons & Hatton, 1961). In 1963, a nursing care clinic was established at the Thomas F. Gailor Out-Patient Clinics, in Memphis, TN, to reduce the excessive workload created by poor, chronically ill patients visiting the hospital outpatient clinics for routine observation and continuation of long-term treatments. Using physician-developed protocols, the nurses independently staffed the clinics, referred patients to specialists, and provided supervision of patients with chronic, stable conditions (Guthrie, Runyan, Clark, & Marvin, 1964). Lewis and Resnick (1964) reported on the nurse clinic established in 1964 at the University of Kansas Medical Center. Their analysis indicated significant reduction in the frequency of complaints, a marked reduction in patients seeking out doctors for minor complaints, and a marked shift in the preference of patients for nurses to perform certain functions. The researchers concluded that the nurses provided competent and effective care to uncomplicated chronically ill patients comparable with that of physicians in outpatient clinics (Fairman, 1999).

Competition and Changing Questions

Many of the reports in the 1970s continued to describe this exciting new nursing role, the various training programs, and touted NPs as an answer to the problem of the lack of PCPs, particularly in underserved populations (Glover, 1967; Martin, 1967; Schiff, Fraser, & Walters, 1969; Walker, Murawski, & Thorn, 1964). And here again, the research questions were socially constructed and designed with an underlying self-consciousness to "prove" to themselves and the rest of the health care world that NPs were safe practitioners in various settings.

A number of reasons accounted for this approach to research questions during this time period. First, physician competence was assumed by other practitioners and the public, based on the strong cultural authority physicians held in the health care system and their professional organizations such as the American Medical Association. Nurses' competence had to be proven over and over, on a case-by-case basis (Fagin, 1992).

Second, health resource demand continued to grow in the 1970s, particularly among the elderly and families with children, while the number of general practice physicians continued to decline as more and more physicians entered specialty practice (Fairman, 1999). In contrast, the number of NPs continued to grow as generous federal funding for nursing education was targeted specifically for NP education beginning in 1971 (Geolot, 1990). Physicians and NPs, due in part to restrictive state practice legislation that required direct physician supervision of NPs, and despite the desperation of overworked PCPs, found themselves in competition for the ownership of skills and knowledge once firmly in medicine's domain (Safriet, 1992).

The 1970s also saw a rise in the number of physician-generated articles, both in the popular press and in organization journals, questioning the ability of NPs to provide quality care, and lending greater support to physician assistants. Articles of this type tended to be polemic, experiential, and opinion pieces. Much of the discussions going on in the professional journals were, in part, a direct response to the competition physicians began to experience from other types of practitioners, such as osteopaths and chiropractors, who achieved reimbursement victories in the late 1960s and early 1970s. Physicians were also undergoing radical and forced changes in their practice philosophies as federal and state health insurance programs began to make the solo practitioner obsolete. The encroachment felt by physicians was perhaps best expressed and forecasted by George E. Ferrar, Jr. (1969), President of the Pennsylvania Medical Society. In an address to Society officers about future challenges, in particular the emerging "doctor assistants," he warned, "this health professional could become the single greatest opposing force that medical doctors have ever faced" (p. 9).

Nurse researchers responded to the growing unease in the medical and nursing press by designing research to show that NPs could, indeed, practice in a qualified, expert manner (Holt, 1998). In the 1970s, more and more studies and reports emerged that indirectly tried to make sense of and legitimize the massive federal investment in NP education, and to enlighten physicians about the roles NPs could play in their practices. Even so, framed by the growing potential for economic and political competition between NPs and physicians, studies comparing physician and NP care in certain venues or for specific populations became the most prevalent form of analysis (Bessman, 1974; Heagarty, Boehringer, Lavigne, Brooks, & Evans, 1973; Russo, Gururaj, Bunye, Kim, & Ner, 1975). The reports generally indicated that NPs could substitute for physicians, and that care provided by NPs was equivalent to, if not better than, care provided by physicians. As early as 1974, the research team of Sackett, Spitzer, Gent, and Roberts (1974) in Ontario, Canada, concluded that NPs were effective and safe, and that it was time to refocus attention to the process of care delivery. Although many comparison studies were simply designed and contained considerable bias, policymakers and the public began to take notice and recognize APNs as legitimate providers of health care.

Initially in the NP professional movement, NPs were conceived as a means to provide health care to underserved populations. Yet few of the early research studies actually addressed the care NPs provided in the context of the patient in underserved areas, nor were the studies designed with a sound theoretical approach. NP researchers of the 1960s and 1970s self-consciously focused on themselves, a trend that continued into the next few decades. Of course, the early research provided valuable support for the fledgling movement and for individual practitioners hungry for legitimization and tools to support their practices. In the end, the studies proved to the NPs themselves that it was safe for them "to think" rather than just follow orders (Fairman, 2008).

ERA II: INNOVATIONS, QUALITY, AND COST, 1975–1995

As we have seen, access to care was a key component in the emergence and use of NPs and other APNs from the 1930s to the 1970s. William Kissick (1994) notes in his book, *Medicine's Dilemmas: Infinite Needs vs. Finite Resources*, that an Iron Triangle between cost, access, and quality of care permeates the U.S. health care system. In the late 1970s, access to care remained a dominant theme in health care policy, leading to research that focused on this domain, but the cost of access and the quality of care began to emerge as issues in health services research in the 1980s. From the late 1970s to the early 1990s, research examining

NP services was driven by health care policy changes, and were clustered around three distinct, but not always novel, themes: (a) cost and quality, (b) comparison and competition with physicians, and (c) innovative nursing practice models.

In the 1970s, U.S. NPs emerged as an important focus of service and research (Levine, 1977). Gaining a better understanding about cost containment for services provided by NPs compared with physicians began to drive new studies in the 1980s. In a purely substitutive model, health policy experts questioned the continued need for NPs in primary care when the physician workforce supply was adequate to meet existing demands (Levine, 1977; Spitzer, 1984). Yet, the recognition that NPs *as nurses* have a vested interest in preventive care, community care, caring for populations at high risk, and emphasizing family and holistic approaches to care, led to testing innovative and emerging health care delivery models in the late 1980s and 1990s. Studies of innovative models in which NPs led care teams or participated in interdisciplinary practice demonstrated cost savings and positive patient outcomes (Lang, Sullivan-Marx, & Jenkins, 1996). In this section, we discuss key research studies over a productive 20-year period in categories related to cost and quality, comparison/competition with physicians, and innovative models.

Cost and Quality

Studies of NP's practice in Era II continued to focus on the structure of NP roles, cost savings or cost-effectiveness of NP practices, productivity or caseloads of NPs compared with physicians, referral patterns, barriers to NP practice, and patient and physician satisfaction with NP care (Levine, 1977; Pender & Pender, 1980; Poirer-Elliot, 1984; Ramsey, McKenzie, & Fish, 1982). LeRoy's (1982) perspective that to determine "cost-effectiveness of NPs, it is necessary to know...whether these services are substitutive or complementary to those provided by physicians" (p. 298) reflected the assumption that NPs were a cost substitute for physicians. Studies were often criticized for their methodological limitations and inability to demonstrate cost effectiveness, yet NP practice research was constrained by both the limited structure and scope of practice barriers facing NPs (LeRoy, 1982; Safriet, 1992).

Feldman and others (1987) reviewed the scientific merit of 248 NP practice documents from the 1970s through the mid-1980s for relevance, clarity, and flaw, resulting in a final list of 56 studies that met scientific merit for examining NP effectiveness. Consistently, NPs demonstrated high quality and effective care (Feldman, Ventura, & Crosby, 1987). Such attention to the value of NPs, as well as physician assistants and midwives, also heightened following the Graduate Medical Education, Nursing, and Allied Professions Commission (GMENAC) report by the U.S. Department Health and Human Services in 1980 on access and quality health care needs. The GMENAC report highlighted the economic perspective that NPs functioned as either complementary or substitutive for physicians (Griffith, 1984; Sox, 1979). Moreover, in the GMENAC report, the federal government acknowledged that nursing had an independent sphere of practice defining NP practice as unique from physician practice, highlighted patient acceptance of NPs, and recommended that NPs and other primary care health professionals should receive direct Medicaid and Medicare reimbursement. This report and other studies focusing on cost and quality were couched in the context of intense discussion in the medical and nursing literature about whom should provide primary care and how the domain of primary care is defined (Pender & Pender, 1980; Prescott, Jacox, Collar, & Goodwin, 1981; Rogers, 1981).

Studies of NPs in the early 1980s indirectly examined cost-effectiveness by focusing on NP referral patterns and types of services provided, to dispel assumptions that NP practice would be more costly due to increased referrals to physicians and specialists. Brodie and Bancroft (1982), however, found no differences between the number and types of referrals provided by NPs and MDs in a comparative study of 395 patients. Weinberg, Lijestrand, and Moore (1983) also found no difference in referrals/consultation requests. Watkins and Wagner (1982) reported that NPs made fewer referrals than recommended by protocol for hypertensive patients in rural areas, yet blood-pressure control outcomes were good.

In 1986, the U.S. Office of Technology Assessment (OTA) issued a landmark report, "Nurse Practitioners, Physician Assistants, and Certified Nurse-Midwives," indicating that NPs could provide 75% of primary care services, 90% of pediatric primary care services, and 65% of anesthesia services (U.S. Congress, 1986). Further, nurse midwives were noted to be 98% as productive as obstetricians in providing maternity services. The summary concluded that the high quality of care, patient satisfaction, and emphasis on health promotion and prevention made NPs an excellent resource for care in managed care. Impediments preventing use of NPs included the lack of physician acceptance, legal restrictions, inaccessible reimbursement, and limited coverage of unique NP services, such as health education and prevention.

Concerns about health costs dominated the health policy arena during Era II, 1975–1995. As NPs' numbers increased, from 16,000 in 1979 to approximately 60,000 in 1995, NP and other nursing organizations moved forward with efforts to gain access to mainstream reimbursement and payment methods at state and federal levels. Questions then raised were about the presumed increases in health care costs by the addition of new providers in the payer mix. Despite opposition, NPs, as well as nurse midwives and nurse anesthetists, made steady, incremental gains in obtaining reimbursement provider status based largely on their ability to meet health care needs for U.S. citizens who were underserved or minimally served. By the end of Era II, NP research demonstrated that innovative practice models led to cost-saving outcomes when NPs were unimpeded in providing their services. Yet, to move toward rigorous NP outcomes research, NPs had to first examine competition and comparison issues within the dominant structure of health care delivery, physician-defined services.

Competition/Comparison

In the late 1970s and early 1980s, descriptive studies focused on the effectiveness of NPs by using physicians as the normal standard and on the acceptance of NPs by patients and physicians (DeAngelis & McHugh, 1977; Runyan, 1975; Weinberg, Lijestrand, & Moore, 1983). One key descriptive study involved a review of NP and physician clinical records in an inner city teaching hospital clinic. The researchers found that NPs and MDs saw equally complex patients, whereas residents' patients were somewhat less complex. NPs in this study focused more on comprehensive and comfort approaches to care than did physicians (Diers, Hamman, & Molde, 1986).

In the 1980s, as the physician supply moved from shortage to surplus, NP research shifted from access and substitution to competition issues. A riveting and challenging editorial in the *New England Journal of Medicine* in 1984 titled "The Nurse Practitioner Revisited: Slow Death of a Good Idea" (Spitzer, 1984), served as a lightning rod for organized nursing to address barriers to NP practice. Interestingly, Spitzer (1984) noted that further repeated "rigorous" studies of NP performance did not seem necessary to prove that NPs are safe and effective, and well received by patients. He noted that NPs were an overstudied health profession and had been for years, in part due to assumptions by leaders and practitioners in both professions that NP care could only be evaluated using physician care as the standard (Lewis, 1975). Interestingly, this issue endures 35 years after the emergence of NP practice (Hooker & McCaig, 2001; Sox, 2000).

Spitzer (1984) raised key questions in 1984 about the continued growth of NPs, namely, will parity of payment between physicians and NPs cancel cost-advantage arguments? Will frustration with barriers to practice escalate in disillusion among NPs? He concludes that, "the prognosis for the long-term viability of the nurse practitioner concept is [was] poor" (p. 1050) and challenged the nursing profession to settle disputes about the role and education of NPs, lest the movement succumb to obsolescence. Despite his provocative questions, research efforts continued to demonstrate NPs' comparability with physicians in patient care, but with a renewed focus on obtaining mainstream payment of health care services (Aiken & Gwyther, 1995; Blendon et al., 1994; Ramsey, Edwards, Lenz, Odom, & Brown, 1993; Sullivan, 1992).

Brown and Grimes (1995) conducted a meta-analysis of NPs, nurse midwives, and physicians in primary care. They concluded that NP and nurse midwifery care was comparable with, and at times, better than, physician care, but controlled trials were needed to make definitive conclusions about the process and outcomes of nurses in primary care. Mundinger and others (2000) conducted a randomized controlled clinical trial of patients assigned to NP or physician care, demonstrating comparable outcomes of care in the two groups of patients. Criticism of methods in Mundinger's study were raised by physician researchers and physician organizations (Sox, 2000), despite the rigor of the study. Both Mundinger et al.'s (2000) and Brown and Grimes' work (1995) failed to settle age-old arguments about comparison and competitiveness between NPs and physicians. Instead, these studies may have encouraged nurse researchers to claim yet again that NP care is effective, but with the acknowledgment that more work is needed on the processes and outcomes in NP care.

Innovative Models

As competition with physicians and a growing concern for escalating cost of health care grew in the 1980s, NP studies focused on clinical success and cost advantages in ambulatory care. As new patient needs emerged and NPs increased in numbers, they moved into new roles in solo practice in primary care and in interdisciplinary teams in long-term care, home care, and hospitals (Brooten et al., 1988; Capezuti, 1985; Kepferle, 1983; Sullivan, 1992; Wanich, Sullivan-Marx, Gottlieb, & Johnson, 1992).

Research that evaluated the unique contributions of NPs began with the inception of the NP role (DeAngelis, Berman, Oda, & Meeker, 1983; Lewis, 1975; Mendenhall, Repicky, & Neville, 1980; Pender & Pender, 1980). Supported by the GMENAC report of 1980, studies of NP care gradually carved niches for NP practice. Health policy analysts and leaders in nursing, however, raised major concerns about the ability to fully demonstrate effects of NP care in a structured delivery system that only paid for and supported traditional medical care, rather than health promotion and comprehensive care approaches (LeRoy, 1982; Lewis, 1975; Prescott, Jacox, Collar, & Goodwin, 1981; U.S. Congress, 1986).

Nursing contributions to care were identified as patient education, coordination of care, holistic and comprehensive approaches to evaluation and management of patient problems, and redefinition of patient problems, with emphasis on the meaning of the situation to patients and their families. Examples of these approaches include NP and APN services focusing on teenage pregnancy, emphasis on quality of life and functional status of older adults, and transitional care. Studies were also conducted to identify the unique contributions that NPs make through examination of established payment databases. Studies demonstrated that NPs and other APNs performed many traditional medical services yet also provided services that addressed patients' needs comprehensively in social and economic areas, taking advantage of opportunities to educate patients and families (Griffith & Robinson, 1992; Robinson, Layer, Domine, Martone, & Johnston, 2000; Sullivan-Marx, Happ, Bradley, & Maislin, 2000). Martin (1995) found that 15% of 181 NPs used nursing diagnoses in their practice to address patients' lifestyles and problems in daily living, such as social isolation and self-care deficit. In another survey of NPs' use of the current procedural terminology (CPT) billing codes, NPs stated that they performed services not identified in CPT codes that addressed comprehensive patient care, attention to social factors, and capturing the teaching moment (Sullivan-Marx, Happ, Bradley, & Maislin, 2000).

In addition to examination of the structure and outcomes of NP practice, analysis of innovative models also included the process of NP care. Johnson's qualitative study (1993) examined the discourse between NPs and patients, compared with physician discourse. She concluded that NP conversation differed from a strictly medical approach by the perceived concern for the patient by the NP. This concern was evident through use of a shared language with patients, by a stance of NP and patient copartnership, and with changes in conversation to establish a connection to the patient through questions, transitions, and brief comments (Johnson, 1993).

APN models emphasizing nursing approaches to patient care problems, rather than physician-centered care, demonstrated improvements in patient outcomes among high-risk and high-need patient groups (Lang, Sullivan-Marx, & Jenkins, 1996). Reduction in the use of physical restraints in nursing homes, prevention of functional loss for hospitalized elderly, reduced hospitalization stays, reduced use of emergency services, and less use of obstetrical anesthesia have been identified in various nursing outcome studies when care is designed, organized, and provided by APN practice models (Brooten et al., 1994; Evans et al., 1997; Jenkins & Torrisi, 1995; Naylor et al., 1994; Wanich, Sullivan-Marx, Gottlieb, & Johnson, 1992).

As we leave Era II, questions remain. Is it necessary to continue to describe and study NP practice from the standard of physician practice when NP care is well established as safe, effective, cost saving, and is well received by consumers and other providers? What models work to best enable NP and APN practice to flourish? What process issues lead to good outcomes that can be replicated and mainstreamed in health care delivery?

ERA III: TAKING STOCK AND MOVING FORWARD, LATE 1990s–PRESENT

As we move into the present, a new constellation of social and economic forces is shaping NP practice and education. Rising health care costs are once again resulting in increased health insurance premiums, and threaten to aggravate long-standing problems with access to care in this country. Deep public mistrust has led many to question whether managed-care strategies are congruent with American social values. Many predict that health care consumers who have purchasing power will increasingly exercise this clout to obtain as much choice and flexibility in their services as possible. Those less fortunate, including millions of Americans for whom employer-provided health insurance may no longer be available, will face a grimmer version of the status quo (Robinson, 2001).

As of 2002, research indicates that NPs have limited impact on health care finance. Insurance companies are reluctant to empanel APNs as independent service providers with billing discretion, except where it has been expedient to do so or has been mandated by state law (Mason & O'Donnell, 2002). The federally subsidized Medicare and Medicaid programs led the way for reimbursement of APNs, and indeed, regulators noted increased billings for Medicare services by NPs and other nonphysician providers since the late 1990s (U.S. Department of Health and Human Services & Office of the Inspector General, 2001). For the moment, the volume of ambulatory care services provided by NPs in the United States remains small (Hooker & McCaig, 2001). However, it is clear that NPs' potential influence in American health care is not fully realized.

New tensions between NPs and the medical profession are building. The American public is becoming increasingly accustomed to NPs. Research findings on acceptability are largely borne out in practice, and across the country, physicians and physician practice groups are incorporating NPs into their teams (Horrocks, Anderson, & Salisbury, 2002). Some physicians perceive NPs as a strong threat and voice concerns that an "uninformed" public may choose providers who are liberal with their time and address psychosocial needs. Physicians, on the other hand, cannot be as generous with their time, due to expectations of high revenue generation for a practice, need to focus on medical problems, and extended training that creates a value perception about their time (Gottlieb, 2001). Organized medicine in the United States continues to finance cross-country lobbying efforts to defend themselves against any further perceived encroachment by nonphysicians on the medical profession's self-claimed territory (Mason, 2000). The rhetoric cites loosely characterized "safety" concerns, but it is clear that individual physicians and their professional associations are fighting diminishing financial prospects (Cooper, Laud, & Dietrich, 1998; Gottlieb, 2001).

The nursing profession that spawned the NP movement is also facing new challenges. A combination of demographic shifts and social forces in the United States resulted in yet another shortage of registered nurses (Buerhaus, Staiger, & Auerbach, 2000). The traditional nursing role in hospitals is seen as a high-pressure, undesirable job (Aiken et al., 2001). Graduate education, always the major vehicle for career mobility in nursing, shifted in a decade from the preparations of educators, managers, and clinical nurse specialists (i.e., advanced training to educate, manage, and support the clinical practice of staff nurses in the traditional role) to the education of NPs. APNs increasingly occupy a large place in nursing practice and education. As traditional staff nurse roles become less attractive to newcomer and veteran nurses alike, tensions develop between generalist nurses, APNs, nurse leaders, and nurse educators regarding professional growth, contribution to society, and resources.

A research agenda for NPs and APNs needs to move beyond amorphous labels identifying APNs as "cheaper, but better" providers of care, substitutes for inaccessible medical care, or holistic, family-focused care managers. Research studies that compare NPs with other providers, characteristic of earlier eras, will continue to be done to fully describe the full enterprise of advanced nursing practice. However, new types of research are now needed to refine and hone the full potential of advanced practice nursing in health care delivery in the United States and throughout the globe.

Outcomes Research: Asking the Right Questions

If Era II's findings and a vast worldwide pool of anecdotal experience are to be believed, stretching the boundaries of traditional nursing practice is both feasible and safe. However, Sox's (2000) critique of Mundinger et al.'s (2000) study (a more expensive and tightly controlled trial of NPs than is ever likely to be conducted again) clearly set an unachievable agenda. Research suggesting equivalence of APNs to physicians would never convince those fundamentally opposed to APN practice. The research achievement represented by the Mundinger study has perhaps taken us to the end of a road.

Benchmarking APN care against physicians on the basis of "hard" outcomes is hindered by a number of factors. First of all, direct comparisons of APN care with physician care are extremely rare, except in research studies. There are often substantial differences in the types of care or the types of patients seen by APNs and physician providers in clinics and hospital settings, due to billing regulations requiring physician oversight. Often for very practical reasons, in many settings, care is organized to assign complex or unstable patients to physicians and primary care aspects of practice to nonphysicians. From a research point of view, the end result is that the natural order provides little opportunity for comparing physician and nonphysician providers' outcomes in providing similar services to similar patient populations. Artificial study conditions are needed to perform the comparisons.

Second, easily tracked hard outcomes, such as mortality and life-threatening complications, may occur so rarely and be so marginally influenced by the process of care that in practice, they are not particularly useful for evaluating APN practice. If direct comparisons of care are intended to highlight or rule out safety problems, they will also always fall short. It is clear that any problems with the outcomes of patients treated by APNs are subtle enough to have escaped detection by the research designs used to date. However, critics are quick to point out that this may reflect shortcomings of the studies, rather than true equivalence of outcomes between physicians and NPs. The lack of routinely collected data in areas that may, in fact, be sensitive to APNs' practice patterns (for instance, fine-grained measures of patient quality of life) is distressing. Although patient quality-of-life measures and rehospitalization rates, to choose two examples, have intuitive appeal as outcomes, connecting these variables to measurable doses of APN care is often extremely difficult. Beyond this, there are often practical issues involved in collecting such data from enough patients over a long enough time for researchers to stand a reasonable chance of showing differences across patient groups treated under different models of care.

Clearly, the search for sensitive outcome measures to illuminate NPs' contributions must continue. However, instead of restricting attention to questions of comparability and safety, perhaps a better strategy involves addressing the contexts of care and circumstances under which NPs are the best choice for meeting client needs. For many employers, NPs are a means of lowering the cost of medical care, rather than a way of providing new or qualitatively different services or addressing the needs of underserved client groups. Outside academic settings and organized nursing groups, scope of practice debates deal with legally permitted tasks and acceptable levels of involvement in the care of different types of patients. A coherent, conceptually defensible role for NPs in meeting the health needs of well-defined populations supported by empirical evidence is lacking.

The role of the NP in acute care grew during Era III to become a certified specialty in the nursing profession, and particularly relevant in tertiary medical centers (Becker & Richmond, 2003) in this book). The research literature evaluating acute care NPs is early, small, and characterized by data-driven descriptions of the NP role in tertiary settings. Some single-site studies have described the cost effectiveness of acute care inpatient medical services provided by NPs in comparison with physician and physician-in-training staff (Howie & Erickson, 2002). Although many of the same methodological issues seen in research on primary care practice also appear in tertiary care studies, the literature to date is clear that implementing the NP role in acute care is quite feasible, and may entail cost savings and improvements in patient satisfaction.

If randomized trials are considered the standard of evidence to define a scope of practice, will a new Mundinger-type study need to be conducted in each setting in which the legitimacy of NP care is questioned? The Mundinger et al. (2000) study suggests that, for a group of mostly medically indigent women with stable chronic illnesses seen in primary care settings, NP care has outcomes indistinguishable from that of physician care. Are the findings of this and other research being extrapolated beyond reasonable limits by NPs in various settings, as some physicians have claimed? Can the findings of Mundinger and her colleagues be used to bolster claims that NP care is safe and effective in tertiary care settings? Can the findings be extrapolated to primary care settings in which caseloads typically involve more episodic and urgent care? Again, this is a question of politics and values as much or more as it is about fact or testable hypotheses. However, researchers may assist in answering it by gathering data about the multifaceted context and outcomes of care, thereby opening up advanced-practice nursing to the inquiries typical of nursing outcomes research (Mitchell, Ferketich, & Jennings, 1998). Specifically, what are the best models of care and the best mix of providers in different settings? Do different models of care produce varying outcomes across clienteles and settings?

Defining a niche that NPs can sell to the public and the health care system as their own (as distinct from those of physicians, physician assistants, and generalist nurses) can only be a positive development.

Even if there are clear areas in which NPs can claim superior outcomes, simple comparisons of cost effectiveness between physicians and other providers cannot factor in complexities of reimbursement and the social and organizational realities of health care. In order to achieve their goals of consolidating and expanding their place in the health care system, NPs must assemble evidence that addresses the factors foremost in the minds of decision makers. Findings from methodologically pristine randomized trials may well fall flat in introducing health care system change without a fully developed evaluation model that takes into account the nature of APN and physician practice and the multiple consequences of differences between them.

Another research option beyond direct comparisons is to go back to some of the approaches characteristic of Eras I and II, but with research tools and perspectives that were previously not applicable or applied. In some respects, recent studies of APNs that examine outcomes using carefully chosen instruments and driven by reflections on the nature of advanced practice (Baradell & Bordeaux, 2001; Hamric, Worley, Lindebak, & Jaubert, 1998) may represent a real advance, even though (or perhaps, especially because) they involve no physician comparison groups and are not randomized trials. A focus on the process of care and patient outcomes, rather than on the caregivers themselves, is sorely needed, and will eventually lead to frameworks that will shape settings of care and the education of NPs. In Era III, researchers will direct their efforts squarely at measuring the outcomes of NP care, but with a clear understanding of the limitations of the much-vaunted "gold standard" of the clinical trial in developing the science of advanced-practice nursing, and in moving advanced-practice nursing's political agenda forward.

Looking Back and Moving Forward: Historical Context

The second major type of research taking shape in Era III deals with broader questions of context. With nearly 40 years of evolution now behind us, it is time to revisit roles of historical, societal, and health system forces in the evolution of the NP movement in the United States and elsewhere. With the growing place of NP education in schools of nursing, and with gathering evidence of yet another shortage of generalist nurses, it is time to examine the ties of the NP movement to the parent nursing profession so that both groups can better chart their futures.

Historical research on the NP movement is providing important insights about the future (Fairman, 1999). Viewed through the lens of professional domination and control, the struggles of APNs are not new or unique—they are the only the latest in a series of gender and class-driven fights that nurses have faced over the past century (Group & Roberts, 2001). Understanding NP practice as an outgrowth of the clinical autonomy that nurses claimed for the good of patients in settings such as critical care and public health connects NPs to the profession and its past, and points NPs and NP leaders to effective solutions for dilemmas they currently face.

In many senses, the NP movement is approaching the end of its stormy adolescence. Many forces will influence whether and how it moves into a more secure "adult" identity. Outcomes research and historical and contextual research that pose "big picture" questions hold great promise for helping NPs take full measure of the accomplishments of the movement and charting its future.

ERA IV: EMBARKING ON QUESTIONS FOR THE FUTURE

NPs and other APNs rose from a need to address access to care, and ensuing practice and research continuously responded to external societal pressures to prove APNs' worth, safety, and cost savings. Yet NPs and others are sometimes puzzled why the plethora of research on the safety and value of NPs has so little impact on their entry to mainstream U.S. health care. Internationally, nurses are employing the U.S. NP model to meet needs in many countries. As the NP literature is used for various purposes, NPs and health policymakers need to be aware that current NPs are educated, motivated, and shaped by a different set of forces within and outside nursing than their historical contemporaries of 20, and even 10, years ago. Research regarding NPs in the past was driven more by the need to defend positions in health care and less by a need to know what constituted optimal patient care. However, the movement continues to encounter barriers that cannot be overcome with findings from well-conducted research studies alone.

These are barriers that involve core societal and health care system values. Questions for the future encompass several key areas: (a) optimal patient care through evidence-based practice, (b) organizational models of APN practice, (c) barriers to APN practice in primary and specialty care, (d) representation of APN practice in public and private databases, (e) translation of U.S. NP models internationally, and (f) historical themes and social context of APN practice.

The questions guiding research in Era IV will be formulated in the context of economic and political arenas, both in the United States and globally, in ensuing years. That there will be a strong and steady market for health care is a certainty, however, the architecture of the system in which patients will receive care in 20 years is not known. Therefore, it is only by articulating a clearer identity and better understanding of the larger context in which they operate that NPs can lay claim to a part of this future. We believe that research using a variety of methods and perspectives can help NPs do this, but that it is not research alone that will determine the movement's future. Nurses have been taught for a half-century to view research as the key to professional emancipation and self-governance for the profession, and to see differences in opinion as being best resolved with empirical data. Perhaps in Era IV, we will start to see a more realistic assessment of what research actually has to offer in an interprofessional struggle. This struggle is as much about economic realities as it is about empirical fact, and is as much (or more) about politics than it is about public safety.

CONCLUSIONS: AN INTERNATIONAL AGENDA

NPs and others turn to historical roots and research to legitimize their practice, and may be puzzled why the research has had so little impact. Further, when they search for an understanding of the present by reading about the origins of the NP movement, they are not always aware that they are educated and motivated differently than physicians or nurses. NPs today are shaped by a different set of forces than their historical contemporaries of 20, and even 10 years ago. Opportunities and barriers on the national and international arena involve core societal and health care system values that may not be overcome with research studies alone.

Well-thought-out arguments that are based on outcomes research evidence and that address political, policy, and financial circumstances are critical to move advanced-practice nursing forward. Determining under what models of care patient and systems outcomes will be better with care provided by APNs will require considerable cooperation between clinicians and researchers. With the spread of the idea of advanced-nursing practice abroad, APNs and NPs in other countries often have training and scopes of practice radically different than in the United States, and can provide some fresh opportunities for gaining insights in this area. In the countries that have attempted to bring in expanded scope of practice for nurses, where is it working well and where is it not? In which countries is a "good" fit being identified between the implementation of APN roles and societal values and health care politics? Where is the U.S.-inspired model encountering serious resistance? Where are other models working better? What are the "outer limits" of roles that can be effectively assumed by APNs under the right circumstances? An ambitious international consortium of researchers, clinicians, and policymakers may one day be able to look across borders and continents to answer research questions involving models of care that for fundamental structural and operational reasons cannot be addressed in the United States. International studies of NPs have an added urgency for other obvious reasons, as well. Government officials and leaders in clinical agencies worldwide are attempting to adapt the NP role to address problems in their health care systems. They read literature on U.S. NPs, and are frustrated by the absence of roadmaps for implementing the expanded roles and being given no insight at all into how the U.S. model may or may not work elsewhere.

Only by articulating a clear identity and better understanding the larger context in which NPs practice can they then lay claim to a part of a global future. We believe that research using a variety of methods and perspectives can help NPs do this, but that it is not research alone that will determine the movement's future. Nurses have been taught for a half-century to view research as the key to professional emancipation and self-governance for the profession, and to see differences in opinion as being best resolved with empirical data. Research will contribute to an understanding of the role of NPs nationally and internationally within a wider context of the players and agenda.

EPILOGUE

Julie A. Fairman and Eileen M. Sullivan-Marx: As editors, it seemed clear to us that the preceding chapter was an excellent contribution regarding the evolution of NPs who support their practice and their place in health care. Since the last edition of this book, researchers have produced great quantities of research examining NPs. Hence, we decided to republish the chapter from the 4th edition and add commentary in this epilogue as a reflection and update on the range of research related to NPs.

Efficacy studies continue to be produced, but new trends have emerged. Studies that evaluate outcomes of particular clinical programs and types of treatments are now more focused on NP practice than comparative effectiveness between nurses and physicians doing the same thing. These types of studies support the paradigm of specific skills embedded in NP practice, rather than documenting how well they can perform traditional medical skills. In addition, NPs have developed research in all areas of nursing science: (a) conducting research that generates new knowledge; (b) translational science; (c) historical research; (d) health services research—comparative effectiveness, workforce, interprofessional collaboration/teams; and (e) programmatic training and curricular education research (Institute of Medicine, 2008).

Conducting studies as principal investigators to examine the full range of nursing phenomena is an important area of growth for NPs. Barbara Resnick, a geriatric NP, has been a leader with a full program of research on exercise science for frail older adults in long-term care, particularly among those with hip fracture (Resnick et al., 2009). Her research is linked directly with her practice, in which she is actively engaged. Barbara Medoff-Cooper, funded by the National Institutes of Health, demonstrates interventions that improve infant development, feeding of high-risk infants, and infant temperament (Medoff-Cooper, Shults, & Kaplan, 2009). Integrating research careers with practice is challenging, although more opportunities to do so are developing in faculty practice career tracks. Translational science will present new opportunities for NPs to be involved with bench-to-bedside research as members of research teams, who not only contribute to the scientific conduct of research, but guide the research questions that must be asked in integrative science teams.

Historical research regarding NPs has served to inform policy and leadership among nursing and other stakeholders. Pioneered by NP Joan Lynaugh, this work has evolved as a lens for examining nursing careers, sociological context of health professions in the United States and elsewhere, and as a foundation for health policy strategies. Examining NPs from an historical standpoint will also provide new explanations about the politics and changes occurring in the health care system in general, issues of gender and work, and the diffusion of ideas and technology.

A new push for comparative effectiveness, as documented by the Institute of Medicine's (IOM) continued work in this area, should and does go beyond the question of which profession can claim ownership of particular procedures or provide particular types of care. Instead, there is much support at both the legislative and practice levels for evaluating different models of care in terms of outcomes, cost, and patient satisfaction. Studies of this sort will have important policy implications that have an impact on NP practice—if it is indeed included as a variable. For example, the Medicare demonstration projects on the medical home will be key for establishing the cost and quality of this model of care. However, NPs are included only as support personnel rather than heads of homes, despite the documented effectiveness of NPs as team leaders in chronic care and other models of care. Continued education of NPs in academic research careers, for example, at the PhD-prepared clinician educator level, will provide a core number of NPs who are qualified to participate in such research.

More analysis is needed across all health disciplines regarding the best curriculum, learning, and types of health professional and interprofessional education to prepare a workforce to meet society's needs. The Carnegie Foundation for the Advancement of Teaching report (Benner, Sutphen, Leonard, & Day, 2010) on undergraduate education is an excellent example of a study that sets forth the foundational expectations that graduate schools of education can build on when designing the best approaches to prepare NPs and assist them in lifelong learning.

Future studies of NPs should focus on comparisons between models of care that are NP-driven and managed, as well as the cost effectiveness of payment that is service oriented rather than practitioner-specific. In this way, research and policy can move beyond the question of who should be reimbursed and provide particular types of services, thus tempering complaints that adding additional types of providers to the payment schemes will be costly. Another area to consider would be research on the various educational models that have emerged. The public should remain assured that nurses are adequately prepared to provide care based on appropriate sets of competencies. Finally, building on the IOM report, *Crossing the Quality Chasm*, different models of interprofessional education should be tested and priced to see whether we can provide more cost-effective and better socialized health care providers (Institute of Medicine, 2001).

Research studies of multiple methods and foci have, over time, provided the foundation for nurses' role expansion and informed patient care. From the analysis in the chapter published in 2003, we can see how research trends developed along disciplinary developmental lines, reflecting the political nature of practice and the clinical needs of patients across particular times and places. The message from the authors still rings true today—critical study of NPs must continue to inform practice and policy. This work will have broad implications for NPs' place in the health care system and across the globe.

REFERENCES

Aiken, L., & Gwyther, M. (1995). Medicare funding of nurse education. *Journal of the American Medical Association, 273*, 1528.

Aiken, L. H., Clarke, S. P., Sloane, D. M., Sochalski, J. A., Busse, R., Clarke, H., et al. (2001). Nurses' reports of hospital care in five countries. *Health Affairs, 20*(3), 43–53.

Baer, E. D. (1997). Values that drove nursing science in the 1960's. *Reflections, 23*(3), 42–43.

Baradell, J. G., & Bordeaux, B. R. (2001). Outcomes and satisfaction of patients of psychiatric clinical nurse specialists. *Journal of the American Psychiatric Nurses Association, 7*(3), 77–85.

Becker, D. E., & Richmond, T. S. (2003). Advanced practice nurses in acute care services. In M. D. Mezey, D. O. McGivern, & E. Sullivan-Marx (Eds.), *Nurse practitioners: Evolution of advanced practice* (4th ed., pp. 135–149). New York: Springer Publishing Company.

Benner, P., Sutphen, M., Leonard, V., & Day, L. (2010). *Educating nurses: A call for radical transformation*. San Francisco: Jossey-Bass.

Bessman, A. N. (1974). Comparison of medical care in nurse clinician and physician clinics in medical school affiliated hospitals. *Journal of Chronic Disease, 27*, 115–125.

Blendon, R., Mattila, J., Benson, J. M., Shelter, M. C., Connolly, F. J., & Kiley, T. (1994, Spring). The beliefs and values shaping today's health reform debate. *Health Affairs, 13*, 275–284.

Brodie, B., & Bancroft, B. (1982). A comparison of nurse practitioner and physician costs in a military out-patient facility. *Military Medicine, 147*, 1051–1053.

Brooten, D., Brown, L. P., Munro, B. H., York, R., Cohen, S. M., Roncoli, M., et al. (1988). Early discharge and specialist transitional care. *Image: Journal of Nursing Scholarship, 20*(2), 64–68.

Brooten, D., Roncoli, M., Finkler, S., Arnold, L., Cohen, A., & Mennuti, M. (1994). A randomized trial of early discharge and home follow-up of women having Caesarean birth. *Obstetrics & Gynecology, 84*, 832–838.

Brown, S. A., & Grimes, D. E. (1995). A meta-analysis of nurse practitioners and nurse midwives in primary care. *Nursing Research, 44*, 332–339.

Buerhaus, P. I., Staiger, D. O., & Auerbach, D. I. (2000). Implications of an aging registered nurse workforce. *Journal of the American Medical Association, 283*(22), 2948–2954.

Capezuti, E. (1985). Geriatric nurse practitioners: Their education, experience, and future in home health care. *Pride Institute Journal of Long Term Health Care, 4*(3), 9–14.

Cooper, R. A., Laud, P., & Dietrich, C. L. (1998). Current and projected workforce of nonphysician clinicians. *Journal of the American Medical Association, 280*, 788–794.

DeAngelis, C., Berman, B., Oda, D., & Meeker, R. (1983). Comparative values of school physical examinations and mass screening tests. *Journal of Pediatrics, 102*, 477.

DeAngelis, C., & McHugh, M. (1977). The effectiveness of various health personnel as triage agents. *Journal of Community Health, 2*, 268.

Diers, D., Hamman, A., & Molde, S. (1986). Complexity of ambulatory care: Nurse practitioner and physician caseloads. *Nursing Research, 35*, 310–314.

Evans, L. K., Strumpf, N. E., Allen-Taylor, S. L., Capezuti, E., Maislin, G., & Jacobsen, B. (1997). A clinical trial to reduce restraints in nursing homes. *Journal of the American Geriatrics Society, 45*, 675–681.

Fagin, C. M. (1992, May): Collaboration between nurses and physicians: No longer a choice. *Academic Medicine, 67*, 295–303.

Fairman, J. (1997). Thinking about patients: Nursing science in the 1950's. *Reflections, 23*(3), 30–32.

Fairman, J. (1999). Delegated by default or negotiated by need? Physicians, nurse practitioners, and the process of critical thinking. *Medical Humanities Review, 13*(1), 38–58.

Feldman, M. J., Ventura, M. R., & Crosby, F. (1987). Studies of nurse practitioner effectiveness. *Nursing Research, 36*, 303–308.

Ferrar, Jr., G. E. (1969). Keynote address, 1969 officers conference, Pennsylvania Medical Society. *Pennsylvania Medicine, 6*, 9–10.

Geolot, D. H. (1990). Federal funding of nurse practitioner education: Past, present, and future. *Nurse Practitioner Forum, 1*(3), 159–162.

Glover, B. H. (1967). A psychiatrist calls for a new nurse therapist. *American Journal of Nursing, 67*(5), 1003–1005.

Griffith, H. (1984). Nursing practice: Substitute or complement according to economic theory. *Nursing Economics, 2*, 105–112.

Griffith, H., & Robinson, K. R. (1992). Current procedural terminology (CPT) coded services provided by nurse specialists. *Image: Journal of Nursing Scholarship, 25*, 178–186.

Group, T. M., & Roberts, J. I. (2001). *Nursing, physician control, and the medical monopoly*. Bloomington, IN: Indiana University Press.

Guthrie, N., Runyan, J., Clark, G., & Marvin, O. (1964). The clinical nursing conference: A preliminary report. *New England Journal of Medicine, 270*(26), 1411–1413.

Hamric, A. B., Worley, D., Lindebak, S., & Jaubert, S. (1998). Outcomes associated with advanced nursing practice prescriptive authority. *Journal of the Academy of Nurse Practitioners, 10*(3), 113–118.

Heagarty, M. C., Boehringer, J. R., Lavigne, P. A., Brooks, E. G., & Evans, M. E. (1973). An evaluation of the activities of nurses and pediatricians in a university outpatient department. *Journal of Pediatrics, 83*(5), 875–879.

Holt, E. (1998). Confusion's masterpiece: The development of the physician assistant profession. *Bulletin of the History of Medicine, 72*(2), 246–278.

Hooker, R. S., & McCaig, L. F. (2001). Use of physician assistants and nurse practitioners in primary care, 1995–1999. *Health Affairs, 20*, 231–238.

Horrocks, S., Anderson, E., & Salisbury, C. (2002). Systematic review of whether nurse practitioners working in primary care can provide equivalent care to doctors. *British Medical Journal, 324*, 819–823.

Howie, J. N., & Erickson, M. (2002). Acute care nurse practitioners: Creating and implementing a model of care for an inpatient general medical service. *American Journal of Critical Care, 11*(5), 448–458.

Institute of Medicine. (2001). *Crossing the quality chasm: A new health system for the 21st century*. Retrieved September 29, 2009, from http://www.nap.edu/openbook. php?record_id=10027&page=1

Jenkins, M., & Torrisi, D. (1995). Nurse practitioners, community health centers, and contracting for managed care. *Journal of the American Academy of Nurse Practitioners, 7*, 1–6.

Johnson, R. (1993). Nurse practitioner-patient discourse: Uncovering the voice of nursing in primary care practice. *Scholarly Inquiry for Nursing Practice, 7*, 143–157.

Kepferle, L. (1983). Projects and demonstrations relating to long-term care. *Journal of Long Term Care Administration, 16*, 54–57.

Kissick, W. L. (1994). *Medicine's dilemma: Infinite needs versus finite resources*. New Haven, CT: Yale University Press.

Lang, N. M., Sullivan-Marx, E. M., & Jenkins, M. (1996). Advanced practice nurses and success of organized delivery systems. *American Journal of Managed Care, 2*, 129–135.

LeRoy, L. (1982). The cost-effectiveness of nurse practitioners. In L. H. Aiken & S. R. Gortner (Eds.), *Nursing in the 1980s: Crisis, opportunities, & challenges* (pp. 295–313). Philadelphia: Lippincott.

Levine, E. (1977). What do we know about nurse practitioners? *American Journal of Nursing, 77*, 1799–1803.

Lewis, C. E., & Resnick, B. A. (1964). Nurse clinics and progressive ambulatory care. *New England Journal of Medicine, 277*(23), 1236–1241.

Lewis, J. (1975). Structural aspects of the delivery setting and nurse practitioner performance. *Nurse Practitioner, 1*, 16.

Martin, K. (1995). Nurse practitioners' use of nursing diagnosis. *Nursing Diagnosis, 6*, 9–15.

Martin, N. (1967). Freeing the doctor from well-baby care. *Medical Economics, 44*(4), 118–119, 123, 127.

Mason, D. J. (2000). Here we go again. Organized medicine launches an attack on nursing. *American Journal of Nursing, 100*(5), 7.

Mason, D. J., & O'Donnell, J. P. (2002). Nurse practitioners and managed care. In T. G. Cesta (Ed.), *Survival strategies for nurses in managed care.* St. Louis, MO: Mosby.

Medoff-Cooper, B., Shults, J., & Kaplan, J. (2009). Early feeding behavior of pre-term infants as a predictor of developmental outcomes. *Journal of Developmental and Behavioral Pediatrics, 30*(1), 16–22.

Mendenhall, R., Repicky, P., & Neville, R. (1980). Assessing the utilization and productivity of nurse practitioners and physician assistants: Methodology and findings on productivity. *Medical Care, 18,* 609–623.

Mitchell, P. H., Ferketich, S., & Jennings, B. M. (1998). Quality health outcomes model. American Academy of Nursing expert panel on quality health care. *Image: Journal of Nursing Scholarship, 30*(1), 43–46.

Mundinger, M. O., Kane, R. L., Lenz, E. R., Totten, A. M., Tsai, W. Y., Cleary, P. D., et al. (2000). Primary care outcomes in patients treated by nurse practitioners or physicians: A randomized trial. *Journal of the American Medical Association, 283*(1), 59–68.

Naylor, M., Brooten, D., Jones, R., Lavizzo-Mourey, R., Mezey, M., & Pauly, M. (1994). Comprehensive discharge planning for hospitalized elderly. *Annals of Internal Medicine, 120,* 999–1006.

Pender, N. J., & Pender, A. R. (1980). Illness prevention and health promotion services provided by nurse practitioners: Predicting potential consumers. *American Journal of Public Health, 70,* 798–803.

Poirer-Elliott, E. (1984). Cost-effectiveness of non-physician health care professionals. *Nurse Practitioner, 10,* 54.

Prescott, P. A., Jacox, A., Collar, M., & Goodwin, L. (1981). The nurse practitioner rating form: Part I—Conceptual development for potential uses. *Nursing Research, 30,* 223–228.

Ramsey, J. A., McKenzie, J. K., & Fish, D. G. (1982). Physicians and nurse practitioners: Do they provide equivalent health care? *American Journal of Public Health, 72,* 55–57.

Ramsey, P., Edwards, J., Lenz, C., Odom, J. E., & Brown, B. (1993). Types of health problems and satisfaction with services in a rural nurse-managed clinic. *Journal of Community Health Nursing, 10,* 161–170.

Resnick, B., Gruber-Baldini, A. L., Galik, E., Pretzer-Aboff, I., Russ, K., Hebel, J. R., et al. (2009). Changing the philosophy of care in long-term care: Testing of the restorative care intervention. *The Gerontologist, 49,* 175–184.

Robinson, J. C. (2001). The end of managed care. *Journal of the American Medical Association, 285,* 2622–2628.

Robinson, K. R., Layer, T., Domine, L., Martone, L., & Johnston, L. (2000). Capturing the workload of advanced practice nurses. *National Academies of Practice Forum, 2,* 223–230.

Rogers, D. E. (1981). Who should give primary care? *New England Journal of Medicine, 305,* 577–578.

Rogers, M. (1972). Nursing: To be or not to be? *Nursing Outlook, 20,* 42–46.

Runyan, J. (1975). The Memphis chronic disease program. *Journal of the American Medical Association, 231*, 130–135.

Russo, R. M., Gururaj, V. J., Bunye, A. S., Kim, Y. H., & Ner, S. (1975). Triage abilities of nurse practitioner vs. pediatrician. *American Journal of Diseases of Children, 129*, 673–675.

Sackett, D. L., Spitzer, W. O., Gent, M., & Roberts, S. R. (1974). The Burlington randomized trial of the nurse practitioner: Health outcomes of patients. *Annals of Internal Medicine, 80*(2), 137–142.

Safriet, B. J. (1992). Health care dollars and regulatory sense: The role of advanced practice nursing. *Yale Journal of Regulation, 9*, 417–488.

Schiff, D. W., Fraser, C. H., & Walters, H. L. (1969). The pediatric nurse practitioner in the office of pediatricians in private practice. *Pediatrics, 44*(1), 62–68.

Sigma Theta Tau International. (1996). *Sigma Theta Tau international research fund grant recipients, 1936-1996.* Indianapolis, IN: Sigma Theta Tau International.

Silver, H. K., Ford, L. C., & Stearly, S. G. (1967). A program to increase health care for children: The pediatric nurse practitioner program. *Pediatrics, 39*(5), 756–760.

Solomons, G., & Hatton, M. (1961). The public health nurse as an objective scientific observer. *Nursing Outlook, 9*, 486.

Sox, H. C. (1979). Quality of patient care by nurse practitioners and physician assistants: A ten year perspective. *Annals of Internal Medicine, 91*, 459–468.

Sox, H. C. (2000). Independent primary care practice by nurse practitioners. *Journal of the American Medical Association, 283*, 106–108.

Spitzer, W. O. (1984). The nurse practitioner revisited: Slow death of a good idea. *New England Journal of Medicine, 310*, 1049–1051.

Sullivan, E. (1992). Nurse practitioners & reimbursement: Case analyses. *Nursing & Health Care, 13*, 236–241.

Sullivan, J. (1982). Research on nurse practitioners: Process behind the outcomes? *American Journal of Public Health, 72*, 8–9.

Sullivan-Marx, E. M., Happ, M. B., Bradley, K. J., & Maislin, G. (2000). Nurse practitioner services: Content and relative work value. *Nursing Outlook, 48*, 269–275.

U.S. Congress, Office of Technology Assessment. (1986). *Nurse practitioners, physician assistants, and certified nurse-midwives: A policy analysis (Health technology case study no. 37).* Washington, DC: U.S. Government Printing Office.

U.S. Department of Health and Human Services & Office of the Inspector General. (2001). *Medicare coverage of non-physician provider services.* Report OEI-02-00-00290. Retrieved May 22, 2002, from http://oig.hhs.gov/oei/reports/oei-02-00-00290.pdf

Walker, J. E. C., Murawski, B. J., & Thorn, G. W. (1964). An experimental program in ambulatory medical care. *New England Medical Journal, 271*(2), 63–68.

Wanich, C. K., Sullivan-Marx, E. M., Gottlieb, G. L., & Johnson, J. C. (1992). Functional status outcomes of a nursing intervention in hospitalized elderly. *Image: Journal of Nursing Scholarship, 24*, 201–207.

Watkins, L. O., & Wagner, E. H. (1982). Nurse practitioner and physician adherence to standing orders criteria for consultation or referral. *American Journal of Public Health, 72*, 22–29.

Weinberg, R. M., Lijestrand, J. S., & Moore, S. (1983). Inpatient management by a nurse practitioner: Effectiveness in a rehabilitation setting. *Archives of Physical Medicine and Rehabilitation, 64,* 588–590.

7 Long-Term Outcomes of Advanced-Practice Nursing

SUSAN W. GROTH, LISA NORSEN, AND HARRIET J. KITZMAN

The development, confirmation, and dissemination of the best possible scientific evidence about outcomes of the advanced-practice nurse (APN) into decision making are critical to the delivery of health care and health policy. Particularly important is evidence about APN interventions that affect long-term change in the developmental trajectory of health and disease. Although all interventions that improve health, reduce disease, and improve the related quality of life are important, interventions whose positive impact continues to grow over time are extraordinarily cost-effective. For example, if a lifestyle intervention reduced or delayed the development of elevated blood glucose, the long-term cost savings would grow each year of delay because treatment of the disease and its complications would be avoided.

By definition, long-term outcomes of APN services are complex, multifaceted, and difficult to detect. The challenge and complexity of research that attempts to quantify APN practice outcomes is made more difficult by the frequently absent, or insufficiently developed, theoretical frameworks, poorly defined and often scientifically weak designs and methodologies, imprecise definitions and selection of outcomes, inaccurate measurement techniques, lack of treatment fidelity, and ambiguous relationships among structures, processes, and outcomes. All need attention if the integrity of the evidence of long-term impact of APN practice on outcomes is to be ensured.

The focus of this chapter is a discussion of research related to long-term outcomes associated with APN interventions. To discuss this emerging field of inquiry, we need to describe long-term outcome research, as well as some of the pilot and more developed work that is associated with interventions performed by APNs, as well as models of care outcomes associated with APN practice.

The length of time that is required for an outcome to be designated *long-term* is variable, but generally refers to outcomes that are not immediately evident following a treatment or intervention, and may include those that evolve over a person's lifetime. In this chapter, we have organized examples of long-term outcomes research based on type of care management: acute care and transitional care, and chronic disease management. Selected research reports are individually reviewed to demonstrate the range of methodologies used to determine long-term outcomes and the diversity of interventions studied. We also describe some of the basic conceptual, methodological, and logistic challenges of conducting long-term outcomes research, and discuss emerging trends.

EXAMPLES OF STUDIES OF LONG-TERM OUTCOMES

Acute Care/Transitional Care

Gracias and colleagues (2008) examined compliance with clinical practice guidelines in a semi-closed intensive care unit (ICU) in which acute care nurse practitioners (ACNPs) were fully integrated into the critical care team. Three separate clinical practice protocols for anemia, stress ulcers, and deep vein thrombosis (DVT) were simultaneously introduced into both the semi-closed and the usual care ICUs. Compliance with guidelines was significantly better in the semi-closed ICU compared with the usual care ICU, but also improved in the usual care ICU when the format was applied in that setting. The authors report that at the time of publication, the model had been expanded and continued to be used successfully in the hospital in which it was implemented and tested. Although these outcomes were short-term in nature, it is reasonable to extrapolate favorable long-term outcomes. For example, compliance with guidelines might shorten length of stay, reduce complications, and reduce cost of care over time.

Although always cognizant of the transition of patients out of acute care, ACNP interventions typically focus on immediate needs with an eye to short-term benefit. One study documenting longer term patient and system outcomes is a randomized controlled trial (RCT) in which geriatric patients were assigned to an added "dose" of NP care (sample size of 326), compared with usual care (sample size of 324) during an emergency room (ER) visit (Mion et al., 2003). The NP performed a comprehensive geriatric assessment before discharge with referral to community agencies when indicated. Although service use (ER visits, hospitalizations) was no different between groups, those patients receiving the geriatric assessment reported higher satisfaction with care and experienced fewer nursing home admissions 30 and 120 days following the ER visit. The authors considered the model "ineffective" for their outcomes, because service use rates were unchanged. However, from another perspective, the outcomes selected may not have adequately captured the effect of the intervention. It is possible that frail elders could not be successfully managed after referral, or the particular outcome indicators could not reflect long-term changes. For example, the number of nursing home admissions might be a better representation of success for this population.

Another example of research related to patient transition from inpatient to a home setting addresses patient anxieties and struggles as they move toward independence and separation from the safety net of regular nursing care. Patients recently discharged from a rehabilitation unit continued to seek care from the nursing staff after discharge (Rawl, Easton, Kwiatkowski, Zemen, & Burczyk, 1998). In response to the apparent patient need, an APN proactive follow-up program was developed and tested using an RCT design with patients (sample size of 100) assigned to the intervention or control group, and compared 4 months after discharge. There were significant differences between groups, with the treatment group experiencing less anxiety, number of calls made to the unit, and amount of time spent with social workers and staff nurses.

Evidence has continued to emerge concerning the importance of quality in discharge planning in the United States and internationally. In a medical center in northern Taiwan, Huang and Liang (2005) used a randomized trial design to study the effectiveness of a nurse practitioner (NP)-based discharge planning intervention in 126 hospitalized elders over 65 years with hip fracture due to falling. Those in the intervention group had shorter lengths of hospital stay, fewer readmissions, improved rate of survival, and improvements on all subscales of the SF-36 quality of life measures and activities of daily living (ADLs).

One of the most important programs of research on transitional care has been conducted by Naylor et al. (2004). In an RCT of 239 elderly patients admitted to hospital with heart failure, they examined the impact of an intervention with APN training using the Quality-Cost Model of AP Transitional Care management strategies. One year after the index hospital admission, when compared with patients in the control usual care group, patients in the transitional care intervention experienced lower readmission rates and co-morbidity-related admissions, and the cost of their care was lower. The group of patients receiving transitional care also experienced fewer deaths.

Chronic Disease Management

Care provider time, energy, and dollars are increasingly directed toward chronic disease management. As the population ages and the obesity epidemic continues unabated, systems and methodologies for chronic disease management are becoming more and more essential.

An important study related to chronic disease was a study comparing outcomes for patients randomly assigned to NPs in a primary care clinic at an urban academic medical center, or to physicians in community-based primary care clinics (Mundinger et al., 2000). Physicians and NPs were subject to the same expectations in terms of productivity, coverage, and number of patients scheduled. Follow-up 6 months and 1 year for 1,316 patients after enrollment found no difference in use, overall satisfaction with care, health status, or physiologic measures for those with asthma and diabetes between NP and physician patients. Patients with hypertension in the NP group had lower diastolic values than their counterparts in the physician group. This large-scale randomized trial strongly supports similar long-term outcomes for NPs and physicians providing primary care (Mundinger et al., 2000).

Using a 5-year RCT that included 309 African American men with hypertension, Dennison et al. (2007) demonstrated the effectiveness of a collaborative effort of NPs, community health workers, and physicians to institute a multifaceted intervention to improve control of hypertension, and thus reduce the negative sequelae of hypertension in this population. The intervention included education and counseling, regular NP visits, need-based home visits by the community health worker, and MD consultation as needed. Blood pressure (BP) was better controlled in the intervention group at 3 years, but was not significantly different between groups at 5 years. A decrease in progression of cardiac damage was evident, as there was significantly less left ventricular hypertrophy in the intervention group, likely reflective of improved BP control over time and the use of an angiotensin-receptor blockade with losartan. The use of patient-centered approaches and team collaboration demonstrates that chronic disease in high-risk underserved populations can be managed over time (Dennison et al., 2007).

Focusing on lipid levels and cost-effectiveness as outcome measures, Paez and Allen (2006) used an RCT design to test the effectiveness of an NP case management intervention for lipid management on patients after revascularization. The NP role as case manager included an initial appointment to establish a plan for lipid management that included counseling, medication, telephone follow-up, and monitoring with medication adjustments as needed. After 1 year, there were significantly lower low density lipoprotein-cholesterol (LDL-C) and total cholesterol levels in the intervention group, and significantly more in that group achieved lipid levels in accordance with the guidelines. NP effort decreased over time, but there were increased costs related to medications, reflective of increased compliance and improved dose titration.

Goessens et al. (2006) compared the effect of using an NP plus usual care model with usual care on risk-factor reduction in vascular disease. The intervention included the establishment of an action plan for lifestyle changes, and reinforcement of the plan with subsequent visits with the NP. The cardiovascular risk profile of 236 patients randomized to either the treatment or control group, and who had two or more modifiable vascular risk factors, was evaluated at 1 year. The intervention group was more successful at achieving treatment goals than the control group, including lower BP, total and LDL-C, and body mass index (BMI) decrease. There was also better compliance with medication usage in the intervention group. This is a demonstration showing that the addition of NP care to usual care improved management of vascular risk factors in participants with symptoms of vascular disease.

The APN role in all three of the studies used increased frequency of appointments or contact with patients, and focused to a large extent on counseling, education, medication management, and support of lifestyle changes. These studies capitalized on what APNs do well and demonstrated that APN practice, when used in this manner, can effect change in long-term outcomes of chronic disease, with a sustained impact on morbidity and mortality related to risk factors that contribute to cardiovascular disease.

A fourth study, somewhat related, randomized 157 patients with hypertension and diabetes to a physician–NP team or physician alone for a 12-month period (Litaker et al., 2003). The NP took the lead on development of treatment plans, patient contact, education, and patient support. The team approach did not result in significantly different outcomes in terms of BP or total cholesterol. However, team-supported patients had improved high density lipoprotein-cholesterol (HDL-C) and small decreases in HbA1c values. Of interest, these improved values disappeared within 12 months after study completion when the participants were no longer under the care of the NP–MD team. Patients under the care of the team had increased contact time with care providers throughout the year, and reported increased satisfaction with care and quality of life. In this study, it is evident that there is an improvement in the level of counseling and patient-centered education when NPs are a part of the care team. This study, albeit small, demonstrates the positive impact on long-term outcomes when using NP–MD collaborative or partnered teams in the management of chronic disease.

A final chronic disease study reviewed is related to Alzheimer's disease and the usage of an APN-led interdisciplinary team to improve quality of care for patients with Alzheimer's disease and their caregivers (Callahan et al., 2006). This was an RCT in which 153 older adults with Alzheimer's disease, along with their caregivers, were randomized to either usual care or collaborative care management over a 1-year period. APNs provided education along with regular visits promoting nonpharmacologic modalities of treatment. If this approach was unsuccessful, the physician and APN included additional team members, such as a psychiatrist, as needed. This collaborative approach improved the quality of care along with decreased behavioral and psychological dementia symptoms that persisted at an 18-month assessment, without an increase in usage of antipsychotics or sedatives. At the same time, caregivers in the treatment group experienced a decrease in stress.

CONCEPTUAL AND METHODOLOGICAL CHALLENGES IN LONG-TERM OUTCOMES RESEARCH

Obtaining Clarity in a Theoretical Framework

The health care system is ever evolving in response to the needs of the population; advanced-practice nursing changes are a part of that process. To conduct research on long-term outcomes of APN care in an ever-changing environment, a theoretical base or conceptual framework is needed that provides a foundation and depicts the posited relationships between the structure, process, and outcomes surrounding the health care phenomena of interest (Donabedian, 1966). This framework needs to focus on clinical practice (Gleeson et al., 1990) and reflect the integral role and unique contribution of APNs to patient care and long-term outcomes. Without a conceptual framework to guide the study, it is difficult to understand and explain the variation in measured long-term outcomes and how they are linked to APN practice.

An example of a framework that aids in understanding process in long-term follow-up studies is an RCT conducted by Dennison et al. (2007), discussed earlier in the chapter. In analyzing the data, they learned that treatment of hypertension reduced the progression of cardiac damage, as evidenced by significantly less left ventricular hypertrophy in the intervention group, compared with the control group. They, therefore, demonstrated a framework whereby treatment of hypertension had a more extensive effect of reducing actual long-term heart damage.

Design and Methods: The Challenge of Outcomes Research

Science is built in phases or steps, at times systematic, and at other times resulting from random serendipitous discoveries (Barber & Fox, 1970). Although serendipitous discoveries may change the direction of study in an area, the process by which the knowledge from this discovery is translated into treatment and tested needs to be deliberate. There are multiple descriptions of the process, one being disseminated by the National Cancer Institute and developed as a five-phase standard efficacy-effectiveness research model. Although seldom implemented in its entirety, it is an elegant, scientifically defensible model. In the first two phases of the model, hypotheses are constructed based on established concepts in a theoretical model, and methods are established and validated. Phase 3 builds on work done in Phases 1 and 2, and consists of carefully controlled intervention trials, during which hypotheses and methodologies are refined. Efficacy trials during this phase determine how well a treatment works in those who actually receive it, under ideal conditions. In Phase 4, the revised intervention is tested in carefully defined subpopulations of the ultimate population targeted. Finally, in Phase 5, through demonstration and implementation studies, the proven intervention is introduced to the community at large, and the health outcomes are measured. Phases 4 and 5, determining how a treatment works in those to whom it is offered, and how it works in the real world, constitute an effectiveness trial. It is reasoned that if the intervention cannot be shown to be effective when actually administered to persons under ideal conditions, there is little need to go further. If an intervention is found to be effective in an efficacy trial, however, effectiveness is not yet ensured and the effectiveness trial is needed. Once the intervention is performed under real-world conditions and the broader target population in effectiveness studies, costs, difficulties with implementation of the interventions, and side effects may be identified that, in turn, render the intervention unacceptable.

Recent national and international emphasis has added support for this basic process in translational research. Emphasis on clinical translational research emerged with the recognition that to date, we know much more about how to prevent, diagnose, and treat disease, but this knowledge is not always "translated" into or used in clinical practice. Translational research is the activity through which knowledge and understanding of mechanisms and techniques generated in the laboratory (either bench or behavioral basic science) are introduced into activities designed to prevent, diagnose, and/or treat disease (Woolf, 2008). Translational research has been described as at least two phases, T1 and T2, with some describing additional levels, T3 and T4; T1 is translation of laboratory-generated mechanisms into prevention, diagnosis and treatment; T2 is the translation of clinical studies into clinical practice; T3 is the translation of this knowledge into practice-based research; and T4 is the translation into population-based studies.

The experimental method, or RCT, is a powerful technique by which the efficacy of interventions can be determined; and it is of particular importance at the efficacy trial phase-3 level. The rigorous

RCT design allows the investigator to make the most scientifically credible statement about the impact of the treatment/intervention. Studies using this design are more easily accepted for publication and receive greater attention in public policy. Although Shrier et al. (2007) have argued for the qualified inclusion of observational studies, the RCT design is frequently considered a necessary criterion for a study to be accepted as evidence in a meta-analysis study. Therefore, the value of evidence from well-conducted randomized trials cannot be overstated.

Nevertheless, much can be learned about the phenomena under investigation, the mechanisms inherent in the treatment-effect process, and the impact of characteristics of the individual (for whom) and the environment (under what conditions) from other methodologies. Mixed methods (qualitative and experimental), which can include mixing philosophies, mixing designs, and mixing data-collection devices (Lawrenz & Huffman, 2006) are increasingly recognized as important in understanding the phenomena and the inferences drawn from trials in health services and nursing research, in which it is difficult to measure the complex interactions of the person, treatment, and environment. The advantages of adding descriptive and qualitative methods to experimental/quantitative research on long-term outcomes are many. The methods help the investigator discover aspects of the environment and the health care system that affect outcomes, they can aid in the understanding of complex social process, and they can uncover characteristics of the individual that affect his or her behaviors and that may affect the acceptance or response to treatment (Curry, Nembhard, & Bradley, 2009). Because of the unique contributions of qualitative methods, investigative teams wishing to move novel interventions through the translation research process are increasingly combining descriptive, qualitative, and experimental/quantitative methods.

Long-Term Outcomes

Outcomes that have a continued effect over time are of significant value due to the trajectory of potentially lifelong changes. If a treatment/intervention reduces distress or improves functioning for a day or week, although important, it is of less value than a similar treatment that improves functioning for a year, or even a lifetime. For example, a nurse home visitor program demonstrated short-term impact on outcomes of pregnancy and a longer term impact on infants during the first 2 years after birth (Kitzman et al., 1997). However, of even greater value was the intervention's effect on the life-course trajectory of the women in terms of improved spacing between pregnancies, decreased use of welfare, fewer arrests, and less substance-abuse impairment during the 15-year period after delivery of their first child (Olds et al., 1997).

One of the primary foci of nursing practice is working with patients to develop strategies to monitor their health status and/or illness and to maintain positive health practices that reduce their risk for, lessen the impact of, or prevent further deterioration from disease, while promoting optimal functioning and quality of life. As a result, nurses have the potential to change the natural history of the person and the disease, and thus affect long-term outcomes.

Because of the potential impact on the person's natural history, when selecting and examining long-term outcomes, it is particularly important to compare change in status, using repeated measures, in the group receiving the APN intervention with the control group that did not receive the intervention. For vulnerable populations, for example, there may not be improvement in the treatment group, and if looked at independently, the investigator may risk concluding no treatment effect, when in reality, the treatment prevented decline. In this instance, treatment effect can only be seen when comparing the no change in the treatment group with the decline in the control group. This, of course, is less critical with random assignment, in which the control and treatment groups can be expected to be similar at intake into a study, than it is in quasi-experimental designs, in which assignment to group at intake is less rigorous.

Although producing improvements in some areas, APN interventions have the potential to disrupt the sensitive balance among ADLs and to affect fragile social connections and processes. As a result, during the design and review of any intervention study, it is important to consider in the model not only the desired primary and secondary outcomes, but also potential unintended effects. For example, interventions designed to improve individual functioning may change the dynamics of delicate family relationships. Using a pre–post pilot study design, a recent study of an APN-directed social ecology and self-efficacy-guided, team-delivered, restorative care intervention was carried out by Resnick, Galik, Gruber-Baldini, and Zimmerman (2009). Using a team approach that included an NP, restorative care nurse, and a registered nurse with expertise in rehabilitation and physical activity, the intervention focused on ongoing assessment and motivation of nursing home residents to engage in physical activity. Despite the small sample size for this pilot study ($n = 14$ residents), residents' time spent in physical activity increased significantly, as did their functional status based on the Barthel Index. Of particular interest, however, is that as social support for exercise from experts increased, social support from family decreased. Although a pilot study that will require further study before it can be evidence for practice, the findings do speak to the importance of the conceptualization of how the intervention was intended to operate, and the need to measure the multiple areas that are likely to be affected.

To determine the impact of a nursing intervention, long-term outcomes selected should be targeted, measurable, and timely to capture the concept thought to be affected by the intervention. It is important not only to consider the potential to accomplish the specific outcomes of interest, but to know whether the intervention affects the individual's risk status in other areas. In some instances, the success of the program in producing the projected outcome, for example, weight reduction, can also be expected to reduce the risk status of the person, for example, cardiovascular disease. In the case of obesity, the short-term outcome of weight reduction is evident, but detection of disease reduction associated with obesity, a long-term outcome, will not be detected in the short term.

Intervention Effectiveness

The degree to which the intervention is provided as planned (fidelity) is critical in research related to treatment efficacy and effectiveness, and in dissemination. Practicing APNs cannot use evidence of long-term outcomes that is produced in one intervention and assume the same outcomes if the intervention was not implemented in the same way and with like populations. Nevertheless, when an intervention has been found to be effective, clinicians are often challenged to provide the intervention to more people and at lower cost. Financial constraints result in continued pressures not only to replace expert APNs doing the intervention with less highly trained personnel, but also to reduce the intensity or duration of the services, thus, allowing more patients to be served. Such replacement and reduction can compromise the integrity of the intervention, rendering it ineffective.

Determining the lowest dose or the amount and quality of treatment/intervention needed to produce the desired long-term outcomes for the populations served and under what conditions is a challenge. The answer to the question about amount needs to be addressed in the original design of a study in which participants are randomized to different doses of an intervention; otherwise, the study needs to be repeated with treatment at a different level. Comparison of those in the treatment group who had full treatment with those who had less than full treatment does not adequately address this question, because the individuals who received less than full treatment are likely different from those who received full treatment.

Nurse researchers are increasingly asked to take the next steps in defining more carefully the "fit" or adequacy of APN interventions, good for whom and under what conditions. Nursing interventions cannot be expected to "fit" or be effective for everyone given the biological, psycho-emotional, and sociocultural diversity of the populations studied and the nature of the interventions themselves. Generally, studies are designed to answer primarily the question about whether the intervention works to the extent that the outcomes of the group receiving the intervention are different from the group not receiving it. Similar to what APNs see in practice, most often, some individual participants improve while others stay the same, and still others decline. This, at times, leads to conclusions that the program is ineffective, when, in reality, it had a positive effect for some, no effect for some, and a harmful effect for some. Researchers often discuss potential individual and contextual moderators of treatment such as psychological, social, and environmental resources, because they want to know the responses of those individuals in the treatment group based on these characteristics.

When examining the long-term outcomes of trials of specific APN interventions, it is often difficult to explain what looks like contradictory evidence. Clinicians examining evidence-based approaches are encouraged to consider carefully the characteristics of research participants and the settings within which the studies take place, attempting to identify the moderators or other unmeasured factors that may be influencing effects.

TRENDS–WHERE EVIDENCE IS NEEDED

There is no question that research about NP-generated long-term outcomes must be done to document APN contribution and influence on patient care. The chaotic nature of national health care underscores the importance of establishing the success and value of APNs in managing long-term outcomes for patients and systems. If APNs cannot fully participate, they run the risk of becoming irrelevant in the inevitable reform of the health care system. Conversely, APNs are uniquely positioned to clearly establish the true magnitude of their contribution if they assume full accountability for their practice and clearly demonstrate the beneficial outcomes of their care (Carroll & Fay, 1997).

Emerging Health Information and Other Technologies

Emerging technologies will aid in the demonstration of long-term outcomes for APN practice. For example, the linked electronic medical record (EMR), a cornerstone of health care reform because it promotes efficient, timely, and accurate information sharing, has the capability to provide data that can be used to facilitate care coordination, as well as document unique long-term APN outcomes. Information related to APN care then can be linked to patient satisfaction, quality of life, costs, and other yet-undetermined outcomes of care provided by APNs. Although the EMR with fully integrated point of care technology has significant potential, great challenges are associated with its introduction. For example, gaining consensus on a uniform system, obtaining consistency of data elements, and managing the associated costs require extensive negotiation. As a result, the full integration of the EMR is likely to be an incremental process. It will be important for nurse researchers to be involved in the development of the linked EMR to help ensure that APN-sensitive indicators are included in databases. By doing so, accurate, comprehensive, aggregate data appropriate to APN practice can become available for ongoing research to capture the contributions of APNs and draw inferences and conclusions about NP practice.

Given the challenging opportunities with health care reform, APNs need to be open to other new technologies to deliver services that have the potential to influence long-term outcomes. For example, currently there is limited research to determine long-term outcomes of the newer telemedicine (*e*-health) technology. Telemedicine (*e*-health) technology may be incorporated at any point of the health and illness continuum from early prevention to complex chronic disease treatment management. Full integration of telemedicine potential is anticipated to allow patients "to receive the appropriate type and level of care they need, in proximity to their homes, from the appropriate provider, and in the appropriate setting" (Bashshur & Shannon, 2009, p. 4). Given the importance of nursing in remote and in-home monitoring of patients, telephone management, and coordinating of care procedures, it is surprising that to date, so little research has been conducted that incorporates and identifies the contributions of APNs in telemedicine (*e*-health). We know little about the capacity of telemedicine (*e*-health) to facilitate the work of the APN, nor about the barriers and facilitators of this care.

The Social Determinants of Health "Equity"

Social determinants of health that include "poverty, education, early childhood education, treatment of women, employment opportunities, and individual empowerment" (Wilensky & Satcher, 2009, p. 194) have a powerful impact on humans' health status and life expectancy (Wilensky & Satcher, 2009). Although extensive efforts have been undertaken to improve equity in access and quality, evidence is increasing that traditional care alone will not eliminate current disparities. Improvement of conditions into which people are born, live, and die will have an impact on health. Although APNs can engage in political efforts to improve context, they also must consider these contextual conditions in their practice, because at the individual level, how people manage their daily lives within the context of limited resources or difficult circumstances is critical. Most of the APN interventions reviewed above place emphasis on preparing people for self-care, which requires consideration of person and context. Evidence from some studies indicates that those with the least personal and social capital gain the most from nurse interventions (Kitzman et al., 1997). There are reasons other than economic ones that make APNs the provider of choice for many populations in which health disparities are the highest. APNs are trained to provide the type of individualized care that considers the person's living conditions and responds to his or her needs for motivation, education, and problem solving to engage in behaviors that have long-term developmental health consequences.

Interdisciplinary Outcomes Research

Because of the type of questions related to long-term developmental health outcomes being pursued, few can be answered by the lone investigator, regardless of background. The questions require the expertise of multiple disciplines using interdisciplinary team methods. This is particularly important as one moves from individual to multilevel interventions involving several levels, including insurers, systems, providers, and consumers. For interdisciplinary teams to reflect the potential long-term contribution of APNs, however, nurse scientists who have expertise and the ability to clearly explain and articulate the unique perspective/contribution of the APN to the question need to be contributing members. They will ensure that questions are addressed that will help to develop the understanding and evidence needed for the continued incorporation of APN practice into the ever-evolving health care system.

The interdisciplinary team will increasingly be the target of long-term-outcomes research. Knowledge about the potential of the interdisciplinary health care team will require study of not only the process by which outcomes are achieved, but also about structure, because it is often the organizational structure that prohibits APNs from fulfilling their promise. This research will be difficult; however, nurse scientists are increasingly members of health services research teams, new information technology will aid in the management of data, and the policy analysts are waiting for what is learned.

Preparation of the APN for Practice and Research

One of the major factors likely to affect trends in APN long-term-outcomes research is the increasing academic and clinical preparation of APNs for their integral place in the management, as well as the delivery, of health care. As well-prepared APNs collaborate as members of interdisciplinary teams, they have the unique opportunity to capitalize on their expert clinical knowledge and the existing evidence to generate creative, innovative solutions to patient care dilemmas. These conceptualized interventions are informed by the literature but grounded in, and arise out of, practice. APNs change or restructure practice based on what is seen to work. After delivery of interventions and with new technologies, APNs have the ability to track the process and explain important nurse-sensitive outcomes. Interventions then can be further developed and tested by nurse researchers to further the evidence needed for intervention, dissemination, and policy development. This ability to bring insights from practice and integrate knowledge gained into practice using all the tools of translation is critical.

CONCLUSIONS

The best possible scientific evidence about APN long-term outcomes is critical to the organization and delivery of health care and to the development of health policy. Particularly important is evidence about APN interventions that affect long-term change in the trajectory of development of health and disease. Nevertheless, evidence about the efficacy and effectiveness of interventions in different populations and under dissimilar conditions does not come without careful planning, thoughtful and informed conceptualization, and rigorous design and methods. Given the trends of emerging health care technology and EMRs, the national charge to reduce health disparities and the enhanced preparation of APNs and nurse scientists, the future is promising. Nurses will increasingly be at the policy table, in the boardroom, or in the interdisciplinary team meeting holding rigorously obtained evidence regarding the potential of APNs in providing care that reduces health disparities and increases the quality and cost-effectiveness of services.

REFERENCES

Barber, B., & Fox, R. (1970). The case of the floppy-eared rabbits: An instance of serendipity gained and serendipity lost. In D. Forcese & S. Richer (Eds.), *Stages of social research: Contemporary perspectives* (pp. 27–38). Englewood Cliffs, NJ: Prentice-Hall.

Bashshur, R., & Shannon, G. (2009). National telemedicine initiatives: Essentials to healthcare reform. *Telemedicine and e-health, 15*, 1–11.

Callahan, C. M., Boustani, M. A., Unverzagt, F. W., Austrom, M. G., Damush, T. M., Perkins, A. J., et al. (2006). Effectiveness of collaborative care for older adults with Alzheimer's disease in primary care: A randomized controlled trial. *Journal of the American Medical Association, 295*(18), 2148–2157.

Carroll, T. L., & Fay, V. P. (1997). Measuring the impact of advanced practice nursing on achieving cost-quality outcomes: Issues and challenges. *Nursing Administration Quarterly, 21*(4), 32–40.

Curry, L. A., Nembhard, I. M., & Bradley, E. H. (2009). Qualitative and mixed methods provide unique contributions to outcomes research. *Circulation, 119*(10), 1442–1452.

Dennison, C. R., Post, W. S., Kim, M. T., Bone, L. R., Cohen, D., Blumenthal, R. S., et al. (2007). Underserved urban African American men: Hypertension trial outcomes and mortality during 5 years. *American Journal of Hypertension, 20*(2), 164–171.

Donabedian, A. (1966). Evaluation of the quality of medical care. *Milbank Memorial Fund Quarterly, 44*(1), 166–206.

Gleeson, R. M., McIlvain-Simpson, G., Boos, M. L., Sweet, E., Trzcinski, K. M., Solberg, C. A., et al. (1990). Advanced practice nursing: A model of collaborative care. *American Journal of Maternal Child Nursing, 15*(1), 9–10.

Goessens, B. M., Visseren, F. L., Sol, B. G., de Man-van Ginkel, J. M., van der Graaf, Y., Group, S. S., et al. (2006). A randomized, controlled trial for risk factor reduction in patients with symptomatic vascular disease: The multidisciplinary vascular prevention by nurses study (VENUS). *European Journal of Cardiovascular Prevention & Rehabilitation, 13*(6), 996–1003.

Gracias, V. H., Sicoutris, C. P., Stawicki, S. P., Meredith, D. M., Horan, A. D., Gupta, R., et al. (2008). Critical care nurse practitioners improve compliance with clinical practice guidelines in "semiclosed" surgical intensive care unit. *Journal of Nursing Care Quality, 23*(4), 338–344.

Huang, T. T., & Liang, S. H. (2005). A randomized clinical trial of the effectiveness of a discharge planning intervention in hospitalized elders with hip fracture due to falling. *Journal of Clinical Nursing, 14*(10), 1193–1201.

Kitzman, H., Olds, D. L., Henderson, C. R., Jr., Hanks, C., Cole, R., Tatelbaum, R., et al. (1997). Effect of prenatal and infancy home visitation by nurses on pregnancy outcomes, childhood injuries, and repeated childbearing. A randomized controlled trial. *Journal of the American Medical Association, 278*(8), 644–652.

Lawrenz, F., & Huffman, D. (2006). Methodological pluralism: The gold standard of STEM evaluation. In D. Huffman & F. Lawrenz (Eds.), *Critical issues in STEM evaluation* (pp. 19–34). San Francisco: Wiley.

Litaker, D., Mion, L., Planavsky, L., Kippes, C., Mehta, N., Frolkis, J., et al. (2003). Physician–nurse practitioner teams in chronic disease management: The impact on costs, clinical effectiveness, and patients' perception of care. *Journal of Interprofessional Care, 17*(3), 223–237.

Mion, L. C., Palmer, R. M., Meldon, S. W., Bass, D. M., Singer, M. E., Payne, S. M. C., et al. (2003). Case finding and referral model for emergency department elders: A randomized clinical trial. *Annals of Emergency Medicine, 41*(1), 57–68.

Mundinger, M. O., Kane, R. L., Lenz, E. R., Totten, A. M., Tsai, W. Y., Cleary, P. D., et al. (2000). Primary care outcomes in patients treated by nurse practitioners or physicians: A randomized trial. *Journal of the American Medical Association, 283*(1), 59–68.

Naylor, M. D., Brooten, D. A., Campbell, R. L., Maislin, G., McCauley, K. M., Schwartz, J. S., et al. (2004). Transitional care of older adults hospitalized with heart failure: A randomized, controlled trial. *Journal of the American Geriatrics Society, 52*(5), 675–684.

Olds, D. L., Eckenrode, J., Henderson, C. R., Jr., Kitzman, H., Powers, J., Cole, R., et al. (1997). Long-term effects of home visitation on maternal life course and child abuse and neglect. Fifteen-year follow-up of a randomized trial. *Journal of the American Medical Association, 278*(8), 637–643.

Paez, K. A., & Allen, J. K. (2006). Cost-effectiveness of nurse practitioner management of hypercholesterolemia following coronary revascularization. *Journal of the American Academy of Nurse Practitioners, 18*(9), 436–444.

Rawl, S. M., Easton, K. L., Kwiatkowski, S., Zemen, D., & Burczyk, B. (1998). Effectiveness of a nurse-managed follow-up program for rehabilitation patients after discharge. *Rehabilitation Nursing, 23*(4), 204–209.

Resnick, B., Galik, E., Gruber-Baldini, A. L., & Zimmerman, S. (2009). Implementing a restorative care philosophy of care in assisted living: Pilot testing of Res-Care-AL. *Journal of the American Academy of Nurse Practitioners, 21*(2), 123–133.

Shrier, I., Boivin, J. F., Steele, R. J., Platt, R. W., Furlan, A., Kakuma, R., et al. (2007). Should meta-analyses of interventions include observational studies in addition to randomized controlled trials? A critical examination of underlying principles. *American Journal of Epidemiology, 166*(10), 1203–1209.

Wilensky, G., & Satcher, D. (2009). Don't forget about the social determinants of health. *Health Affairs, 28*, 379–386.

Woolf, S. H. (2008). The meaning of translational research and why it matters. *Journal of the American Medical Association, 299*(2), 211–213.

Regulatory and Policy Environments

The efforts of individuals, professional organizations, state boards of nursing, and shifting coalition memberships engaged over time to advance the role and recognition of nurse practitioners (NPs) could not be better documented than in the first-person participant voices found in these four chapters.

The current health care reform effort is brought into sharp focus through O'Rourke's description of NPs' efforts to gain legislative approval for a bill recognizing NPs as primary care providers; despite the demand for more primary care providers, the Massachusetts Coalition of Nurse Practitioners had to fight vigorously to gain recognition, demonstrating both political and policy savvy in their successful legislative battle.

For new and veteran NPs who have followed the efforts of regulatory agencies and professional organizations to create consistency in licensure, accreditation, certification, and educational requirements for APNs, the chapter by Johnson, Dawson, and Brassard provides the clearest and most cogent description of the proposed regulatory model and how it was constructed through consensus. This chronicle of extraordinary efforts, supported by representatives of state boards of nursing and more than 30 organizations, captures the recent history of the NP movement and points to the regulatory and educational route

111

forward. It also shows the possibilities of coalitions and consensus, characteristics not always common in nursing's history.

Through their case studies, Mackey and Woolbert, followed by Sampson, give insiders' views and analyses of special interest groups tenaciously battling advanced-practice nurses (APNs), and NPs in particular, attempting to limit any expansion of scope of practice despite the desperate need for primary care providers. Mackey and Woolbert detail the events in Texas that mark the back and forth in the regulatory battles to expand and provide access to NP practice. One state's legislative description of practice is brought to life through their recounting, and serves as both a cautionary and optimistic tale about perseverance and commitment. Sampson also chronicles the Texas experience, though more narrowly focused on prescriptive authority, and contrasts it to the very different jurisdictional scenario of New Hampshire, noting that "place matters." These descriptions give credence to the admonition to become involved, articulate, and persistent in achieving big goals.

Frederick Douglass is quoted as saying, "Power never conceded without a demand, it never did, and it never will." These chapters are testimony to the commitment and diligence of individual nurse leaders and organizations to challenge power and effect the changes that could improve access to health care and strengthen the preparation and practice of NPs across the country.

State Health Care Reform: The Role of Nurse Practitioners in Massachusetts

NANCY O'ROURKE

BACKGROUND

Health care costs are rising at a dramatic rate, and the number of uninsured individuals continues to rise. Overall, the expenditures for health care in the United States have increased by approximately 10% over the last 20 years, and are predicted to consume 20% of our gross national product by 2020 (Kaiser Family Foundation, 2006, p. 1).

Currently, health care spending exceeds our economy's growth by 2.5% and lack of insurance presents serious financial consequences if illness occurs (Kaiser Family Foundation, 2006, p. 1). The need for a new perspective is clear, and the roles of providers and health insurers, as well as quality, access, and cost, must be examined in any health reform effort. The federal government recognized this, and in 2006, began to negotiate reform at the state level. The first of such initiatives was to encourage states to control health care spending and direct more monies to primary care, as opposed to tertiary facilities. In this context, Massachusetts was forced to rethink how the Commonwealth funded the free care pool.

Massachusetts health care was suited to this type of reform, as the state had a large proportion of employer-based insurance programs and a relatively low uninsured population, as compared with other states in the nation (Massachusetts Division of Health Care Finance and Policy, 2008). Massachusetts developed the option of directing the funding to subsidize low-income health insurance, rather than reimbursing institutions for the free care pool. This new model of "universal health care" was the result of cost containment and quality improvement efforts in Massachusetts.

CHAPTER 58

Massachusetts has been long noted for revolutionary thinking, and true to our historical form, Governor Mitt Romney signed into law Chapter 58, *An Act Providing Access to Affordable, Quality, Accountable Health Care* (MGL 176R) (Massachusetts General Courts, 2006). A Common Health Connector Authority was created to work with major insurance carriers to create affordable insurance plans for all residents by using insurance reforms, subsidization, and tax benefits. The Connector would then write policies and oversee these subsidized insurance programs. Chapter 58 requires employers to offer health insurance to employees or to pay a "fair share" contribution to the state to help subsidize the uninsured. Individuals who can afford health insurance, but opt not to purchase it, are subject to state tax penalties (Gabel et al., 2008).

Since the passage of this legislation, Massachusetts health care reform has been the focus of national media attention. Overall, Chapter 58 is the most ambitious health care reform legislation in the nation, and sets precedent by mandating health care for all Massachusetts residents. A recent article in the *New York Times, A Lesson on Health Care From Massachusetts,* (Sack, 2009) discusses the challenges that Massachusetts faces in the implementation and sustainability of Chapter 58. Mandating universal coverage before addressing the rising costs of health care was both innovative and risky. Economic downturns, inaccurate estimates of the numbers of uninsured, and rising enrollments in the subsidized health plans have strained the state's budget, creating a deficit that must now be addressed. And the daunting task of controlling health care costs must be the next agenda item for Massachusetts if the universal health care program is to survive.

This groundbreaking legislation, the first of its kind in the nation, required all citizens of Massachusetts to be enrolled in a health care plan or face penalties. Consequently, Massachusetts citizens were now mandated to have health insurance, and employers were required to offer health care choices and subsidies or face financial penalties. Individual citizens who did not comply by signing up for health insurance would be required to forfeit their state income tax refunds. These "penalty funds" would be funneled back into the tax base and used as a means of supporting health care reform.

TRANSFORMATIVE EFFECT ON HEALTH CARE

Though it remains controversial because it challenges Employee Retirement Income Security Act (ERISA) federal laws and mandates universal health care before addressing cost-containment issues, this legislation has changed health care in Massachusetts in several ways. The number of uninsured in Massachusetts has fallen by one-half (Long, 2008). At this time, 439,000 once-uninsured people now have health care coverage, and care provided by the free care pool has decreased by 37% (Massachusetts Division of Health Care Finance and Policy, 2008). The Urban Institute reported that uninsured rates in Massachusetts had fallen from 13% to 7% after the implementation of Chapter 58 (Long & Masi, 2008). The most dramatic results were among young adults, whose uninsured rates fell from 23% to 13%. The report also showed improvements in access to care and preventative health care use (Long & Masi, 2008).

Improved access to health care created an increased demand for primary care providers (PCPs). In 2005, the Massachusetts Coalition of Nurse Practitioners (MCNP) anticipated that the proposed Chapter 58 legislation could be an opportunity to recognize nurse practitioners (NPs) as PCPs, thus improving access to care through the use of NPs, and yield measurable data about outcomes of NP care. Prior to this legislation, NPs worked within a physician's patient panel and did not have a distinct panel of their own, limiting access to care and maintaining the invisibility of NP practice. In 2005, the MCNP filed legislation to gain recognition as PCPs.

At the same time, a coalition including physicians, hospitals, and insurance carriers filed legislation requesting a uniform credentialing process specific to physicians and excluding other health care providers. The MCNP and lobbyists Craven and Ober Policy Strategists, LLC, while monitoring the progress of Chapter 58, recognized that this credentialing legislation excluded NPs and likely posed a barrier to NP practice. Policy strategists, as representatives of the MCNP, conferred with the American Academy of Nurse Practitioners and the American College of Nurse Practitioners, and researched testimony on barriers to advanced-practice nurses presented to the United States Department of Justice by the American Nurses Association (Pearson, 2000). Based on these discussions and findings, the legislation was thought to have potential implications regarding anti-trust laws, and would lead to a competitive disadvantage for NPs in the health care marketplace. To ensure that patients in Massachusetts had access to the services of NPs, the MCNP communicated with key legislators about the problems associated with any exclusive physician-credentialing legislation. The chronology of these events are in Appendix 1, and show how this dialogue with legislators and the attorney general, which continued through the remainder of the legislative session, ultimately and successfully blocked the progress of a potentially restrictive and harmful version of physician-credentialing legislation.

Initially, in the 2005–2006 legislative sessions, the MCNP's bill to gain PCP status passed through the Senate without issue. In the House, however, the bill met opposition from the Massachusetts Medical Society and was not signed into law.

As Chapter 58 was adapted, interested parties came together to determine the best way for our overburdened health system to absorb the projected 500,000 uninsured who would now be seeking health care in Massachusetts. Governor Romney, wanting inclusion of all providers, appointed an NP (Nancy O'Rourke) to the Health Care Cost and Quality Council. This council is the Advisory Board to the Health Connector Authority, and was charged with the daunting task of improving access and quality of care within a given structure of cost containment.

The primary care system was bursting at the seams, and most primary care practices were closed to new patients. Patients were waiting an average of 50 days for a primary care appointment, and 42% of practices were not accepting new patients (ACP Advocate, 2008; Kowalczyk, 2008). Emergency departments, feeling the burden of increasing visits and providing urgent care to the uninsured population, and now facing the loss of state funding from the free care pool, wondered how the primary care system would or could absorb this number of patients. Chapter 58 however, was embraced by all as the answer to the uninsured crisis (McDonough, Rosman, Butt, Tucker, & Kaplan Howe, 2008).

As this health care dilemma unfolded, a company that provided urgent care in retail pharmacies, The Minute Clinics, recognized the opportunity to develop their business model in the Massachusetts market. Because all citizens were covered under Chapter 58, there now was a greater demand for access to primary and urgent care. Minute Clinics petitioned the Massachusetts Department of Public Health (DPH) to change regulations regarding physical facilities so that Minute Clinics could operate in a variety of retail spaces. The open regulatory hearings enabled a full public discussion not only about physical space, but also the role of the NPs staffing the Minute Clinics. The Massachusetts Medical Society vehemently opposed changing the regulations and allowing this new delivery model to develop in Massachusetts. Their concerns centered on lack of continuity of care and NPs providing care in "unsupervised" settings.

The Department of Public Health (DPH) called on the MCNP to educate both the department officials and the public about the role of NPs, and to provide expert guidance regarding the scope of NP practice in Massachusetts. This was the first time in history that DPH had recognized the Coalition in a public forum.

LEGISLATIVE EFFORTS

With the background of Chapter 58 implementation and the DPH discussion of needed state regulatory changes around limited-service clinics, the MCNP sensed change on the horizon. The contribution and value of NP practice had found its way into the spotlight, and those who previously ignored NPs were inviting opinions and involvement in discussions regarding the future of health care in Massachusetts. Despite the unsuccessful attempt to gain recognition as PCPs in 2005, the MCNP, with Representative Jennifer Callahan as sponsor, re-filed the legislation, Senate Bill 2526. This bill duplicated the previous legislation, asking that all insurers be statutorily required to recognize NPs as PCPs and allow them to manage their own panel of patients.

The lobbying strategy of the NPs was built on previous platforms: to improve access by increasing the numbers of PCPs exponentially and to promote quality care. Using the principles that health care reform must enable value-based competition among health care providers, and that such a system embraces patient choice (Porter & Olmsted-Teisberg, 2006), the NPs argued that 30 years of outcome data demonstrated their expertise in providing primary care and clearly demonstrated their cost effectiveness. Patient choice, a driving force in the creation of Chapter 58, and efforts to control costs and quality through NP care, were the key talking points that the MCNP presented to legislators.

Health insurance plans opposed Senate Bill 2526, believing that the language was "any willing provider" and would force insurers to contract with and credential any NP practicing in Massachusetts. The MCNP demonstrated to the legislators that this was not the case, and only required insurers to recognize NPs who were already contracted providers within the health plans.

Over a 2-year period, 2006–2008, NPs worked closely with legislators, specifically, Representative Callahan and Senate President Therese Murray. The Senate President saw the value in Senate Bill 2526 and recognized the contributions of NPs. Because she was developing a comprehensive health care package to address multiple concerns, including cost containment, surrounding Chapter 58, Senator Murray incorporated the NPs' language of Senate Bill 2526 in her health care proposed legislation, Chapter 305 of the Acts of 2008, *An Act to Promote Cost Containment, Transparency and Efficiency in the Delivery of Quality Health Care*. Believing that there must be incentives to attract providers to primary care, and that NPs are a part of the solution to health care reform in Massachusetts, Senator Murray extended a financial incentive developed for primary care physicians to NPs, as well. Her support for NPs was a result of the strong relationship that had developed between Senator Murray and the MCNP, and was evidenced by her commitment to NPs throughout the development of the total health reform legislation.

On the last day of the legislative session, the physician assistant (PA) group tried to amend the NP section of the bill with language that would require insurers to recognize PAs as PCPs and to reimburse them at the physician rate. As written, the NP section of the bill was budget neutral. This amendment would have added dollar cost to the bill, effectively killing that section of the bill. Some legislators felt that PAs should be included. Representative Callahan, at the last hour, fought hard, taking the unpopular stand of supporting the NP language and not adding the physican assistant on at this late time. Her persuasive arguments, that passing this NP language in its current form was the right thing for legislators to do for their constituents, proved successful. After tense dicussions in the House and Senate and continued opposition of insurers to the NP language included in Senator Murray's legislation, the bill was successfully passed.

Recognizing NPs as PCPs creates tremendous opportunity in Massachusetts. For the first time in Massachusetts' history, insurers are mandated to recognize the NPs they contract with as PCPs and offer patients the option to choose them. The outcomes of quality measures will be reported for NPs, as well as for physicians, and the opportunity for them to be included in the medical home demonstration project now is a reality. These political gains are only the beginning. There are many more areas that will be open to challenge as this legislation, Chapter 305, is implemented and as Chapter 58 continues to unfold. NPs will need to be cognizant of opportunities as they arise. Negotiations with individual insurers to implement Chapter 305 in their internal regulations may result in changes in data collection, and ultimately may affect reimbursement. Insurers will be more inclined to contract with individual NPs now, and not just with those practitioners involved in physician practices. This legislation brings NPs out of the proverbial closet and makes us visible and accessible to patients.

Whether or not Chapter 58 becomes the panacea of health care reform it is touted to be remains to be seen. But the opportunities it has afforded and the political gains it created for NPs are evident. The potential for further advances in practice remain an interesting and exciting question.

REFERENCES

The ACP Advocate. (2008, October 22). *Primary care shortage spawns innovation.* Retrieved August 12, 2009, from http://www.healthbanks.com/PatientPortal/My-Practice.aspx?RemovedHBCode=RemovedValue&LType=11&UAID=%7BA83090 7D-8345-4AA5-A0D5-F8776BBC08BB%7D&TabID=%7BX%7D&ArticleID=620361

Gabel, J. R., Whitmore, H., Pickreign, J., Sellheim, W., Shova, K. C., & Bassett, V. (2008). After the mandates: Massachusetts employers continue to support health reform as more firms offer coverage. *Health Affairs, 27*(6), 566–575.

Kaiser Family Foundation. (2006). *Snapshots: Health care costs: Comparing projected growth in health care expenditures and the economy.* Retrieved August 12, 2009, from www.kff.org/insurance/snapshot/chcm050206oth2.cfm

Kowalczyk, L. (2008, September 22). Across Massachusetts, wait to see doctors grows. Access to care, insurance law cited for delays. *Boston Globe*. Retrieved January 28, 2010, from http://www.boston.com/news/health/articles/2008/09/22/across_mass_wait_to_see _doctors_grows/

Long, S. K. (2008, June 3). On the road to universal coverage: Impacts of reform in Massachusetts at one year. *Health Affairs*, w270–w284. Retrieved August 12, 2009, from http://www.commonwealthfund.org/Content/Publications/In-the-Literature/2008/Jun/On-the-Road-to-Universal-Coverage—Impacts-of-Reform-in-Massachusetts-at-One-Year.aspx

Long, S., & Masi, P. (2008). How have employers responded to health reform in Massachusetts? Employers' views at the end of one year. *Health Affairs, 27*(6), 576–583.

Massachusetts Division of Health Care Finance and Policy. (2008, August). *Health care in Massachusetts: Key indicators quarterly report, August 2008*. (Publication number: 09-189-04 HCF.) Retrieved August 12, 2009, from http://www.mass.gov/Eeohhs2/docs/dhcfp/r/pubs/08/key_indicators_0 808.pdf

Massachusetts General Courts. (2006). *Chapter 58 of the Acts of 2006, An Act providing access to affordable, quality, accountable health care (MGL 176R)*. Retrieved January 28, 2010, from http://www.mass.gov/legis/laws/seslaw06/sl060058.htm

McDonough, J., Rosman, B., Butt, M., Tucker, L., & Kaplan Howe, L. (2008). Massachusetts health reform implementation: Major progress and future challenges. *Health Affairs, 27*(4), w285–w297.

Moran, D. W. (2005). Whence and wither health insurance: A revisionist history. *Health Affairs, 24*(6), 1415–1425.

Pearson, L. (2000). Physician attempt to remove antitrust exemptions stalled. *Nurse Practitioner, 25*, 23–24.

Porter, M., & Olmsted-Teisberg, E. (2006). *Redefining health care: Creating value-based competition on results*. Boston: Harvard Business School Press.

Sack, K. (2009, March 28). A lesson on health care from Massachusetts. *New York Times*. Retrieved August 18, 2009, from http://www.nytimes.com/2009/03/29/weekinreview/29sack.html?_r=1&r ef=politics

The ACP Advocate. (2008, October 22). *Primary care shortage spawns innovation*. Retrieved August 12, 2009, from http://www.healthbanks.com/PatientPortal/MyPractice.aspx?RemovedHBCode=RemovedValue&LType=11&UAID=%7BA83090 7D-8345-4AA5-A0D5-F8776BBC08BB%7D&TabID=%7BX%7D&ArticleID=620361

CHAPTER 8 APPENDIX

The following chronology of the efforts of individual NPs, the MCNP, the MCNP-Political Action Committee (PAC), and their lobbyists, Policy Strategists is a condensed version of an extraordinarily intense and focused campaign. Activities included grassroots efforts, relationships established with and recognition of legislative leaders, and timely use of policy and legal consultants. A true success story achieved by individual NPs and their professional organization.

Fall 2004

- Identified practice issues of greatest need for policy change through research and meeting with MCNP members
- Used the AANP Strategic Plan for 2003–2004 as framework
- Identified need to have NPs recognized in statute as PCPs
- Researched drafting of legislation to meet identified goal and strategized legislators' commitment to serve as bill sponsors.

2005

- Filed bill with five sponsors in both House and Senate
- Developed plan to use news media and *The Boston Globe* articles to assist the cause
- Communicated anti-trust concerns re: physician credentialing legislation for the remainder of the session
- Discussed PCP status with representatives of the Division of Insurance
- Omnibus health care bill released with physician credentialing provisions; MCNP requested inclusion as PCP in the Omnibus Bill
- Met with Massachusetts Business Round Table
- Established MCNP-PAC

- Received communication from Federal Trade Commission (FTC) indicating claims for anti-trust violations in credentialing bill were legitimate
- Testified before Health Care Financing Committee re: S2042, *An Act Providing for Health Access, Affordability and Accountability*
- Examined statutory PCP language in both Maine and Pennsylvania
- Developed "tool kit" for grass roots action
- Testified at hearing on bill before Joint Committee on Public Health, opposed by Massachusetts Medical Society and Joint Committee on Financial Services
- Offered marked-up version of credentialing bill to Senate President and Committees on Public Health and Health Care Financing
- NP bill is released from Joint Committee on Public Health indicating support.

2006

- Met with key lawmakers and representatives of health plans who were forced to establish Health Care Administrative Simplification, or "HCAS," of credentialing applications to address administrative goals in lieu of statutory mandate on physician-only credentialing
- Demonstrated that some health plans provide consumer choice of provider type
- Bill recognized as budget neutral and released from Joint Committee on Health Care Financing
- Governor appointed Nancy O'Rourke to Health Care Quality and Cost Council, Advisory Committee.

2007

- **PCP bill and the physician credentialing bill re-filed for the new session**
- Hearing dates for testimony on PCP and other nursing issues successfully moved from October to May by

MCNP and Policy Strategists; bill favorably released in June by Joint Committee on Public Health and by Joint Committee on Health Care Financing in October

■ MCNP testified in support of limited-service clinics
■ Systematic and widespread grassroots lobbying preserved the bill in the face of opposition by Massachusetts Medical Society and health plans
■ Met with Division of Insurance and Group Insurance Commission to inform them about the bill
■ Opponents of the bill lobbied intensely to change provisions of what is now the Omnibus Healthcare Reform II draft
■ MCNP retained legal counsel to combat language of opponents who tried to weaken bill's intent; PCP bill language incorporated into Health Care Reform Part II (S. 2683)
■ Lobbying intensified to retain PCP language and gain passage by the end of session with language intact
■ House released bill with change to language related to PCP and primary care workforce; education incentives stripped of all NP references
■ Amendments accepted; however, PAs injected into text: in the face of great pressure from opponents, including the Massachusetts Association of Health Plans, both sides attempt to revise bill language to the end of the last day of the session
■ The House and Senate passed PCP (Section 28) in the new S.2683 on the last day of the formal session, July 31, 2008.

9

Consensus Model for Advanced-Practice Nurse Regulation: A New Approach

JEAN JOHNSON, ELLEN DAWSON, AND ANDREA BRASSARD

INTRODUCTION

Nursing regulation exists to protect the public, and as such, regulation is often viewed as the work of state boards of nursing. Yet regulation has a much broader definition, including not only licensing, but also accreditation and certification. Regulation of nurse practitioners (NPs), as well as other advanced-practice registered nurses (APRNs), establishes a minimum standard of competence. The process of NP regulation has become very complicated. There has been significant variability in how states recognize NPs, as well as a breakdown in coordination among the regulatory entities. As a result, a new regulatory model, called the Consensus Model for APRN Regulation, has been proposed and endorsed by organizations representing APRNs. This chapter will: (a) provide an overview of recent history of regulation leading to a new regulatory model; (b) present the new regulatory model; and (c) present background information regarding certification, accreditation, and licensure of nursing, including a discussion of how the new model relates to these regulatory arms.

BACKGROUND

Historically, an attempt to rationalize regulation occurred during the mid- to late 1970s. In 1974, the American Nurses Association (ANA) House of Delegates voted to study the accreditation process. A study was commissioned in 1975 by the ANA, who a year later appointed the Committee to Study Credentialing in Nursing (CSCN). As a result of the work of the CSCN, a paper titled, *A Study of Credentialing in Nursing: A New Approach*, was published (ANA, 1979). This report called for a national nursing credentialing center. Ultimately, the idea of a national credentialing center was dropped for lack of support (Joel, 2003). However, a very useful conceptual model emerged from the work undertaken by the CSCN in the 1970s. The concept of the three prongs of certification, accreditation and licensure forming the framework for regulation, was proposed by Styles (2008). Expanding upon Styles' concept, Figure 9.1 illustrates how these functions relate to education and practice.

The certified NP (CNP) is prepared with the acute care CNP competencies and/or the primary care CNP competencies. At this time, the acute care and primary care CNP delineation applies only to the pediatric and adult–gerontology CNP population foci. Scope of practice of the primary care or acute care CNP is *not setting-specific*, but is based on patient care needs. Programs may prepare individuals across both the primary care and acute care CNP competencies. If programs prepare graduates across both sets of roles, the graduate must be prepared with the consensus-based competencies for both roles, and must successfully obtain certification in both the acute and the primary care CNP roles. CNP certification in the acute care or primary care roles must match the educational preparation for CNPs in these roles.

Complexities in the regulatory environment exist in every aspect. There are multiple certifying and accrediting bodies, as well as 51 separate boards of nursing. Table 9.1 provides information on the various regulatory bodies. Regulatory processes and requirements vary from state to state, adding yet another layer of complexity to an already complicated regulatory environment. Some states certify NPs, others license them. Some states review the details of each NP curriculum, whereas others do not. There is also variability in educational programs, with some adhering to the American Association of Colleges of Nursing's (AACN), *The Essentials of Master's Education for Advanced Practice Nurs-*

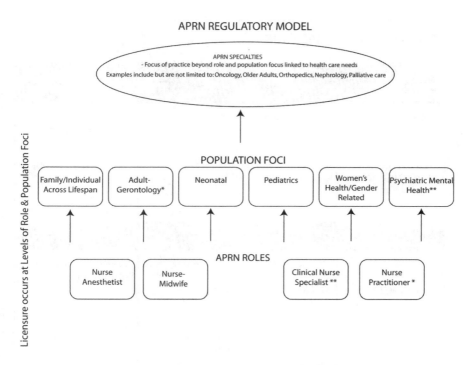

Figure 9.1 Clinical career pathway: Levels of practice and corresponding educational preparation.

ing closely, whereas others incorporate the *Essentials* to a less degree. Some educational programs have opted to prepare individuals in narrowly defined clinical areas, whereas others have decided to do so from a broad perspective. Further adding to the complexity is definitional variation, with NPs calling one area of practice a "specialty," and other NPs call it a "subspecialty." These incongruities have created confusion within nursing and among the public.

Throughout the 1980s and 1990s, standards for NP educational programs and practice continued to change, driving evolution in certification and accreditation. Certifying bodies refined and strengthened their approaches to creating examinations to ensure that the examinations were psychometrically sound, legally defensible, and met nationally recognized standards. Accrediting organizations continued to accredit schools, but not specifically NP or clinical nurse specialist

Table 9.1

REGULATORY ORGANIZATIONS

ACCREDITATION OF EDUCATIONAL PROGRAMS	FOCUS	WEB SITE
Collegiate Commission for Nursing Education	Baccalaureate and higher-degree nursing education programs	http://www.aacn.nche.edu/accreditation/
National League for Nursing Accrediting Commission, Inc.	Accredits practical, associate, bachelor's, and master's programs	http://www.nlnac.org/home.htm

CERTIFICATION ORGANIZATIONS		
American Academy of Nurse Practitioners	Provides a valid and reliable program for entry-level NPs to recognize their education, knowledge and professional expertise—adult, family, and gerontological NPs	http://www.aanp.org/Certification
American Nurses Credentialing Center	Certifies NPs in the areas of acute care, adult, family, gerontological, adult psychiatric and mental health, pediatric, family psychiatric and mental health, and school NPs	http://www.nursecredentialing.org/#
Pediatric Nursing Certification Board	Certifies primary care pediatric, acute care pediatric NPs	http://www.pncb.org/ptistore/control/index
National Certification Corporation	Certifies women's health care NPs	http://www.nccwebsite.org/default.aspx

LICENSING BOARDS		
National Council of State Boards of Nursing	Provides an organization through which Boards of Nursing act and counsel together on matters of common interest and concern affecting the public health, safety and welfare, including the development of licensing examinations in nursing	https://www.ncsbn.org/index.htm

(CNS) programs. Although the 1980s and 1990s marked a time when several important elements of regulation were strengthened, coordination of efforts by regulatory bodies was not a hallmark of this period.

A NEW REGULATORY MODEL

In 2004, spurred by growing discontent among nursing organizations regarding the lack of uniform approaches to regulation, the AACN convened a meeting of approximately 70 organizations representing NPs, CNSs, certified registered nurse anesthetists (CRNAs), and certified nurse midwives (CNMs). The discontent centered on the misalignment of the regulatory triad. Accredited nursing programs were preparing people for roles that were not recognized by some state boards of nursing. For instance, the Texas Board of Nursing did not recognize palliative care NPs, yet these programs were offered by accredited schools. Certifying agencies set up curriculum review processes to ensure that people sitting for an exam completed a legitimate program. In addition, many state boards also set up curriculum review processes because the accreditation bodies did not specifically review NP or CNS programs. The CRNA and CNM programs had a separate accreditation process that the state boards recognized. State boards were facing an increasing number of requests to recognize narrowly focused NP specialties, concentrating on body systems and diseases such as incontinence or diabetes, rather than on the care of the person as a whole. Adding to the rising level of confusion was the varied criteria that state boards used to license NPs. The organizations participating in the 2004 meeting felt it was imperative to resolve the discrepancies and create a regulatory model for the future.

As a result of the 2004 meeting, the major concerns about the current regulatory environment included the lack of a standard definition of advanced-practice nursing and definition of a specialty and subspecialty, the proliferation of narrowly defined education and practice at the APRN level, and the lack of common legal recognition across states. Representatives from 23 of the organizations that participated in the 2004 meeting formed the APRN Consensus Work Group to address these issues. After nearly 2 years of work, a final paper was published. Concurrent with the work of the APRN Consensus Group, a group convened by the National Council of State Boards of Nursing (NCSBN)

Exhibit 9.1

ORGANIZATIONS PARTICIPATING IN THE JOINT DIALOGUE GROUP

American Academy of Nurse Practitioners Certification Program

American Association of Colleges of Nursing

American Association of Nurse Anesthetists

American College of Nurse-Midwives

American Nurses Association

American Organization of Nurse Executives

Compact Administrators

National Association of Clinical Nurse Specialists

National Council of State Boards of Nursing

National League for Nursing Accrediting Commission

National Organization of Nurse Practitioner Faculties

NCSBN APRN Advisory Committee Representatives (5)

was also generating a document concerning regulation of APRN practice. The two documents were very dissimilar. In order to avoid the potential for significant confusion with the release of the two papers, representatives from the NCSBN and the APRN Consensus Work Group came together as the Joint Dialogue Group to resolve differences between the two papers and publish one paper. See Exhibit 9.1 for a list of organizations participating in the Joint Dialogue Group.

All of the previously referenced work sought to develop a regulatory model that would protect the public and address a myriad of issues facing the APRN community. In addition, the groups were committed to ensuring that the policies put forward would do no harm to currently practicing nurses. Finally, there was a commitment to be future-oriented, so that the regulatory model would be flexible enough to support nursing's mission to meet the future health care needs of the public, and be rigorous enough to protect the public.

The overall work to create a new regulatory model resulted in the development of several important elements of a definition that supports the model. These elements are presented in Exhibit 9.2. An important element of this definition is that APRNs provide direct, hands-on care. This element of the definition differentiates APRNs from other groups of nurses who have graduate preparation in areas such as management, informatics, and public health. The preparation of nurses in these areas is vitally important, but does not require state licensure.

Figure 9.1 presents the new APRN regulatory model. This model recognizes levels of practice ranging from broadly defined roles to the narrowly defined specialties. There are four APRN roles, including NPs, CNSs, CNMs, and CRNAs. Preparation for each role requires content in physical assessment, pathophysiology, and pharmacology across the life span—referred to as the "3Ps." These three courses provide the foundation for the APRN role.

Each role has a population focus for practice. The population focus includes six areas: family/individual across the lifespan, adult/gerontology, neonatal, pediatrics, women's health/gender-related, and psychiatric/mental health. Existing certification exams already offer testing covering these populations and much of the role content. Certifying bodies will need to review their exams to ensure appropriate coverage of the education related to the role, as well as the population focus. State boards will license APRNs only at the role and population focus levels.

Specialty practice builds on the role and population focus as defined previously. The definition of a specialty is based on the ANA Criteria for Recognition as a Nursing Specialty (American Nurses Association, 2004). This document outlines 14 different criteria in recognizing a nursing specialty. Specialty practice focuses on special populations, such as individuals with diabetes, or specific patient needs, such as palliative care. Nursing specialties will not require review or licensing by a state board. Professional organizations will develop standards and establish competency requirements for specialties. A specialization cannot expand an APRN's scope of practice beyond the role and population focus as presented in the regulatory model. Specialization provides more in-depth knowledge and skills within the scope of a particular role and population focus. Examples of specialty practice include oncology, palliative care, pain management, cardiovascular, and diabetes care. Not requiring licensing for specialties allows flexibility for nursing to meet new areas of need. If these areas develop beyond a specialty level, the process to become a population focus or a role can be implemented. The identification of a new role would require the establishment of standards, as well as recognition by all of the regulatory arms.

Exhibit 9.2

ELEMENTS OF THE DEFINITION OF APRN

■ Completion of an accredited graduate-level education program preparing him/her for one of the four recognized APRN roles: CRNA, certified nurse-midwife (CNM), CNS, or CNP

■ Passed a national certification examination that measures APRN, role, and population-focused competencies, and maintains continued competence as evidenced by recertification in the role and population through the national certification program

■ Acquired advanced clinical knowledge and skills preparing him/her to provide direct care to patients, as well as a component of indirect care; however, the defining factor for all APRNs is that a significant component of the education and practice focuses on direct care of individuals

■ Practice builds on the competencies of RNs by demonstrating a greater depth and breadth of knowledge, a greater synthesis of data, increased complexity of skills and interventions, and greater role autonomy

■ Educationally prepared to assume responsibility and accountability for health promotion and/or maintenance, as well as the assessment, diagnosis, and management of patient problems, which includes the use and prescription of pharmacologic and nonpharmacologic interventions

■ Has clinical experience of sufficient depth and breadth to reflect the intended certification

■ Has obtained certification to practice as an APRN in one of the four APRN roles (NP, CNS, CNM, and CRNA)

(American Nurses Credentialing Center, 2009, p. 6.)

The APRN regulatory model generally follows the options for NPs that now exist, with two exceptions. Adult and gerontology have been distinct areas of practice with certifying exams available in each area. However, in the new model, adult and gerontology have been combined for the following reasons:

■ There is a great need for NPs who have the knowledge and skills to take care of elderly patients. Enrollment in gerontology NP programs has been limited, and many programs have already combined their adult and gerontology programs. Concern about an adequate workforce to care for our aging population was a critical factor.

■ Confusion for state boards of nursing in knowing when someone is practicing outside of his or her scope based on age. Examples of state boards of nursing limiting adult NPs from caring for the elderly, and gerontology NPs caring for younger adults, began to emerge as anecdotes.

■ Confidence that standards and guidelines could be developed so that the gerontology content in adult–gerontology programs would be as extensive and strong as in current gerontology programs.

The second exception is that psychiatric/mental health NP practice is defined as a population focus. A CNS or an NP could select psychiatric/mental health nursing as a population focus. Within the new model, these nurses will need to complete the required coursework for the "3Ps" and then take courses for the psychiatric/mental health population focus.

CERTIFICATION

Historic Perspective of Certification

The word "certification" has been used in a variety of ways over the years. In the early days of NP certification, only experienced NPs could take the exam. Certification evolved from validating expert practice to controlling entry. Certification through testing by a national board became the basis for recognition by state boards of nursing to allow practice and prescriptive authority in most states. Certification ensures the public of entry-level competency for safe NP practice. Certification recognizes the clinical competence of nurses and APRNs in various practice areas. Although certification for NPs is voluntary, the majority of states require national certification as a condition of licensure (Bednash, Honig, & Gibbs, 2005).

The first national certification exam was administered by the American Association of Nurse Anesthetists (AANA) in 1945. Twenty-five years later, the American College of Nurse-Midwives (ACNM) established a certification program (Fickeissen, 1985). Although certification was conceived by the ANA in the mid 1950s, the ANA certification program was not established until 1973. The American Nurses Credentialing Center (ANCC), a subsidiary of the ANA, currently certifies nurses in 26 different areas, with over 75,000 nurses being certified (American Nurses Credentialing Center, 2009). Within the certification programs, ANCC certifies NPs in nine clinical areas: acute care, adult, adult psychiatric and mental health, advanced diabetes management, family, family psychiatric and mental health, gerontology, pediatric, and the newest certification exam, school NP. The American Academy of Nurse Practitioners (AANP) began certifying NPs in the 1990s, and currently certifies adult, family, and gerontological NPs.

Two other specialty organizations certify NPs. The National Certification Corporation (NCC) for the Obstetric, Gynecological, and Neonatal Nursing Specialties offers certification exams for two NP specialties: neonatal and women's health care. The Pediatric Nursing Certification Board (PNCB) offers certification as a pediatric NP in primary care or acute care.

These four certifying bodies, ANCC, AANP, NCC, and PNCB, follow criteria established by the NCSBN to determine the suitability of advanced-practice certification examinations for regulatory purposes (National Council of State Boards of Nursing, 2002b). Test items are reviewed for content validity, cultural bias, and correct scoring. All exams are required to be psychometrically sound and legally defensible.

Content validity of certification exams is measured through job or task analyses, also known as role delineation studies. Role delineation studies are large national surveys that collect specific data about work activities performed by practicing NPs. Now Web-based, these surveys are conducted at least every 5 years. For instance, the ANCC's 2003 survey asked NP respondents to rate work activities in three areas: how often they performed the task (daily, weekly, monthly, seldom, or not performed); expectation of when they were expected to be able to perform the task (within the first 6 months of working as an NP, after the first 6 months of working as an NP, or never expected to perform this activity); and consequence (incorrect performance of this activity could cause the patient little or no, moderate, or severe physical or psychological harm). NP panels of experts review task analysis results and revise the test content outlines to reflect current practice.

A similar practice analysis of adult, family, and gerontology NPs was conducted for the AANP Certification Program in 2006. NPs were surveyed regarding tasks and knowledge areas. NPs were asked how often during a clinical day they performed the task, and how important each task is to protect patients from harm. NPs were asked how frequently they used each knowledge area in their clinical practice, and how important it is for a new NP to possess this knowledge (Professional Examination Service, 2006).

Certification Within the New Regulatory Model

Certification for entry into NP practice is a prerequisite for most states now, and will continue to be within the new regulatory model. States will recognize certification in the six population foci of the model. Although there are six populations, there will actually be eight exams available, because the adult/gerontology and pediatrics populations will have both an acute care and primary care exam. The adult and gerontology exams will be combined into one exam that will equally test content relevant to both areas of practice. In addition, the psychiatric mental health exam will cover practice across the life span. An additional, critically important element of the new model is that certification will recognize specialty practice, but specialty practice will not be regulated by state boards of nursing. As noted above, certification for specialty practice will be the responsibility of professional associations.

One example of certification as a specialty currently available is the exam to test the specialty of comprehensive care. There has been exponential growth in the number, currently 91, of academic programs offering a Doctor of Nursing Practice (DNP) degree. One model of DNP education focuses on developing the capacity of NPs to provide care across settings and populations. In order to fit into the new regulatory model, a new certifying body, the American Board of Comprehensive Care (ABCC), established by the Council for the Advancement of Comprehensive Care (CACC), located on the Columbia University School of Nursing campus in New York City, agreed that any exam in "comprehensive care" would be a specialty exam, and therefore, would not be the basis for licensure by a state board of nursing. The certifying body contracted with the National Board of Medical Examiners to administer an exam to be available to individuals who have completed the DNP and are licensed in an NP role and population. Test questions have been derived from the test pool of the United States Medical Licensing Examination (USMLE) Step 3 Exam for MD licensure. Graduates of

DNP programs will continue to take an exam in one of the recognized populations in the model, and then take the "comprehensive care" specialty exam to demonstrate specialty competence. The first DNP exam was administered by ABCC in November 2008.

ACCREDITATION

Historic Perspective on Accreditation

Accreditation is a voluntary, self-regulated process conducted by an accrediting body for an academic institution, and serves the public interest by assessing the educational programs against nationally acceptable standards. Accreditation indicates that the program has met the minimal standards established by the accrediting body. Graduating from an accredited school is important, as many employers and graduate programs only accept candidates from an accredited school. Graduation from an accredited NP program is necessary to sit for national certification exams (Overby & Aaltonen, 2001). There are two nationally recognized accrediting agencies: the National League for Nursing Accrediting Commission (NLNAC) and the Commission on Collegiate Nursing Education (CCNE). Both organizations are recognized by the United States Department of Education as accrediting agencies.

In the early 1900s, the National League of Nursing (NLN) created a standard curriculum for schools of nursing and by 1938 initiated accreditation for registered nurse (RN) programs (National League for Nursing Accrediting Commission, 2008). In 1997, the NLNAC was founded, and became responsible for all of the accreditation work that was previously done within the NLN. NLNAC remains a subsidiary of NLN, and is accountable to the Board of Governors of NLN.

In 1995, AACN convened a task force to explore the feasibility of another accrediting agency to further emphasize a continuous quality-improvement approach to evaluating educational programs for nurses. The CCNE, which evolved from this task force, identified four standards for nursing education: (a) mission and governance, (b) institutional commitment and resources, (c) curriculum and teaching–learning practices, (d) student performance and faculty accomplishments (Commission on Collegiate Nursing Education, 1998).

By 1997, NLNAC had incorporated standards for APRN programs. Whereas NLNAC is recognized as an accrediting body for all levels of nursing, including DNP programs, they primarily accredit the associate degree programs. At the same time, CCNE provides accreditation for 4-year college and university-based programs, including baccalaureate, master's, and DNP programs. Both accrediting bodies require schools to have an active self-regulatory, voluntary assessment that is submitted to the accrediting body prior to having a site visit team comprised of peers.

Broad steps have been taken over the past decade to establish standards and competencies for NP education and practice to provide the foundation for accreditation. Competencies have been established for acute care, adult, family, gerontological, pediatric, and women's health, as well as competencies for psychiatric and mental health NPs (National Organization of Nurse Practitioner Faculties [NONPF], 2002, 2003, 2004).

With the development of the DNP, AACN developed the *Essentials for Doctoral Education for Advanced Practice Nurse Practitioners* (National Organization of Nurse Practitioner Faculties, 2002). In 2003, AACN and NONPF sponsored a forum with other APRN organizations to discuss the DNP competencies. As a result, NONPF created entry-level competencies specific to NPs for the DNP, which enhanced the broad competencies developed by AACN (American Association of Colleges of Nursing, 2006; Nurse Practitioner Roundtable, 2008). The CNSs have also identified criteria for education and practice, and created a document for guidance, *Statement on Clinical Nurse Specialist Practice and Education* (National Association of Clinical Nurse Specialists [NANCS], 2004). Since then, NACNS has refined the competencies.

In 2002, the NONPF worked in collaboration with AACN to bring all NP organizations together to develop evaluation criteria for NP education. The evaluation criteria were last updated in 2008. The criteria were developed to assist programs in organizing information that would be needed for accreditation. A concerted effort was made to negotiate with CCNE and NLNAC to incorporate the evaluation criteria into their accreditation process. CCNE incorporated the criteria into their process, and NLNAC recommends the incorporation of the criteria.

Accreditation Within the New Regulatory Model

A major change in the accreditation process occurred in the early 2000s, when CCNE required the participation of APRNs as part of a site visit team. The accreditation process includes a review of NP programs and integrates the NP evaluation criteria into the process. NLNAC's process recommends use of the criteria. The new regulatory model strongly supports integration of the criteria into accreditation.

Licensure

Licensure for NPs has changed as nurse practice acts have evolved (Porcher, 2003). Since 1992, the NCSBN has recommended that all state boards require two levels of licensure for NPs: licensure as an RN and licensure as an APRN. At this time, 14 states have 2 licenses or a separate NP license (Pearson, 2009). Licensure for NPs includes regulation of prescriptive authority. Prescriptive authority for NPs was first granted in the mid 1970s in several states (Buppert, 2008).

Since 1989, *The Pearson Report* has provided state-by-state information on NP licensure and scope of practice regulations, and variations between the states. With each passing year, the number of states that permit NPs to practice independently, without physician involvement, has increased. NPs in all states may prescribe, but many states have some degree of physician involvement in prescriptive practice, ranging from collaboration to direct supervision. NPs in all states diagnose and treat illness, but in more than half of the states, physicians are involved in NP diagnosing and treating.

Boards of nursing in all states govern NPs, but in a handful of states (seven states in 2009), NP regulations are controlled by joint boards of nursing and boards of medicine (Pearson, 2009). NCSBN has been a strong advocate for uniformity in state licensure laws and regulations for APRNs (National Council of State Boards of Nursing, 2002a). For initial licensure/authority to practice in a recognized APRN role and title, NCSBN requires: (a) an unencumbered RN license, (b) graduation from or completion of a graduate-level APRN program accredited by a national accrediting body congruent with the APRN role and title, and (c) certification by the national certifying body in the APRN specialty appropriate to educational preparation.

The NCSBN APRN uniform nurse practice act for multistate advanced-practice privilege does not include prescriptive authority. NCSBN defers to state practice laws any requirements imposed by states to grant APRN prescriptive authority (National Council of State Boards of Nursing, 2006).

Licensure Within the New Regulatory Model

Within the new regulatory model, only the four roles and population foci will be regulated. Boards of nursing will not regulate any APRN specialties. State boards will "license" APRNs, thus mandating a second licensure. Although some states currently have a second license, this is not a uniform practice, and states use different terminology to recognize APRNs. For instance, some states license and others certify. The official titling of APRNs that will appear on licenses will be APRN, followed by the role designation. An example would be: APRN, CNP. An NP can also include the population focus on a name badge, in addition to the APRN and role, such as APRN, CNP, Pediatric. The recommendations that are part of the model include a statement that each state board should have at least one APRN member, as well as an APRN advisory group, to ensure that each of the four roles has input into board decisions. The state boards face a significant challenge in implementing the proposed regulatory model to create a uniform approach to licensing because of the uniqueness of each state and their boards of nursing.

IMPLICATIONS FOR EDUCATION PROGRAMS

When adopted, the new regulatory model will force significant changes in NP education to accommodate standardization across the nation. Over the years, NP educational programs have responded to federal and private funding opportunities and targeted population needs, leading to variation in how curriculum and specialty-focused education was organized. Flexibility within nursing education is vital to responding to changing demands, nevertheless, narrowly focused programs have emerged that have created problems for state boards. The proposed APRN regulatory model supports flexibility at the specialty level and maintaining broad-based education for initial preparation. Education in a specialty will be developed and overseen by professional organizations. The current model of certification for specialty practice will remain, and likely expand. Professional organizations will continue to develop standards for the specialty, as well as implement a method for assessing competency.

A significant consequence of the new regulatory model is the merger of the adult and gerontology populations that requires education for

NPs in both adult and gerontology. Standards related to the integration of the two populations will guide the expectations of programs. A joint initiative supported by The John A. Hartford Foundation with the AACN and organizations that set standards for clinical expertise in these two populations is underway to create competencies for graduates of what will become joint adult and gerontology NP programs. Combining the two populations should increase the number of NPs who are competent to care for older adults. Certification in the specialty care of the most frail and vulnerable older adults by APRNs can be established through professional organizations and certifying bodies. NPs graduating from the integrated program will know how to care for complex older adults with significant functional disability and comorbidities, as well as the older adult with stable chronic illness. The combined program will be longer than either the adult or gerontology programs are, and will require significant clinical experience in geriatric settings.

Finally, the psychiatric/mental health NP will be required to meet the broad-based educational requirements, including pathophysiology, pharmacology, and physical assessment, and then will move into his or her psychiatric mental health content. This approach will facilitate having more psychiatric mental health NPs available to meet the growing need for a comprehensive approach to care.

CONCLUSIONS

Regulation is a complex, multi-pronged process to enhance the probability of having safe providers, regardless of the discipline. The components of the nursing regulatory system include licensure, accreditation, and certification, that are intended to work together to keep patients safe. The new APRN model of regulation is intended to clarify issues that have created confusion in the past, and to ensure effective communication among the entities in the future. Much work remains to implement the model by 2015, the recommended date to have the model in place. An organizational structure will need to be developed to bring all aspects of regulation together to continue to enhance communication and work through issues of concern. The new regulatory model has been created through a long and thoughtful process, and with the endorsement of many nursing organizations, the time has come for the model to move forward.

REFERENCES

American Nurses Association. (1979). *A study of credentialing in nursing: A new approach.* Washington, DC: Author.

American Nurses Association. (2004). *Recognition as a nursing specialty.* Washington, DC: Author.

American Nurses Credentialing Center. (2009). *About ANCC.* Retrieved May 1, 2009, from http://www.nursecredentialing.org/FunctionalCategory/AboutANCC.aspx

APRN Consensus Group and National Council of State Boards of Nursing APRN Advisory Committee (2007). *Consensus model for APRN regulation: Licensure, accreditation, certification and education.* Retrieved August 28, 2009, from http://www.aacn.-nche.edu/Education/pdf/APRNReport.pdf

Bednash, G., Honig, J., & Gibbs, L. (2005). Advanced practice nursing: Emphasizing common roles. In J. M. Stanley (Ed.), *Formulation and approval of credentialing and clinical privileges* (2nd ed.). Philadelphia: F.A. Davis.

Buppert, C. (2008). *Nurse practitioner's business guide and legal guide* (3rd ed.). Sudbury, MA: Jones and Bartlett.

Commission on Collegiate Nursing Education. (1998). *Mission statement and goals.* Retrieved April 30, 2009, from http://www.aacn.nche.edu/accreditation/

Fickeissen, J. L. (1985). Getting certified. *American Journal of Nursing,* 85(3), 265–269.

Joel, L. (2003). *Major studies of the nursing profession. Kelly's dimensions of professional nursing* (9th ed., pp. 71). New York: McGraw-Hill.

National Association of Clinical Nurse Specialists. (2004). *Statement on clinical nurse specialist practice and education.* Atlanta, GA: Author.

National Council of State Boards of Nursing. (2002a). *Uniform advanced practice registered nurse licensure/authority to practice requirements.* Retrieved May 13, 2009, from https://www.ncsbn.org/149.htm and https://www.ncsbn.org/Uniform_Advanced_Practice_Registered_Nurse_ Licensure_Authority_to_Practice_Requirements.pdf

National Council of State Boards of Nursing. (2002b). *Requirements for accrediting agencies and criteria for APRN certification programs.* Retrieved August 26, 2009, from https://www.ncsbn.org/149.htm and https://www.ncsbn.org/Requirements_for_Accrediting_Agencies_and_t he_Criteria_for_Certification_Programs.pdf

National Council of State Boards of Nursing. (2006). *Model nursing act and rules.* Retrieved May 4, 2009, from https://www.ncsbn.org/312.htm

National League for Nursing Accrediting Commission. (2008). *Standards and criteria.* Retrieved April 30, 2009, from http://www.nlnac.org/manuals/SC2008.htm

National Organization of Nurse Practitioner Faculties. (2002). *Primary care competencies in specialty areas: Adult, family, gerontological, pediatric, women's health.* Retrieved May 1, 2009, from http://www.nonpf.org/finalaug2002.pdf

National Organization of Nurse Practitioner Faculties. (2003). *Psychiatric-mental health nurse practitioner competencies.* Retrieved May 1, 2009, from http://www.nonpf.org/finalcomps03.pdf

National Organization of Nurse Practitioner Faculties. (2004). *Acute care nurse practitioner competencies.* Retrieved May 1, 2009, from http://www.nonpf.org/ACNPcompsfinal20041.pdf

National Organization of Nurse Practitioner Faculties. (2006). *Practice doctorate nurse practitioner entry-level competencies.* Retrieved May 1, 2009, from http://nonpf.com/ NONPF2005/PracticeDoctorateResourceCenter/CompetencyDraftFInalApril2006. pdf

Nurse Practitioner Roundtable. (2008, June). *Nurse practitioner DNP education, certification and titling: A unified statement.* Retrieved August 26, 2009, from http://www. aanp.org/NR/rdonlyres/D751E805-2F41-4189-8263-FB19EE68A1AD/2657/DNP.pdf

Overby, J., & Aaltonen, P. (2001). A comparison of NLNAC and CCNE accreditation. *Nurse Educator, 26*(1), 17–22.

Pearson, L. (2009). *The Pearson report.* Retrieved May 4, 2009, from http://www.webnp. net/downloads/pearson_report09/ajnp_pearson09.pdf

Porcher, F. K. (2003). Licensure, certification, and credentialing. In M. D. Mezey, D. O. McGivern, & E. M. Sullivan-Marx (Eds.), *Nurse practitioners: Evolution of advanced practice* (4th ed., pp. 415–430). New York: Springer Publishing Company.

Professional Examination Service. (2006). *Report of the practice analysis of adult, family, and gerontology nurse practitioners prepared for the American Academy of Nurse Practitioners Certification Program.* New York: Author.

Styles, M. (2008). Advanced practice nursing: Framework for discussion of issues, goals, and options. In M. Styles, M. J. Schumann, C. Bickford, & K. M. White (Eds.), *Specializing and credentialing in nursing revisited: Understanding the issues, advancing the profession.* Silver Spring, MD: American Nurses Association.

10 Politics of Organized Opposition: A Case Example

THOMAS A. MACKEY AND LYNDA FREED WOOLBERT

REGULATION OF NURSE PRACTITIONERS IN TEXAS

The Texas Board of Nursing (BON) has sole authority to regulate nurse practitioners (NPs) and other advanced-practice nurses (APNs) in Texas. However, that authority has met with challenges. The BON first adopted rules on APN education in 1978, and rules on APN eligibility and practice in 1980. The Texas Hospital and Texas Medical Associations filed law suits in 1981 challenging the BON's authority to adopt such rules. Despite the defeat of legislation granting the BON specific authority to regulate APN practice in 1979 and 1981, the courts found in favor of the BON in 1986. Although many challenges to APN practice in Texas have long since been resolved, others remain.

The BON regulates Texas NPs under its general authority to regulate the practice of professional nurses, as well as the specific authority granted in §301.152, Texas Occupations Code, titled, *Rules Regarding Specialized Training* (Texas Occupations Code, 1999). The cryptic title symbolizes the legislative challenges NPs face in Texas. Due to opposition by medical organizations to recognizing APNs in legislation, the words "advanced-practice nurse" or "nurse practitioner" never appeared in the Texas Nursing Practice Act until 1995, even though some NPs gained prescriptive authority 6 years earlier.

PRESCRIPTIVE AUTHORITY

Legislation to grant APNs prescriptive authority was first filed in 1989, when an economic incentive prompted Texas legislators to act. Federal legislation creating rural health clinics (RHCs) required them to employ an NP, nurse midwife, or physician assistant (PA) who had authority to prescribe medications. To take advantage of funds available for RHCs, stakeholders negotiated language allowing physicians to delegate prescriptive authority to APNs and PAs in medically underserved sites. The language was included in the Texas 1989 Omnibus Rescue Health Bill, 71st Regular Texas Legislative Session, House Bill 18 (Acts of the 71st Regular Texas Legislative Session, 1989).

Thus began the legislative trail to one of the most complex laws on prescriptive authority in the United States. Although NPs in Texas enjoy autonomy in many aspects of practice, such as ordering and interpreting diagnostic tests, the opposite is the case in prescribing. Prescriptive authority must be delegated by a physician and is site-specific. Each site has peculiar requirements including the amount of time a delegating physician must be on-site with the NP, ranging from no face-to-face time in some primary practice sites, to 20% of the time the NP practices in alternate practice sites.

Changes in prescriptive authority occurred in 1995, 1997, 2001, and 2003. The change in 2003 gave physicians the authority to delegate prescriptive authority for controlled substances, Schedules III–V, to NPs, other APNs, and PAs. Changes in other years simply added additional sites at which physicians could delegate prescriptive authority, or allowed the medical board to waive some requirements, such as the amount of time the physician had to be on-site or the percentage of charts the physician must review. Although changes enabled additional NPs to have prescriptive authority, it also made the law progressively more difficult to interpret and regulate.

Consequently, for the first time in 14 years, APNs in Texas mounted a strong legislative effort in 2009 to end delegated, site-based prescriptive authority. Efforts centered on the National Council of State Boards of Nursing model APRN language to allow APNs to diagnose and prescribe as part of the APN's scope of practice granted by the Texas Nursing Practice Act (Texas Nursing Practice Act, 2009). Unfortunately, this legislation was unsuccessful. The bill the Texas Legislature passed was based on negotiations between some convenient care clinics and the medical associations. The bill ultimately included some amendments that APNs wanted, but failed to end site-based prescriptive authority.

DEVELOPMENT OF PROFESSIONAL ORGANIZATIONS

The first statewide organization for NPs emerged at the same time NPs were gaining prescriptive authority. Texas Nurse Practitioners (TNP) held its first annual meeting in July 1989. Organizational development of TNP was an integral step in uniting NPs and advancing the profession in Texas. As a founding member of the Coalition for Nurses in Advanced Practice (CNAP; n.d.), TNP also built political power for NPs.

Leaders of the statewide organizations representing NPs, nurse anesthetists, and nurse midwives realized success at the Texas Capitol required pooling resources to hire representation for APNs. NP leaders quickly learned legislation beneficial to NPs could potentially harm other groups of APNs, such as nurse midwives and nurse anesthetists. The CNAP became the legislative and regulatory arm of its member organizations.

Today, CNAP has eight member organizations representing the four APN roles, plus additional organizations representing specialties that have unique interests, such as neonatal, gerontological, and pediatric NPs. Representatives from member organizations set the legislative agenda for APNs in Texas. The primary agenda is set at a retreat that includes the leadership of CNAP member organizations representing a cross-section of practices. Consequently, the agenda includes concerns important to the practice of specialty groups in various practice settings. CNAP has an excellent working relationship with Texas Nurses Association (TNA), and both organizations support mutual legislative efforts (CNAP, n.d.) Although CNAP leads the legislative efforts on behalf of APNs, TNA spearheads other issues related to nursing in Texas. Negotiations with medical organizations always include APNs representing TNA, CNAP, and the four statewide CNAP member organizations of NPs: clinical nurse specialists (CNSs), certified registered nurse anesthetists (CRNAs), and certified nurse midwives (CNMs).

MEDICAID AND OTHER REGULATORY EFFORTS

Full-time political representation by CNAP means APNs are profession-ally represented in legislative matters. Equally important is the represen-tation before state agencies that operate such programs as Medicaid. Through consistently submitting comments on new regulations pub-lished weekly in the *Texas Register*, APNs are included in many state agency rules.

Prior to 1992, only family NPs (FNPs), pediatric NPs (PNPs), nurse anesthetists and nurse midwives were reimbursed under the Texas Medicaid Program. CNAP's first action in 1992 was a successful lobbying effort at the Department of Human Services to expand and increase Medicaid reimbursement for all APNs. The reimbursement rate was raised to 85% in 1992 and 92% in 2004. The Texas Medicaid Program also allows NPs to be primary care providers in Medicaid-managed care plans, although not all the plans take advantage of that option.

APNs now face new challenges. In 2008, CNAP petitioned the Texas Health and Human Services Commission to update many outdated Medicaid rules to allow APNs to order durable medical equipment, physical therapy, and other services for Medicaid clients. Unfortunately, the Texas Medical Association (TMA) continues its historic position, and opposes such changes, stating APNs do not have authority to order such services. TMA's current position conflicts with the BON, so the conflict could escalate.

EDUCATION AND PRACTICE ISSUES

Like most states, Texas faces extraordinary challenges related to the supply and education of nurses. The demand for full-time registered nurses in Texas in 2009 exceeds supply by 22,000 (Texas Team, 2008). To date, there are no estimates for the number of NPs needed to fill the gap for acute and primary care provider/service shortages. However, schools of nursing are increasing the number of Doctorate of Nursing Practice (DNP) programs geared toward producing qualified clinicians and teachers. The University of Texas, School of Nursing at Houston, started the first DNP program in 2006, with three stipulations by the Texas Higher Education Coordinating Board (THECB): (a) all students must be post-master's, (b) the program must be part time, and (c) the majority of the curriculum could not be on-line. The THECB was concerned that master's-prepared NPs would be eliminated if all NPs were educated at the doctoral level, and a full-time program would necessarily eliminate many nurses needing to work full time. Despite such restrictions, demand for DNP education continues to increase. Since 2006, three other DNP programs began, and others are planned. The THECB is relatively silent regarding a decision to comply with the American Association of Colleges of Nursing's recommendation to have all APNs educated at the DNP level by 2015.

TMA, initially opposed the DNP, testified before the THECB against starting the first DNP program in Texas, and was the architect of the 2005 House of Delegate resolution to study the scope of practice of limited-license practitioners, such as NPs. TMA followed with an American Medical Association (AMA) resolution in 2006 to deny practitioners other than a doctor of medicine, osteopathy, or dentistry the right to use the title *doctor*. A physician, also a state representative, filed a similar bill in the Texas House in 2007 that was defeated. TMA has been relatively silent on the subject since.

CHALLENGES CONTINUE

In 2007, Texas enacted legislation joining the APRN Compact. In preparation for implementing the compact on November 14, 2008, the BON adopted a rule amendment changing APN authorization to APRN licensure. In comments on the BON's rule amendment, TMA stated that calling the advanced-practice approval process "licensure" exceeds its [the BON's] statutory authority. The BON rejected TMA's assertion, but such challenges are likely to increase before they come to an inevitable end.

WHERE DO WE GO FROM HERE?

Despite past and present challenges, setbacks, and roadblocks, NPs are providing outstanding care to thousands of Texans on a daily basis. The future for NPs in the State of Texas is bright. CNAP is a strong organization addressing the issues most important to NPs, and speaking with one voice for a large number of organizations and individuals.

Others (educational institutions, professional organizations, state agencies) are equally devoted to evolving the regulation, prescriptive authority, education, and practice issues of tomorrow. Although the current practice climate in the State of Texas is not ideal for NPs, we are clearly optimistic about the future.

REFERENCES

Acts of the 71st Regular Texas Legislative Session. (1989). Retrieved January 28, 2010, from http://www.legis.state.tx.us/tlodocs/74R/analysis/html/HB01520H.htm
Coalition for Nurses in Advanced Practice. (n.d.). Retrieved August 5, 2009, from http://www.cnaptexas.org/
Rules Regarding Specialized Training, Texas Occupations Code §301.152 (1999).
Texas Nursing Practice Act. (2009). Retrieved August 9, 2009, from http://bon.state.tx.us/nursinglaw/npa.html
Texas Team. (2008). *Texas nursing: Our future depends on it.* Retrieved August 9, 2009, from http://www.dshs.state.tx.us/chs/cnws/TexasTeam/TexTeamFact.pdf

11

The Idiosyncratic Politics of Prescriptive Authority: Comparing Two States' Legislative Negotiations

DEBORAH A. SAMPSON

In 1965, health care in the United States was in crisis. Access to primary care, particularly for people of color and the poor in urban and rural areas, was unavailable because of a lack of primary care physicians who were willing to work in certain geographic areas. Fewer and fewer medical students were willing to pursue careers in primary care medicine. Large numbers of United States citizens were uninsured and unable to afford more and more costly health care services. Hospital care was becoming more and more expensive as hospitals expanded in response to population growth, technological and scientific advances, and expanding demand from consumers and specialist physicians alike.

During this time of profound change in U.S. society, President Lyndon B. Johnson's administration and Congress responded with the Great Society initiatives, which included innovation to relieve the pressing crisis in American health care aimed at ensuring that all citizens were able to afford and had local community access to health services. The most well known of the initiatives of this time were Medicare and Medicaid, insurance programs aimed at society's most vulnerable people, such as the elderly and the poor. Less well known was an initiative, developed and supported not only by government, but by nursing, medical, health policy, and community leaders, to provide substantial federal funds and training programs aimed at educating nurses to fill the primary care physician void in geographically, economically, and racially underserved communities throughout the United States. The concept was based on the idea, documented in prior community health demonstration projects, that nurses with a bit more education could safely provide at least 80% of primary care services without physician oversight. The agenda for change was put in motion, beginning an initiative that would result in millions of dollars earmarked for nurse practitioner (NP) education grants in programs across the country over the next several decades. The concept was met with enthusiasm by nurses, individuals, and communities alike. However, when applied at the state level, the idea that nurses should prescribe met with varying degrees of success in the actual implementation. Because state laws regulate health professions practices, the laws in all states needed to change to allow these nurses (now called NPs) to practice without direct physician supervision, a necessary process if these NPs were to realize the mandate of the national agenda and people's health needs (Fairman, 2008; Sampson, 2008).

Prescribing rights became the crucible within which NPs in many states would clash, primarily with organized medicine, but also, in some cases, with pharmacists. As Keeling (2007) describes, the right to have nurses prescribe through legislative initiative is to legally sanction what has already been occurring for a very long time. In truth, of course, nurses have always "prescribed" and managed medications, regardless of geographic location or site of patient care, whether in the home, clinic, or hospital, and have done so using their own knowledge and judgment. But nurses' legislative prescribing initiatives often stimulate physician and pharmacist opposition activity that is more imbued with professional authority, control, and economic concerns than a focus on patient need. "Patient safety" rhetoric, rather than concrete data, often serves as a rationale for opposing NP prescribing rights by both pharmacists and organized medicine. How and when this opposition occurs (whether in the actual legislative process or in subsequent rule-making), the voracious initiatives of opposition and the process and duration of time until prescriptive authority rights are won by NPs varies so much by state that each United States state and territory has an idiosyncratically crafted NP prescribing law.

The politics of prescription and the shape of NP legislation are formed not only by the commitment of those individuals and groups determined to see their legislative agenda win, but also by the culture, legislative structure, and mechanisms of political influence in each state. Place matters, and the culture, geography, and history of each state is unique and affects the shape of NP legislative initiatives. Comparative analyses of legislative processes in different states, in this case, New Hampshire and Texas, helps identify some characteristics peculiar to the place and also reveals similarities. Geographically, demographically, and culturally very different, these states also have dissimilar practice acts, histories, and health disparity problems, providing an opportunity to reveal nuances of the legislative process.

NEW HAMPSHIRE

An early adopter of the NP idea, the state of New Hampshire passed an addition to the Nurse Practice Act in 1973, specifically designating a new category of nursing, advanced registered nurse practitioners (ARNPs), who could "perform any task for which they had been educated and could demonstrate competency" (*New Hampshire Board of Nursing Education and Registration Newsletter*, 1973, p. 2). No part of the nursing or medical practice act required physician collaboration or supervision of NPs. Additionally, a large citizen legislature and small geographic area meant that much of the state population knows and has easy access to state senators and representatives. Legislative campaigns often cost no more than a few thousand dollars, so political action contributions are often quite small, and lobbying influences are often more personal than financial. New Hampshire NPs negotiated in a state in which personal freedom is part of the state culture. Undoubtedly, these state characteristics affected the outcome of NP legislation (Sampson, 2008). This law was supported by two state bureaucrats, Board of Nursing Executive Director and nurse Marguerite Hastings and physician Maynard Myers, Executive Director of the New Hampshire Public Health Department. Both believed in nurses' ability to ameliorate many unmet primary care needs and supported NP practice. Moreover, both recognized that NPs had requisite knowledge to prescribe, and perhaps knew that NPs were already finding ways to meet patients' medication needs. As nurses have often done, the NPs made medication decisions independently by calling prescriptions into a pharmacy using a physician's name, using prescriptions presigned by a physician, or signing a physician's name to the prescription. The physician, who often had a long professional relationship with the NP, agreed to this arrangement, trusting the NP to make sound judgments. Therefore, the trust and mutuality of the individual physician/nurse relationship was the foundation for this prescribing process.

Because of increasing pressure from federal and law enforcement agencies, in 1977, the Board of Pharmacy investigators began meticulous scrutiny of retail pharmacy adherence to federal Drug Enforcement Agency law, and effectively put an end to this prescribing practice. Suddenly, the NPs found themselves unable to prescribe using any mechanism, and as Myers and Hastings worked behind the scenes, the NPs were thrust into the legislative theater to negotiate a prescribing addendum to the Nurse Practice Act. With the support of other state nursing organizations, the newly formed New Hampshire Nurse Practitioner Organization embarked on a journey to win legal prescribing rights for NPs.

The NPs lost the first legislative initiative. Myers, who was also a powerful ex-officio member of the Board of Medicine, and Hastings would only be in their positions for a few more years, and were unavailable for subsequent legislative sessions. In spite of mounting hostility from the Board of Medicine after Myers left, vehement ongoing opposition from the Board of Pharmacy, surprise last-minute prescribing bill amendments that included physician supervision requirements, and shifting political sentiments toward social initiatives, the NPs finally achieved victory in their third legislative attempt in 1984.

The lessons learned from failures enabled NPs to strategize successfully with the support of a powerful and nurse friendly state senator, Susan McLane. The final prescribing law required NPs to collaborate with (but not be supervised by) physicians, an activity that had always been part of their practice anyway.

TEXAS

In the previous chapter, Tom Mackey and Lynda Woolbert describe the chronology of Texas NPs' regulation and oppositions to advanced practice. NPs in Texas, as elsewhere, have worked long and hard to win the right to prescribe under Board of Nursing regulation without physician oversight. In Texas, NP prescribing, however, can only be delegated by physicians, and even this physician delegation right in Texas has endured several legislative revisions, resulting in rather draconian and complex rules. They are certainly difficult for either nurses or physicians to interpret or implement in a way that meets patient needs. Moreover, in Texas, the law not only confers exclusive "ownership" of medication prescribing to physicians, but also states that only physicians may diagnose disease. Physicians, then, are assumed to be the only legitimate authorities of referent critical knowledge to identify disease and determine medication treatment under the law. Of course, the actual practice of patient care in Texas and elsewhere demonstrates quite the opposite.

Although specialist advanced-practice nurses had long worked independently in Texas, the majority were nurse anesthetists or nurse midwives, who often were also Catholic nuns working in poor rural communities' clinics. For the most part, these two advanced-practice groups have always worked without direct supervision of physicians who specialize in anesthesia or obstetrics, but complied with the law by working with other physicians or surgeons (who arguably had less knowledge of anesthesia or pregnancy and birth than the nurses) to "supervise" nurses' practice under the law.

NPs did not appear to be present in significant numbers until the 1980s, even though the geospatially huge state of Texas had, and still has, one of the highest proportions of underserved populations, more primary care provider vacancies in poor areas than any other state, and some of the worst health disparities in the nation (Texas State Department of Health, 2005; U.S. Department of Health and Human Services, 2008). By the early 1990s, however, NPs were becoming more numerous and prominent in Texas, perhaps because of the increase in academic programs in the state and private Texas colleges. Even in the early 1990s, both Governor Ann Richards, an active and vocal supporter of nurses, including NPs, and later, then-Governor George W. Bush, supported NP practice and legislation so much so that there is currently an NP positioned in the Texas State House who provides care to elected officials and their staffs.

Prior to 1992, the Texas Nurses Association was involved in NP legislative negotiations, even filing a partially successful bill for direct insurance payment to NPs. The Texas Medical Association (TMA) blocked the inclusion of Medicaid, the state-funded insurance for the poor, effectively preventing nurses from being paid for services to the very group that the national initiative intended they would serve. This glitch, and the Texas Nurses Association's need to attend to a myriad of other nursing concerns, were the stimuli for NPs, psychiatric clinical specialists, nurse midwives, and nurse anesthetists to form the Texas Coalition for Nurses in Advanced Practice (CNAP). This group focused solely on passing independent prescribing and practice legislation in direct opposition to the agenda of the self-proclaimed TMA "legislative juggernaut" (Hinchey, 2007).

The CNAP raised money, mostly from the state nurse anesthetists' organization and individuals, hired a lobbyist, an absolute necessity in Texas politics, organized nursing organizations members, and filed legislation in each of the seven legislative sessions from 1993 to 2009, trying to win advanced-practice nurses both practice and prescribing rights without physician oversight requirements. Small incremental successes occurred with each attempt, as legislative health committee members, the Board of Nursing, lobbyists for CNAP, and the Texas Nurses Association, Hospital Association, and Association of Community Health Centers negotiated, sometimes together, against the Medical Association for NPs to have medication management latitude that would ensure care for underserved Texas residents. Conspicuously absent from the fray and silent about the issues, unlike in New Hampshire, are the Texas Boards of Medicine and Board of Pharmacy.

Today, Texas NPs have the right to prescribe, but only under a complex system of laws contained both in the Medical and Nursing Practice Acts that include varying amounts of onsite physician supervision, even at the most remote geographic clinics, and requirements that individual NPs maintain written protocols and practice supervision plans kept on file with the Board of Medicine. Further, The Texas Medical Practice Act states that diagnosing of disease is a medical act, and nonphysicans can "diagnose" only when delegated to do so by a physician (Texas Board of Medical Examiners, 2008). NPs won a significant victory in 2003 when, along with physician assistants, they were granted legal authority to prescribe some of the less addictive narcotics in hospitals under written physician-delegation protocols. This ensured that nurse midwives and nurse anesthetists were able to care adequately for hospitalized patients, but provided little relief for the care of patients in primary care and outpatient settings. There was a heavy price to pay for this victory, however. The TMA agreed to concede and not fight this provision if nurse organizations declared a moratorium on initiatives for expansion of any nursing practice until 2009. The nurses, painfully and reluctantly, agreed to the moratorium, reasoning that they now had 6 years to strategize and gather money to try for independence again in 2009 (Acosta, 2009; CNAP, 1992, 1993, 2000, 2003, 2008; Texas Administrative Code, 2003; Texas Board of Nursing, 2003; Texas Board of Medical Examiners, 2008).

Texas political machinations are odd, as any fan of the late Texas journalist, Molly Ivins, can attest ("Syndicated Columnist," 2007). In Texas, the legislature meets for only 140 days every 2 years, actually voting only during the last 60 days or so, although special sessions are often added. Year round, special-interest lobbyists spend considerable time and enormous sums of money meeting with legislators to influence votes on bills. It is not unusual for a lobbyist to pay upwards of $1000 to attend a legislator's birthday party. The TMA Political Action Committee (TEX-PAC) is the second highest contributor to legislative campaigns, with an annual contribution war chest of over one and a half million dollars, five times more than the whole annual operating budget for the CNAP. The wealthy TMA, which includes almost 100% of the 50,000 Texas licensed physicians and medical students, has relentlessly lobbied to prevent any law sanctioning NP practice without some legal mechanism requiring direct physician involvement. The TMA simply outspends everyone else in a system in which expensive lobbying efforts hold sway over state legislators, and the population's health needs are an afterthought. Moreover, the TMA has waged an all-out campaign to discredit NPs and ensure that no individual physicians support NP-friendly legislation. The TMA has openly notified individual physicians who support NP legislation that their support is unacceptable. They were responsible for the wide circulation of an image of a duck in a nurse's cap and stethoscope, intended to suggest that NPs were "quacks" (CNAP, 1992, 1993). It is no small miracle that the Texas nurses have achieved as much as they have.

CONCLUSIONS

First, although nurses often have conflicts among each other, in this case, in each state sometimes seemingly disparate nursing groups worked together to help a special interest nursing group achieve success. Although the level of success varied in each place, undoubtedly coopera- tion among different groups of nurses in the public arena was important. Nurses cooperated in both states, in spite of the personal and career demands and, in the case of Texas, the need to communicate and negotiate across a vast geographic area.

Second, organized medicine and individual physicians often do not have the same perspective concerning NP abilities. When individual NPs and physicians work together, physicians trust and value the NP's diagnostic and prescribing skill (Fairman, 2008), and individual physi- cians in positions of power may be committed to support, such as Maynard Myers was in New Hampshire.

Third, although organized medicine may have significant resources to oppose nursing legislation, cohesive, committed, and determined nurses can succeed, in spite of having comparatively miniscule finances. Money is only one factor, and often not the deciding factor, at that, in winning legislative battles. In politics, having significant funding for a battle may help, but a strong cohesive state-wide nursing community and grassroots legislative constituency and patient support is more important. Strong support from legislators and other stakeholders for NPs' legislative initiatives is often important to counterbalance orga- nized medicine's vocal and sometimes very well-funded opposition. Success will cost money, time, and energy, but it can be achieved, although often incrementally over time, rather than occurring in one legislative session.

Fourth, it is important to have an insider in the legislative commit- tees who can help prevent last-minute bill changes, or, at the very least, keep the changes from being a surprise. Nurses in Texas had an insider lobbyist, and were never surprised about a bill's final language. Nurses in New Hampshire did not have a "mole" inside the legislative machine, and were forced to strategize at the last minute when bills unexpectedly contained unacceptable language.

Finally, and perhaps most obviously, place matters. National health policy is conceptualized to alleviate national problems, but implement- ing the national agenda on a local level is another thing indeed. This study of the trials and tribulations of the legislative process reveal differences in state-specific factors, such as the structure of state govern- ment, stakeholder interests, and the timing of any initiative. State-level negotiations occurred within the context of unique geography, space, and time, and reveal much about the complexities of interprofessional space, boundaries, and tasks. The roles and authority of nursing and medicine varies in the legal definitions from state to state. How the controversy about who should prescribe and who controls medicine and nursing plays out in different states with different cultures, geographies, and populations says much about how patient needs get lost in the battle over the "contested terrain" of professional authority and boundaries.

Unchanged from the 1960s, adequate numbers of primary care providers are persistently unavailable in many rural and urban areas, yet many states continue to prohibit legislation that would permit NPs to alleviate the primary care provider shortage. This shortage disproportionately affects preventable morbidity and mortality in racial and ethnic minorities. Currently, 36 states' laws prohibit NPs from fully practicing to their fullest extent (Phillips, 2008). Many states still have significant populations in urban and rural areas without access to affordable community-based care.

In spite of rhetoric, the health needs of a state population, particularly those without financial or political power, are not necessarily the overarching focus in the legislative arena. Professional turf wars consume enormous resources and are often fueled, or at least supported, by the idiosyncrasies of state politics. Although cause and effect cannot be assumed, the cost of these wars may actually be neglected health care for the most vulnerable and needy people in the state, the very thing the national NP initiative was crafted to alleviate.

REFERENCES

Acosta, M. (2009). *TexPac scores more victories.* Retrieved January 27, 2009, from http://www.texpac.org

Coalition for Nurses in Advanced Practice (CNAP). (1992). *Meeting minutes and attachments.* (Available at the CNAP headquarters, West Columbia, TX).

Coalition for Nurses in Advanced Practice (CNAP). (1993). *Meeting minutes and attachments.* (Available at the CNAP headquarters, West Columbia, TX).

Coalition for Nurses in Advanced Practice (CNAP). (2000). *Meeting minutes and attachments.* (Available at the CNAP headquarters, West Columbia, TX).

Coalition for Nurses in Advanced Practices (CNAP). (2003). *Meeting minutes and attachments.* (Available at the CNAP headquarters, West Columbia, TX).

Coalition for Nurses in Advanced Practice (CNAP). (2008). *Meeting minutes and attachments.* (Available at the CNAP headquarters, West Columbia, TX).

Fairman, J. (2008). *Making room in the clinic: Nurse practitioners and the evolution of health care.* New Brunswick, NJ: Rutgers University Press.

Hinchey, W. W. (2007, October). A legislative juggernaut: TMA refines its advocacy process. *Texas Medicine, 103*(10), 2–3.

Keeling, A. W. (2007). *Nursing and the privilege of prescription, 1893–2000.* Columbus, OH: The Ohio State University Press.

New Hampshire Board of Nursing Education and Registration Newsletter. (1973, September). Archival records, Newsletter April 1966–December 1979. *New Hampshire Board of Nursing Education and Registration Newsletter. 8*(1).

Phillips, S. J. (2008).Legislative update: After 20 years, APNs are still standing together. *Nurse Practitioner, 33*(1), 10–13.

Sampson, D. A. (2008). Alliances of cooperation: Negotiating New Hampshire nurse practitioners practice boundaries. *Nursing History Review, 17,* 153–178.

Syndicated columnist Molly Ivins dies at 62. (2007, January 21). *MSNBC online.* Retrieved July 21, 2008, from http://www.msnbc.msn.com/id/16910834

Texas Administrative Code, Advanced Practice Nurses with Prescriptive Authority Rules, Title 22, part 11 § 222.1-12 (2003). [electronic version]. Retrieved January 30, 2009. from http://info.sos.state.tx.us/pls/pub/readtac$ext.TacPage?sl=T&app= 9& p_dir=P&p_rloc=105994&p_tloc=&p_ploc=1&pg=6&p_tac=&ti=22&pt=11& ch= 222&rl=6

Texas Board of Medical Examiners, Rules, Regulations and Guidelines. (2008). *Standing delegation orders Chapter 193.1-193.12193.6, Delegation of the carrying out or signing of prescription drug orders to physician assistants and advanced practice nurses* [electronic version]. Retrieved July 4, 2009, from http://www.tmb.state.tx.us/rules/ rules/193.php#f

Texas Board of Nursing. (2003). *Nursing Practice Act 2003.* Retrieved September 30, 2008, from http://www.bon.state.tx.us/nursinglaw/npa.html

Texas Department of State Health Services. (2005). *Healthy people 2000: Health status indicators by Texas public health regions and race/ethnicity, 1990-2000.* Retrieved July 4, 2009, from http://www.dshs.state.tx.us/chs/pubs/healthy/hpin2000.pdf

U. S. Department of Health and Human Services. (2008). *Medically underserved areas/ populations.* Retrieved July 4, 2009, from http://bhpr.hrsa.gov/shortage/

Integration of Nurse Practitioners in the Health Care Environment

The authentic and expert voices of practice included in this section are instructive in terms of primary and specialty care, and the political, legislative, and fiscal implications of various types of service delivery. McGivern sketches the current environmental factors shaping nurse practitioner (NP) practice; the context is being determined by the degree of provider activism, understanding of the opportunities and obstacles in the current delivery structure, and the ability to communicate aspects of the innovative models demonstrated in some systems and for specific populations.

King and Hansen-Turton, experts in the area of nurse-managed centers, provide the fullest explication of the history, funding, advantages, requirements, and obstacles to the use and expansion of this source of primary care. The expansion of nurse-managed clinics and federally qualified health centers has been included in the 2009 stimulus/reform discussion. Understanding the future development that is associated with community-based care centers will be facilitated by the grounding this chapter provides.

The descriptions of specialty practice with diabetic children, families with elderly members, the evolution of HIV practice, and the range of system innovations provide a glimpse of the universe of possibilities and contributions of NPs. Lipman demonstrates one of the important elements of the practitioner description: participation in and use of research, in this case, studies of best management of physiologically, socially, and developmentally complicated pediatric conditions. Kirton's exemplar on HIV/AIDS reflects another important commonality, NPs taking the lead in orchestrating models of care, while at the same time working successfully with health care teams to address complex needs of populations that have changed significantly over time in terms of demographics, treatment, and chronicity.

The extraordinary change in our population profile and subsequent need to prepare NPs to serve broader segments of the adult population is brought to life by Taylor and Bradway. Their clinical case study documents the need for the educational and credentialing changes that combine adult and gerontologic preparation, in order to meet the needs of intergenerational families and expanding numbers of the elderly that are now consistent with recommendations of advanced-practice nurse (APN) certification and regulation in Johnson's chapter earlier in this book.

The Veterans Administration is the rare U.S. national example of a large enterprise able to reconfigure itself, support innovation, and promote the contribution of nurses and NPs in a kaleidoscope of geography, patient demographics, and complex needs of recent veterans. Robinson's chapter provides a glimpse into the array of innovations led and supported by NPs in quite diverse settings.

Ulrich and Zeitzer's discussion of the ethical issues surrounding advanced practice resonate with the experiences portrayed in these exemplars and the experiences of many APNs. Increasing autonomy, more complex care issues, reimbursement policies, and practicing with a multidisciplinary team of providers create an increasing number of ethical challenges for which NPs, among others, feel unprepared. The authors make an extremely convincing case for expanded education in ethics and ethical decision making as part of graduate preparation for practice.

12

Environmental Factors Shaping Advanced Practice

DIANE O. McGIVERN

INTRODUCTION

The 4-decade evolutionary tale of advanced-practice nursing has been characterized by growth in practitioner numbers, expanded legislative and regulatory recognition, and changing reimbursement policies. There is, however, one continuous theme, the ongoing interdisciplinary tension focused on which profession will determine nurse practitioners' (NPs) level of autonomy, oversight of practice, appropriate compensation, and access to reimbursement.

Many factors shaping current and future practice include the active health care reform dialogue, obstacles to reimbursement, unequal supply and demand for providers, efforts to achieve standardization of licensing, accreditation, certification, and education for advanced practice, and the profession's relative position in an integrated delivery system.

The drive behind advanced-practice role development and expansion is frequently presented in the simplest terms. Most contemporary literature notes that the NP role arose solely to compensate for the lack of physician services, giving credence to the view of NPs as substitutes or extenders, as opposed to providers of both necessary and unique services. This linear connection between physician supply and development of advanced practice from nursing is inconsistent with Loretta Ford's vision, and diminishes the powerful nursing dialogue that guided NP role development and the strong holistic perspective that distinguishes NPs' contribution from medicine (Fairman, 2008).

The development of the NP role has been rich in research, debate, and innovation. The current and potential contributions of NPs have been documented by important and independent observers (Safriet, 1992; U.S. Department of Health and Human Services, Health Resources and Services Administration [USDHHS, HRSA], 2004; U.S. Office of Technology Assessment, 1986). At the same time, however, this recognition is countered by the continued struggle for provider recognition by third-party payers, and a sustained sense of competition and attempts at outside control expressed as concern for quality and patient safety.

Whereas the environmental factors discussed here have roots in earlier decades, these issues of reform, reimbursement, provider availability, standardization of preparation, and practice and delivery integration may now result in better outcomes for consumers and NPs. In contrast to several decades ago, the advantages of greater numbers of advanced-practice nurses (APNs), more politically savvy practitioners and organizational leaders, instant access to information and networks—all suggest that the opportunities at hand can be exploited positively in ways only partially realized since the 1960s.

The environmental factors discussed here, including health care reform, regulatory reform and reimbursement changes, provider availability, drive to standardization, and the integration of providers in new models are in such a fluid state that the ultimate outcomes of any of these developments are difficult to predict with any certainty.

HEALTH CARE REFORM

The current debate about the shape of health care reform highlights the concern regarding the unsustainable current and projected costs of care, desire for improved outcomes, proven efficiency and efficaciousness of interventions, effective professional collaboration, and accessible, affordable insurance coverage. Although the policy debate tries to balance cost, access, and quality, most observers agree that unless cost is controlled and spending slowed, the other two goals of reform will be sabotaged.

Health care costs and the weakened national and global economies are driving reform efforts. Health care spending is projected to reach 19.5% of the gross domestic product (GDP) by 2017, with growth in Medicare spending as the baby boomer generation qualifies. This is expected to be accompanied by limited expansion of private health and out-of-pocket spending through 2017, but accelerated spending on prescription drugs, due to the continued introduction of new drugs and an emphasis on early pharmacologic interventions in the face of problems associated with aging and chronicity (Center for Medicare and Medicaid Services, Office of the Actuary, 2008).

NPs' competencies are clearly compatible with all aspects of health care reform. Their skills in primary care and coordination, chronic care management, contributions to acute care, and accessibility and affordability have long been established (Mundinger et al., 2000). Although the goals of health care reform dovetail with the contributions of NPs, the defined future role that all providers will play, specifically NPs, is being temporarily subordinated by the larger cost and coverage debate. Although nursing has been visible in the public commentary about reform (White House, July 15, 2009), the outlines of system change, the relative weight of input from hospital associations, insurance corporations, medicine, big and small businesses, and state governments have yet to play out clearly or with any degree of commitment (Abelson, 2009a, 2009b; Kirkpatrick, 2009; Krugman, 2009; Pear, 2009a). Indeed, in anticipation of legislative proposals, special interest groups are waging extremely costly television and radio campaigns reminiscent of the attacks on the Clinton plan in the early 1990s (McInturff & Weigel, 2008; Pear, 2009b).

While federal legislators crafted health care reform proposals and compromises, several elements routinely surfaced in the policy debates that have implications for NPs, including emphases on primary care and care coordination, infrastructure that includes physician and non-physician primary care providers supported by information technology, demonstrable quality outcomes, expansion of existing public insurance programs, access to coverage via national insurance cooperatives, and a reimbursement system that recognizes provider collaboration and accountability (American Nurses Association, 2008; Clarin, 2007; Commonwealth Fund, 2009).

However, in the complicated process of reform, reference to advanced-practice registered nurses (APRNs) and their contributions are uneven; the current legislative proposals include funding support for NPs, nurse-led innovations, and nurse education (HR 3200), but in other instances, references are modest. For example, the Senate leader on reform (Baucus, 2009) notes in relation to comprehensive care management that, "careful consideration should be paid to the role of non-physician providers such as NPs and home health aides" (p. 39).

The several states that initiated programs of greater access and insurance coverage were anticipated to serve as demonstration projects that could inform the larger federal reform (Benson, 2007). Massachusetts reached a large percentage of the previously uninsured population but encountered problems that made headlines, including the lack of primary care physicians and associated increased waiting times for appointments of up to 100 days. More people reported a source of care, but an increasing number of people were unable to afford treatment or find a willing primary care physician, leading to continued use of emergency departments (Sack, 2009). National media coverage did not include the idea that primary care NPs could play a significant role in expanding the primary care capacity of the state. Despite the Massachusetts Association of Nurse Practitioners' (MANP) successful legislative efforts to gain recognition of NPs as primary care providers, the extent to which this effective political and policy work will influence other jurisdictions remains to be seen (see chapter 8 in this book). Unlike Massachusetts, the national dialogue and states already committed to access emphasize primary care, but do not discuss or promote non-physician providers in a substantive way.

The national dialogue, if not the outcomes of proposed reform, should accelerate NPs' positions as care providers, care coordinators, collaborators with other professionals, and as community resources. The organizations representing nursing's interests have been actively engaged in the political and policy debates at the highest level. President Obama publically recognized nurses in his summit of health care leaders (Vallina, 2009). The next step is to use his recognition of nurses to sway policymakers at the state and federal levels; this will be the most important task for NPs and their constituent organizations.

Ultimately, if the reform movement results in expanded access to care and the recommended primary care priorities, then demand for NPs' services will increase; if the cost imperative dominates and special interests decelerate the reform effort and system change is unresolved, then demand will be depressed, and recognition of NPs may not experience the anticipated boost. Whatever the short- and long-term outcomes of the current reform effort, nursing and advanced practice have reached a watershed of voice and presence on the national scene (Bonsall & Cheater, 2008; Ginsberg, Taylor, & Barr, 2009; Mullinix & Bucholtz, 2009).

RECOGNITION AND REIMBURSEMENT

The States' Environments

The states' regulatory and reimbursement environments have a direct impact on consumers' access to services and practitioners' autonomy of practice. The uneven nature of state statutes, annual legislative changes, obfuscating language, lack of central sources of legal and regulatory clarity and guidance, and the intricacies of insurance laws and managed care policies make the practice environment difficult. The cross-currents of federal and state agencies' authority that also impact NPs' practice add to the complexity of the practice environment.

Although states' legislative, regulatory, and policy developments regarding NP practice have, on balance, been deemed "progressive" by several analysts, there is steady pressure by physicians and others to contain NP autonomy. According to Phillips, Harper, Wakefield, Green and Fryer (2002), some states are reporting initiatives to restrict physician collaboration with NPs, and there are other indications of organized resistance to NP practice, including the resolution to restrict the title of "doctor" and "residency" (Pearson, 2009). Several physician organizations have taken this position, and cautioned against substitution of NPs for physicians. Seven states have statutory restrictions against NPs with doctorates being addressed as "doctor" (Pearson, 2009).

A study commissioned by the USDHHS, HRSA (2004) examined the professional practice of NPs, physician assistants, and nurse midwives across the 50 states. Among the key findings of the 1992–2000 data were the significant increase in the number of professionals and expansion of their scopes of practice; however, no states provided the optimal practice environment for these three professions. The USDHHS, HRSA study attempted to quantify the factors that lead to the resultant degree of optimal practice environment conducive to professional autonomy, by state. The study's basic assumption was that legal status largely determined the other important drivers, namely, reimbursement and prescriptive authority.

Comparison of the 1992 and 2000 practice environments, using these indices, supported the conclusions that as expectations for practice have increased, so have the legal scopes of practice. There has been greater standardization of the professional practice environment, and there is a positive relationship between the environmental indices and the number of NPs in the jurisdiction. The improved indices are "associated with broader functions, more autonomous practice environments and greater opportunities to prescribe controlled substances" (p. 46). In addition to better options for consumers and increased number of practitioners in states resulting from more positive legal environments, the indices were also significantly positively correlated with managed care penetration. From this data, the researchers suggested that managed care influences the regulatory environment.

Lugo, O'Grady, Hodnicki, and Hanson (2007) also examined states' environments to determine how conducive they were to consumer access and practitioner autonomy, including diagnostic and prescriptive authority, by assigning a numerical score and letter grade. Arizona scored 100 or A for a state "exemplary for patient choice," whereas Alabama rated a 35 or F for a state that "severely restricts patient choices."

Ironically, the eight states judged to have the best grade A ranking are some of the least populated, and combined have only 6.9% of NP preparatory programs, producing a limited number of practitioners available to practice in the best environments. The 11 states graded F because of strict limitations on patient choices and regulatory restriction on practice have greater populations, and claim more than 27% of the preparatory programs. There is limited anecdotal evidence that these environmental indices influence NP distribution. Although environmental scans are reviewed by practitioners, other professional and personal factors weigh more heavily (L. Pearson, personal communication, August 7, 2009).

An overview of NP scopes of practice released in 2007 by The Center for the Health Professions highlighted the wide range of variation produced by state and federal regulations (Christian, Dower, & O'Neil, 2007). Examination of the statutes, regulations, and ambiguous language revealed policies that limit NPs from demonstrating their competencies, support obstacles to reimbursement and malpractice insurance, and ultimately discourage providers and payers, limiting consumers' access to services.

The scopes of practice vary widely in the degree of physician involvement, requirements of practice protocols, authority to diagnose, order diagnostic tests, or make referrals to other providers and services. The states and the District of Columbia practice acts also differ in prescriptive authority, including degree of physician oversight, types of drugs that can be prescribed, and the allowable quantities within the respective schedules.

Some states recognize degrees of shared authority between the Board of Nursing, the Board of Medicine, or a combined entity. The majority include the requirement for national certification.

Christian, Dower, and O'Neil (2007) identified a number of ambiguities that confound the legal parameters of practice, including definitions of what constitutes physician supervision, practice protocols, or even "independent" practice. NP titles also vary by state; for example, in Hawaii it is "advanced practice registered nurse," and in Nevada, "advanced practitioner of nursing." These inconsistencies among state laws, and in some cases, within the state, are compounded by the lack of transparency about the full complement of the laws and regulations within each state that govern practice, and the absence of information about how to access all relevant law from one identifiable source. The researchers conclude that this lack of clarity limits optimum practice environment, limits consumer choice, provides rationale for managed care organization policies, and "constrains the uniform expansion of NP services" (p. 15).

The annual Pearson Report, which profiles the legislative, regulatory, and political changes by state, provides an extremely timely analysis of jurisdictional practice environments. The 2009 Report notes that of the 51 jurisdictions, 18–20 (with several states' pending changes) have expanded the NP scope of practice during 2008 (Pearson, 2009). Tracking annual changes informs practitioners and policymakers, and also prompts active participation by NPs and others for proactive change leading to greater autonomy.

The central issues for NPs have moved beyond prescription authority and legal NP/physician practice obligations to empanelment by third-party payers, and specifically, obtaining provider numbers to secure reimbursement. Standardized, transparent, and readily accessible practice law and regulation facilitate recognition by managed care organizations (MCOs). Recognition by managed care organizations and insurance carriers allows NPs to be more visible and to serve previously underserved communities.

Managed Care Environment

If managed care organizations were required or encouraged to recognize NPs, MCOs would serve patients with greater autonomy, resulting in lowered costs and improved access (USDHHS, HRSA, 2004). Such recognition would also support a more definitive estimation of NP services currently being documented as physician-generated. These findings were supported by Hansen-Turton and colleagues (2006, 2008), who examined the managed care policies affecting primary care NPs; many managed care entities refused to credential NPs as primary care providers, and others reimbursed NPs at lower rates than physicians. These and other MCO policies discriminate against APNs despite protective state and federal laws. Surveyed at 2-year intervals, the researchers concluded that MCO policies continue to vary widely, although the percentage of the organizations that credentialed primary care NPs rose from 33 to 53%.

Hansen-Turton, Ritter, and Torgan (2008) examined federal and state antidiscrimination statutes that protect classes of providers, and found these laws by and large do not protect primary care NPs, nor do they have any significant influence on managed care credentialing policies. In 2006, The Centers for Medicaid and Medicare Services reported that 42 states enrolled a significant number of Medicaid and Medicare beneficiaries in managed care plans presumably influenced by federal regulations that prevent provider discrimination. However, Hansen-Turton, Ritter, and Torgan (2008) found that whereas 73% of MCOs with large percentages of Medicaid enrollees recognized NPs as primary care providers, only 43% of those with predominantly commercial, and 33% of those with predominantly Medicare, enrollees recognized NP primary care providers. One of the assumptions from these two surveys is that Medicaid beneficiaries have more limited access to primary care, and hence, their need is met by primary care NPs.

Recognition by MCOs is the key to continued evolution of advanced-practice nursing, prompting NPs to look for underserved communities and population niches, and permit more transparency about what services are provided. However, access to and by larger populations is based not only on recognition, but on adequate reimbursement (USDHHS, HRSA, 2004).

Federal and State Agencies

Reimbursement via Medicare and Medicaid also has ramifications for quality care, as well as access. Intrator et al.'s (2005) study of nursing homes found that facilities with higher Medicaid reimbursement rates were more likely to employ NPs and physician assistants, and as demonstrated elsewhere, NPs contribute to quality, as evidenced by reduced hospital admissions and emergency department use.

Because state law regulates insurance, whether NPs qualify for reimbursement depends, in part, on state law. Since 1989, Medicaid payments are required for pediatric and family NPs, although some states reimburse all NPs, though at varying rates (Buppert, 2008; see chapter 3 in this book).

In summary, there is wide variation in the states' environments that determine scopes of practice (Christian, Dower, & O'Neil, 2007; USDHHS, HRSA, 2004; Lugo et al., 2007; Pearson, 2009). States create laws and regulations of the individual jurisdictions, which are overlaid by the federal agencies responsible for areas that influence health care, including the Drug Enforcement Agency, The Food and Drug Administration, and the Occupational Health and Safety Administration. The lack of consistency and clarity in law, difficulty in appreciating effects on individual practice, and practitioners' access to information and interpretation make the policy and regulatory environment difficult to understand and manipulate.

DEMAND AND SUPPLY

Demand

Conventional wisdom indicates that the demand for NPs will be accelerated by the country's changing demographics and increasing chronicity, need for primary care but shortage of primary care providers and facilities, acute care demands, increasing recognition of the contributions of providers, and reform proposals that include additional funding for preparation and practice locations for NPs. Although potential demand is only one factor influencing role expansion, the following are significant areas of need compatible with NP competencies.

Demographics and Chronicity

The expanding proportion of older adults in the country suggests a wide range of service needs ranging from health education, to disease and pharmacologic management, and transitional care to home and community to counter the system's incentives for institutionally based care.

The social and economic impact of chronic care is reflected in the debates related to costs, Medicare and re-hospitalizations, Medicaid spending on chronic illness (Krauss, 2009), and lack of capacity to care for the projected number of people with chronic diseases. The frequent references to the impact of chronic illnesses have almost inured Americans to the facts; one of two adults has at least one chronic illness, and 70% of deaths annually, or 1.7 million, are the result of chronic disease and contribute to 75% of health care costs (Centers for Disease Control and Prevention, 2009). For example, half of all Medicaid dollars have been expended on only 4% of Medicaid enrollees, prompting disease management to be introduced initially through commercial vendors.

Billings and Mijanovich's (2007) study of Medicaid fee-for-service clients in New York City demonstrated that high-risk, high-cost patients could be identified, and interdisciplinary interventions such as the chronic care model could reduce costs and readmissions through the use of NPs in disease management, case management, and NP-led multidisciplinary teams (Billings & Mijanovich, 2007; Watts et al., 2009;). Bodenheimer, Chen, and Bennett (2009) examined three approaches to chronic care: specialists, primary care physicians, and interdisciplinary teams. They endorsed team care that emphasized a combination of public health measures, nurse case management and education, and efforts that rely less heavily on face-to-face encounters and physician time (Yarnall et al., 2009).

Primary Care Needs

Primary care needs are frequently couched in terms of lack of access, inconvenience because of practice hours and waiting times, growing numbers of uninsured and underinsured, limited numbers of physicians (Connelly, 2009; Laurant et al., 2008), NPs, and physician assistants in primary care, and modest reimbursement for primary care services. Many of these problems are being addressed by the introduction of new sites and models of care. Several community-based developments may highlight NPs' capacity to meet primary care needs, including retail and other nurse-managed clinics and projects. These capitalize on NP competencies and consumers' desire to address minor health problems in a convenient and less costly manner.

The anticipated growth of retail clinics is viewed by state health policymakers as both an opportunity to improve access and control costs in meeting primary care needs (Scott, 2007). Not surprisingly, the growth of retail clinics raises the expected interprofessional competitive issues of fragmentation, lack of physician oversight, and possible competition with other community-based practices (Takach & Witgert, 2009). Consumer media publications favorably describe retail clinics as an alternate source of lower cost primary care provided by NPs, "registered nurses who have advanced training and can prescribe drugs" (Consumer Reports on Health, 2009). Most retail clinics are staffed by NPs and are expected to grow from over 1,000 sites to 6,000 in the next few years (Scott, 2007). The growth of these clinics and corresponding visibility of NPs will depend on the array of state regulations, opposition from organized medicine, and the economic advantages gained by the host retail chains.

Acute Care Need

Acute care needs are also driving the demand for NPs, including hospital-based team care and reduced resident staff hours, hospitalists' roles, reduced capacity of emergency departments and physicians in emergency medicine, and satellite acute and urgent care centers. The emphasis on reducing cost of care, length of stay, and readmissions, and meeting requirements for residents' work rules has created a variety of roles for NPs in acute care. Although the acute care practitioner role was well established in hospital acute care settings, it was highlighted when the American Council of Graduate Medical Education initiated the 80-hour-work-week rule in 2003. Use of acute care NPs in lieu of house or attending staff or as part of a multidisciplinary team has demonstrated reduced length of stay and cost (Cowan et al., 2006). However, this most recent area of role expansion and settings raises the issue again of NP as physician substitute or collaborator in acute care.

Other developments support the idea that NPs should be used in alternate acute care settings, (Haan et al., 2007) including emergency departments (Ray, 2008), outpatient clinics, and subacute facilities, all which have experienced increased volume due to fewer emergency departments, fewer physicians in emergency care, and diminished access to primary care services offered in the community.

Supply

Whereas demand is well established, the potential supply of NPs is deemed to fall far short well into the future. Several factors will operate to constrain supply, and the solutions are dependent on significant professional, educational, and public and private funding proposals that will be difficult to achieve and sustain. Factors limiting future NP production include the overall nurse shortage and the dominant pre-licensure preparation in associate degree programs, the limited capacity of educational programs, and the lack of significant funding to support aid to students and educational institutions.

The continued imbalance of baccalaureate- to associate-degree-prepared nurses is limiting the pool of nurses prepared to undertake graduate education. Aiken, Cheung, and Olds (2009) note the limited percentage of associate degree program graduates who earned master's or doctoral degrees (5.8%) versus baccalaureate nurses (19.7%). If this prelicensure education pattern continues, the potential pool of master's/doctoral-prepared nurses will preclude any APN increase, whether in the faculty or NP role.

Educational programs' capacity to admit and graduate generalists and APNs is limited by past enrollment cycles that forced faculty losses, the aging of the current faculty cohort, anticipated faculty retirements, institutional budget constraints and most nursing programs' complete reliance on tuition revenue, and difficulties ensuring appropriate levels of clinical competencies for both baccalaureate and master's students.

The estimated 41,000–99,000 applicants qualified but not accepted by pre-licensure programs have been widely discussed (Cleary, McBride, McClure, & Reinhard, 2009; Rother & Lavizzo-Mourey, 2009). Ironically, the negative experience of baccalaureate-prepared nurses, leading to a 25–27% turnover among nurses in the first year of practice (Pricew-aterhouseCoopers' Health Research Institute July 2007 report at www.pwc.com), may lead to higher advanced-practice program enrollment. Beginning nurses' perception of the autonomy and independence of the NP role, in contrast to the hospital staff nurse positions with its perceived stress, hostile work environment, and limited autonomy, may lead to greater numbers of NPs and fewer bedside nurses (American Association of Colleges of Nursing [AACN], 2008a).

The master's program enrollment and graduation picture is equally dire. As of fall 2008 (Pearson, 2009), 762 baccalaureate and higher degree nursing programs offered master's and postmaster's certificate NP preparation. Master's programs report that NPs students represented over 42%, or 29,323, of all graduate program enrollees, and over 44%, or 7,613, program graduates. Of the more than 29,000 enrollees, most were in family (56.7%), adult primary (14.6%), adult acute care (8.1%), and pediatrics (6.4%), heavily weighting the primary care preparation and focus. The increasing number of adult–geriatric and post-master's geriatric programs also expand the primary care preparatory focus of graduate programs (Fang, Tracy, & Bednash, 2009).

Enrollment in master's level programs increased by only 8.7% in 2008 (AACN, 2008b), a lower increase than reported in 2007 (11.7%) and 2006 (18.1%). Graduations increased by 10.6% in 2008, compared with 12.3% in 2007 and 9.7% in 2006. Consistent with enrollment figures, the numbers of NP graduates fell from 8200 (1998) to 6000 (2005), and there is a further decline expected by 2015 to an approximately 4000 annual graduations, despite the increasingly varied demand by role and setting (Bodenheimer, Chen, & Bennett, 2009). Proposals to boost the supply chain of NPs include significant public and private funding for scholarships, loan forgiveness, and capitation to attract student enrollment and institutional expansion. Other suggestions to expand supply have included more competitive faculty salaries, greater educational program efficiencies, accelerated programs linking associ-ate-degree preparation with baccalaureate/master's degrees acquisition, and incentives for community colleges to be granted charters to award baccalaureate degrees to expand the pool of graduate program appli-cants. Although some of these proposals have been discussed at length, the implementation has been limited (Cleary, McBride, McClure, & Rein-hard, 2009).

Students in master's and doctoral programs are predominantly part time, dependent on tuition benefits, and balancing full-time employment and course work.

Lack of significant public and private funding for graduate education ensures that NP students will be part time, and upon graduation may stay in the same agency or institution in positions with titles that may or may not indicate practitioner preparation.

Increased funding for nursing education has been included in the stimulus American Recovery and Reinvestment Act of 2009. Other avenues for support of postlicensure education could be redirection of Medicare funds that currently support hospital nurse training programs (Aiken, Cheung, & Olds, 2009), or plans to establish Medicare reimbursement for advanced-practice students, similar to graduate medical education (GME) funding. Sources of funding for other possible solutions, including competitive faculty salaries, greater technologic innovation, as well as clinical simulations, consortia development, new clinical site development, and faculty role development for clinicians, are more elusive. The slow economic recovery will delay private donations, local and state government contributions, and/or a substantial increase in institutional support. Programmatic changes that lead to accelerated degree attainments through charter changes, program compression, and flexible scheduling for full-time workers and career changers may be less resource-intensive, but take extended time, as well.

PROGRAM DIVERSITY

At the same time that professional organizations are advocating standardization efforts in licensure, accreditation, certification, and education (LACE) (Stanley, 2009, p. 103), other educational programs and certifications are being introduced, including the Doctor of Nursing Practice (DNP), the Comprehensive Care certification examination, the Clinical Nurse Leader (CNL), and the CNL certification examination. Over 84 DNP programs are admitting students, and over 50 additional schools are considering similar curricular proposals (AACN, 2009). In contrast to the practice-focused doctorate, the 74 CNL programs are master's-level programs that purport to prepare advanced generalist clinicians eligible to take the CNL Certification Examination overseen by the Commission on Nurse Certification, a subsidiary of the AACN

(AACN, 2009). How these new degrees and titles will renew or reconfigure graduate program enrollment, tuition benefits, and revenue remains to be seen.

REGULATION AND STANDARDIZATION

Governmental and organizational efforts to regulate and standardize all aspects of preparation and certification of advanced practice are not new. Rozella Schlotfeldt in the 1970s called for greater standardization. However, as pressure is brought to bear by insurers, competing professions, nursing's professional organizations, and education programs, the shape of NP practice is being drawn toward more consistent and rigorous standards. Most states require NPs to be nationally certified, and in 2000, the APRN Compact for NPs was developed to achieve some degree of standardization and practitioner mobility. However, only three states are included at this date.

The USDHHS, HRSA study of the three nonphysician provider groups (2004) noted that NPs have become "professionalized" over the last 2 decades, a process that includes increasing standardization of the body of knowledge required for practice, and creating certification requirements that validate the knowledge base (p. 13). Although the emphasis is on standardization, there is static in the system created by variation in states' legislative requirements and the singular influence of a few innovative educational programs. Despite the intense efforts by many relevant professional organizations, there has always been institutional proclivity for making signature or "brand" additions to curricula, reflecting faculty expertise, institutional, and geographic/demographic demands.

State legislative changes are documented annually, tracking the enhanced, limited, or status quo. Generally, these changes in NP practice have been positive, enhancing diagnosis, treatment, and prescribing functions, though not making significant changes in the requirement for physician supervision/collaboration. State statutory changes are influenced by the density of NP populations, the insurance laws related to reimbursement and provider panel listings. Pearson (2009) reports that 22 states report expanded scope of practice (p. 11).

Four years of negotiation between the Alliance APRN Consensus Work Group and the National Council of State Boards of Nursing APRN

Committee and their offspring, the APRN Joint Dialogue Group, resulted in guidelines for current and future education and practice requirements (Stanley, 2009). The regulatory model recognizes the four advanced practice roles and six population groups that each state board of nursing would, in turn, license and designate the professional as an APRN, with a particular population focus optionally identified. The regulatory model endorses the previously configured three-tiered curriculum model, and requires education programs to be approved by "the accrediting body prior to admitting students." APRN program graduates will take one of the state licensing board's recognized certification examinations that measure APRN competencies and the population focus.

LINKS TO OTHER PROFESSIONS

Service delivery that produces effective practice and rational use of resources is based on recognition of complementary practices of health professionals weighed with their competing interests (USDHHS, HRSA, 2004).

The interprofessional discourse focuses on improved access and outcomes, controlled costs, and limited references to NPs or physicians practicing in "integrated delivery systems" with other health professions (Commonwealth Fund Commission on a High Performance Health System, 2009). The players cited in reform proposals as posing the greatest challenges include public and private insurers. For public and private systems to compete, each would need a "selection of provider networks, utilization management, and benefit design." On the other hand, Phillips et al. (2002) and Pearson (2009) report recent examples of state legislation that expands NPs' regulatory and prescriptive authority, a few examples of state laws that facilitate reimbursement, and some laws that expand functions in psychiatric mental health, allow for certification of disability, and in Maryland, certification of births and deaths.

Shortage of other primary care providers may again provide the opportunity for NPs' acceptance, role expansion, and recognition by fiscal intermediaries.

The projected shortage of physicians, continued emphasis on specialty practice over primary care practice, and disincentives to practice as a primary care provider limits the number of primary care physicians.

Paradoxically, organized medicine continues to try to control primary care services, while acknowledging the primary care physician shortage and the availability of other providers to provide the necessary services. Although a body of literature has focused on the need for physician supervision as a "patient-protection issue," the tone of these position statements varies. A recent statement by the American College of Physicians (ACP; Ginsberg et al., 2009) recognized the anticipated ongoing shortage of primary care physicians, and noted that whereas NPs have the ability to meet 60–90% of patients' primary care needs and improve access, health care costs and quality may not necessarily be improved. The ACP "opposes any policies or regulations that have the consequence of replacing or substituting NPs for physicians" (p. 13).

Although NPs are demonstrating the ability to meet primary care needs, other professions are also advancing their primary care bona fides, including physician assistants, physical therapists, and pharmacists. In New York State, the Association of Physical Therapists has introduced a bill to be recognized as primary care providers, which would reduce the $50 "specialist" co-pay. Patients already have direct access without referral to physical therapists for 10 visits or 30 days (P. Vanbrevan, personal communication, June 3, 2009). The American Pharmacists Association, in testimony regarding several of its initiatives examining the pharmacist's role in preventing medication misuse, particularly its Partnership to Fight Chronic Disease, "included pharmacists when it listed primary health care providers who are 'instrumental' to the cause of disease prevention" (Posey, 2009, p.1). Many of these practitioners are arguing that essential services are unavailable to consumers because access is funneled through the primary care physician.

The Center for the Health Professions study (Christian et al., 2007) examined the evolution and "professionalization" of NPs, physician assistants, and certified nurse midwives recognized that several important elements were associated with an increased number of APNs; states deemed more favorable were associated with more autonomous practice and better choice for patients (Pearson, 2009; USDHHS, HRSA, 2004). The introduction of NPs into underserved areas is limited by the distribution of collaborating physicians. However, to the extent that legislation allows for remote supervision/collaboration, it is important to recognize that current and proposed technology supports distance collaboration and consultation among providers.

Whereas many reasons support the uncoupling of NP practice from physician collaboration/supervision, including potentially improved access, recognition of research validating quality and cost-effectiveness, and recognition of professional autonomy, only 23 jurisdictions, including the District of Columbia, do not require physician consultation. The efforts to modify the legal and reimbursement linkages between NPs and physicians will have to be replaced by a fully collaborative practice culture that includes a wide range of health professions, many of which are successfully forging ahead to establish their own autonomy. The integrative model of the future will be necessary to produce the primary, transitional, acute, and rehabilitative care central to the reformists' view of our delivery system.

SUMMARY

In summary, reform efforts, regulatory and reimbursement changes, provider availability, and drive to standardize education and credentialing seem to advance NPs' participation in the delivery system. However, the environment shaping NP practice is kaleidoscopic and noisy; but unlike earlier periods, much of the noise and color is coming from nursing leadership, and progress is being charted in all the areas that will lead to autonomy, continued effectiveness, and greater visibility.

REFERENCES

Abelson, R. (2009a, June 3). Health insurers balk at changes for small business. *New York Times*, pp. B1, B8.

Abelson, R. (2009b, April 2). Study finds many Medicare patients are rehospitalized, raising costs. *New York Times*, p. B2.

Aiken, L., Cheung, R., & Olds, D. (2009). Education policy initiatives to address nursing shortage in the United States. *Health Affairs, 28*(4), w646–w656.

American Association of Colleges of Nursing. (2009). *AACN update on the new comprehensive care certification exam.* Retrieved March 7, 2009, from www.aacn.dnpcert.org/pdf/AACN_Statement

American Association of Colleges of Nursing. (2008a). *Nursing shortage fact sheet.* Retrieved March 7, 2009, from www.aacn.nche.edu/Media/shortageresource.htm

American Association of Colleges of Nursing. (2008b). *Enrollment growth in U.S. nursing colleges and universities hits an 8-year low.* Retrieved March 7, 2009, from www.aacn.nche.edu/IDS

American Nurses Association. (2008). *ANA's health system reform agenda*. Silver Springs, MD: Author.

Baucus, M. (2009). *Call to action: Health reform 2009*. Retrieved July 18, 2009, from www.finance.senate.gov

Benson, E. (2007). Recent developments in health law: States lead the way on health insurance reform. *Journal of Law, Medicine & Ethics, 35*, 329–332.

Billings, J., & Mijanovich, T. (2007). Improving the management of care for high cost Medicaid patients. *Health Affairs, 26*(6), 1643–1655.

Bodenheimer, T., Chen, E., & Bennett, H. D. (2009). Confronting the growing burden of chronic disease: Can the U.S. health care workforce do the job? *Health Affairs, 28*, 64–74.

Bonsall, K., & Cheater, F. (2008). What is the impact of advanced primary care nursing roles on patients, nurses and their colleagues? A literature review. *International Journal of Nursing Studies, 45*, 1090–1102.

Buppert, C. (2008). *Nurse practitioner's business practice and legal guide* (3rd ed.). Sudbury, MA: Jones and Bartlett Publishers.

Centers for Disease Control and Prevention. (2009). *Chronic diseases: The power to prevent, the call to control*. Retrieved September 24, 2009, from http://www.cdc.gov/nccdphp/publications/AAG/chronic.htm

Center for Medicare and Medicaid Services, Office of the Actuary. (2008). Retrieved February 27, 2010, from http://www.slideshare.net/commonhealth/national- health-spending-in-2007-presentation

Christian, S., Dower, C., & O'Neil, E. (2007). *Overview of nurse practitioners scopes of practice in the United States—Discussion*. University of California, San Francisco: The Center for the Health Professions.

Clarin, O. A. (2007). Strategies to overcome barriers to effective nurse practitioner and physician collaboration. *Journal for Nurse Practitioners, 3*(8), 538–548.

Cleary, B., McBride, A. B., McClure, M., & Reinhard, S. (2009). Expanding the capacity of nursing education. *Health Affairs, 28*(4), w634–w645.

The Commonwealth Fund Commission on a High Performance Health System. (2009). *The path to a high performance U.S. health system: A 2020 vision and the policies to pave the way*. New York: Author.

Connelly, J. (2009, April 2). More doctors are opting out of Medicare. *New York Times*, p. A9.

Consumer Reports on Health. (April, 2009). *When you need care fast* (p. 6). New York: Consumers Union.

Cowan, M. J., Shapiro, M., Hayes, R. D., Afife, A., Vazirani, S., Ward, C. R., et al. (2006). The effect of a multidisciplinary hospitalist/physician and advanced practice nurse collaboration on hospital costs. *Journal of Nursing Administration, 36*(2), 79–85.

Fairman, J. (2008). *Making room in the clinic: Nurse practitioners and the evolution of modern health care*. New Brunswick, NJ: Rutgers University Press.

Fang, D., Tracy, C., & Bednash, G. D. (2009). *2008-2009 enrollment and graduations in baccalaureate and graduate programs in nursing*. Washington, DC: American Association of Colleges of Nursing.

Ginsburg, J., Taylor, T., & Barr, M. (2009). *Nurse practitioners in primary care* (American College of Physicians Policy Monograph). Philadelphia: American College of Physicians.

Haan, J. M., Dutton, R. P., Willis, M., Leone, S., Kramer, M. E., & Scalia, T. M. (2007). Discharge rounds in the 80 hour work week: Importance of the trauma nurse practitioner. *Journal of Trauma, Injury, Infection, and Critical Care, 63*, 339–343.

Hansen-Turton, T., Ritter, A., Rothman, N., & Valdez, B. (2006). Insurer policies create barriers to health care access and consumer choice. *Nursing Economics, 24*(4), 204–212.

Hansen-Turton, T., Ritter, A., & Torgan, R. (2008). Insurers' contracting policies on nurse practitioners as primary care providers: Two years later. *Policy, Politics, & Nursing Practice, 9*(4), 241–248.

Intrator, O., Feng, Z., Mor, V., Gifford, D., Bourbonniere, M., & Zinn, J. (2005). The employment of nurse practitioners and physician assistants in U.S. nursing homes. *The Gerontologist, 45*(4), 486–495.

Kirkpatrick, D. (2009, August 9). Democrats say no to cap for drug manufacturers. *New York Times*, p. A 11.

Krauss, C. (2009, August 7). Trickle down costs. *New York Times*, pp. B 1, B 4.

Krugman, P. (2009, June 5). Keeping them honest. *New York Times*, p. A23.

Laurant, M., Reeves, D., Hermens, R., Braspenning, J., Grol, R., & Sibbald, B. (2008). *Substitution of doctors by nurses in primary care (review)*. New York: John Wiley.

Lugo, N., O'Grady, E., Hodnicki, D., & Hanson, C. (2007). Ranking state NP regulation: Practice Environment and consumer healthcare choice. *American Journal for Nurse Practitioners, 11*(4).

McInturff, W. D., & Weigel, L. (2008). Déjà vu all over again: The similarities between political debates regarding health care in the early 1990s and today. *Health Affairs, 27*(3), 699–704.

Mullinix, C., & Bucholtz., D. (2009). Role and quality of nurse practitioner practice: Policy issue. *Nursing Outlook, 57*, 93–96.

Mundinger, M., Kane, R., Lenz, E., Totten, A., Tsai, W-Y., Cleary, P., et al. (2000). Primary care outcomes in patients treated by nurse practitioners or physicians: A randomized trial. *Journal of the American Medical Association, 283*(1), 59–68.

Pear, R. (2009a, May 18). Health care leaders say Obama overstated their promise to control costs. *New York Times*, p. A20.

Pear, R. (2009b, May 28). Warring sides on health care carry their fight to TV and radio ads. *New York Times*, p. A14.

Pearson, L. (2009). The Pearson report. *American Journal for Nurse Practitioners, 13*(2), 8–82.

Phillips, R. L., Harper, D. C., Wakefield, M., Green, L. A., & Fryer, G. E. (2002). Can nurse practitioners and physicians beat parochialism into plowshares. *Health Affairs, 21*(5), 133–142.

Posey, L. M. (2009, May). *APhA, Chronic Disease Partnership file comments with Senate Finance Committee*. Retrieved June 2, 2009, from http://www.pharmacist.com/AM/Template.cfm?Section=Home2&TEMPLATE=/CM/ContentDisplay.cfm&CONTENT ID=19678

PricewaterhouseCooper (July, 2007). *Health Research Institute*. Retrieved July 17, 2009 from www.pwc.com.

Ray, M. M. (2008). Advanced practice registered nurse policy issues in today's health care climate. *Journal of Emergency Nursing, 34*, 555–557.

Rother, J., & Lavizzo-Mourey, R. (2009). Addressing the nursing workforce: A critical element for health reform. *Health Affairs, 28*(4), w620–w624.

Sack, K. (2009, May 28). Massachusetts, model for universal health care, sees ups and down in policy. *New York Times*, p. A19.

Safriet, B. (1992). Health care dollars and regulatory sense: The role of advance practice nursing. *Yale Journal on Regulation, 9*, 417–488.

Scott, K. K. (2007). *Health care in the express lane: Retail clinics go mainstream*. Oakland, CA: California Health Care Foundation.

Stanley, J. (2009). Reaching consensus on a regulatory model: What does this mean for APRNs? *Journal for Nurse Practitioners, 5*(2), 99–104.

Takach, M., & Witgert, K. (2009). *Analysis of state regulations and policies governing the operation and licensure of retail clinics*. Washington, DC: National Academy for State Health Policy.

United States Department of Health and Human Services, Human Resources and Services Administration, Bureau of Health Professions. (February, 2004). *A comparison of changes in the professional practice of nurse practitioners, physician assistants, and certified nurse midwives: 1992 and 2000*. Retrieved September 29, 2009, from http://bhpr.hrsa.gov/healthworkforce/reports/scope/scope6-7.htm

United States Food and Drug Administration. (2004). *Guidance to the industry-consumer directed broadcast advertisements*. Rockville, Center, MD: Author.

United States Office of Technology Assessment. (1986). *Nurse practitioners, physician assistants, and certified nurse-midwives: A policy analysis. Health technology care study 32*. Washington, DC: Author.

Vallina, J. (2009). ANA joins President Obama at White House in call for health care reform. *American Nurse, 41*(4), 1, 16.

Watts, S., Gee, J., O'Day, M., Schaub, K., Lawrence, R., Aron, D., et al. (2009). Nurse–practitioner led multidisciplinary teams to improve chronic care. *Journal of the American Academy of Nurse Practitioners, 21*, 167–172.

White House, Office of the Press Secretary. (2009, July 15). Remarks by the President on Health Care Reform. Retrieved February 27, 2010, from http://www.whitehouse.gov/the_press_office/Remarks-by-the-President-on-Health-Care- Reform/

Yarnell, K., Ostbye, T., Krause, K., Pollack, K., Gradison, M., & Michener, L. (2009). Family physicians as team leaders: Time to share the care preventing chronic disease. *Public Health Research, Practice and Policy, 6*(2), 1–6.

13 Nurse-Managed Health Centers

EUNICE S. KING AND TINE HANSEN-TURTON

There are an estimated 250 nurse-managed health centers (NMHCs), including primary care and wellness centers, throughout the United States (Hansen-Turton, 2005). Broadly defined, nurse-managed centers are sources of care for people provided by nurses using a professional nursing framework to design, implement, and sustain health care for the community. Approximately 112 are community-based centers operated as independent nonprofits or as hospital outpatient clinics. One hundred thirty-eight are academic-based and affiliated with university-based schools of nursing (Institute for Nursing Centers, 2004). Of the 250 NMHCs, 150 provide primary care services; the remaining are considered wellness centers, and provide health promotion and disease prevention services, but not primary care.

Collectively, the 150 nurse-managed primary care centers handle over 2.5 million annual client visits (Hansen-Turton, 2005). The U.S. Congress has praised NMHCs, stating that, "nurse-managed health centers serve a dual function in strengthening the health care safety net by providing health care to populations in underserved areas and by providing the clinical experiences to nursing students that are mandatory for professional development" (U.S. Senate Appropriations Committee, 2005). Unfortunately, most of the general public is largely unfamiliar with nurse-managed centers. However, with the onset of retail-based clinics staffed primarily by nurse practitioners (NPs), their heretofore relatively anonymous existence is changing, as nurse-managed centers have been described as the precursor to the retail clinic movement (Hansen-Turton, Ryan, Miller, Counts, & Nash, 2007).

WHAT IS A NURSE-MANAGED PRIMARY CARE HEALTH CENTER?

NMHCs are health care centers in which a nurse occupies the chief management position; accountability and responsibility for client care and professional practice remain with nursing staff. Advanced-practice nurses (APNs) are the primary providers for clients visiting the center (Matherlee, 1999). Health problems or potential health problems are not viewed in isolation, but within the context of societal, environmental, and cultural influences that have affected the client's past and present health and that have the potential to influence future health. Patients are connected with resources that address and correct the forces that have a negative impact on their health (King, 2005). Patients, their families, and their communities become the focus of care, and the centers are often managed in partnership with the communities served.

NMHCs provide primary care, health promotion, disease prevention, and disease management for clients across the lifespan. Specific services vary by center, but often include primary care, prenatal care, laboratory and diagnostic tests, access to free or low-cost pharmaceuticals, family planning, midwifery, behavioral health, and dental care on site, and referrals to specialists, hospital services, and radiologic services via contracts. The centers are open minimally 20 hours a week, offering some weekend and evening hours, along with 24/7 on-call services (Hansen-Turton, 2005). They address health disparities by providing accessible and affordable comprehensive primary care and community health programs aimed at health promotion and disease prevention, in addition to behavioral health, and sometimes, home-care services (Coleman & Hansen-Turton, 2003).

Enabling services, in other words, those that facilitate clients' access to the health care system and assist in the maintenance of their health, are often provided in NMHCs to complement primary care. They may include transportation to and from the health center or specialty appointments, outreach services, assistance with applying for Medicaid or pharmacy programs, cash and/or housing assistance, case management, eligibility assistance, environmental risk reduction, health education, interpretation and translation services, home visiting, and parenting education (Hansen-Turton, 2005).

Funding for NMHCs comes from a variety of sources, depending upon the populations served, the administrative structure, services provided, and affiliations. Specific examples include foundation grants; local, state, or federal grants and/or contracts; in-kind or cash subsidies from the parent or cooperating institution (e.g., college, university, hospital, or housing authority); reimbursement from third-party payers for services provided; fees collected from clients; and individuals' and corporations' contributions to the centers.

HISTORICAL BACKGROUND

The philosophy of nurse-managed centers has its origin grounded by the work of Lillian Wald, who, in the late 19th century, established the Henry Street Settlement to administer to the health care needs of New York City's poor. Like NMHC, the Henry Street Settlement was an example of nurse-delivered health care that resided outside the traditional health care system of the day (Glass, 1989) and was followed by others, such as the rural clinics established by Mary Breckinridge in Hyden, Kentucky, in 1925 (Bartlett, 2009). Many of these early, nontraditional models of nurse-managed care were eventually replaced by public health nursing departments or divisions within municipal or county departments of public health that focused primarily on providing maternal child health care. It was not until the development of educational programs to prepare nurses for expanded roles, the emergence of public and private support in the mid 1960s–1970s allowing NPs to provide primary care, and the availability of funding to support development of models of care for the underserved, that NMHCs could emerge as they did in the mid 1980s.

DIVISION OF NURSING

The history of today's NMHCs is a chronicle of collaborating entities working toward a shared vision, and a convergence of timely events and circumstances that enabled a new model of health care to emerge. Nationally, one of the most important entities was the Division of Nursing, an organizational unit within the Bureau of Health Professions, one of the four divisions within the Health Resources and Services Administration (HRSA) of the U.S. Department of Health and Human Services. Historically, the Division of Nursing was the federal agency responsible for providing the national perspective on the nursing workforce, nursing practice, and nursing education. In the late 1960s, the Division of Nursing funded an evaluation of the innovative NP program developed by Loretta Ford and Henry Silver at the University of Colorado, which documented NPs' competence and acceptance by patients, parents, and other health professionals. This report was one of the catalysts for federal legislation passed in 1968 that was renewed several times, continuing through to the present day, and that has enabled the Division to fund NP education (Starbecker, 2000).

With the emergence and growth in NP programs in nursing schools, it became imperative for program faculty to demonstrate expert clinical competence. Thus, some schools established clinics run by NP faculty, simultaneously providing a site for faculty practice and research, a clinical practice site for NP students, and fulfillment of a community-service mission (Boettcher, 1996; Zachariah & Lundeen, 1997). The first Division of Nursing grants were made in the late 1970s, and the Division's Special Projects program (Clear, Starbecker, & Kelly, 1999; Starbecker, 2000), created through Section 3 of the Nurse Education Amendments of 1985 and subsequent amendments, has continued to support the establishment of NMHCs by academic schools or departments of nursing through to the present day.

Among the funding criteria that had to be met by the academic-based nurse-managed centers were that: (a) they improve access to primary care in medically underserved areas, (b) they be operated and staffed by faculty and students in the affiliated school of nursing, and (c) the center be under the administrative aegis of the school of nursing. Initially, grants made under this program were 5-year awards and were not designed to be renewed, as this period was considered adequate for allowing a center to become credentialed by third-party payers, to cultivate other sources of funding, and to build the practice with sufficient numbers of patients to enable it to become financially self-sustaining. Unfortunately, this was not the case with many centers. Some struggled to sustain themselves, and others were forced to close primarily for financial or financial-related reasons (Barger, Nugent, & Bridges, 1993; Campbell, 2003; Sullivan, Fields, Kelly, & Whelan, 1993).

INDEPENDENCE FOUNDATION

In the Philadelphia area, the Independence Foundation was an important partner for many nurse-managed centers (King, 2005). A private philanthropy in Philadelphia, Pennsylvania, the Independence Foundation in 1993 designated community-based nurse-managed health care as one of its primary funding initiatives, consistent with its mission of supporting programs that provide services to those who do not ordinarily have access to them. Over the next decade, the Foundation awarded grants to a number of Philadelphia-area NMHCs, including four that were academic-based, one hospital-based, and the remaining five operated by nonprofit health and human service organizations.

The Foundation's role in supporting nurse-managed centers in the Philadelphia region was multifold. Grants to the centers helped them weather the rough financial periods until they could develop strategies for becoming more financially secure. Cooperation among centers was fostered informally through the convening of NMHC leaders two-to-three times a year for networking and conversation with a prominent nurse leader. Additionally, in 1996, an Independence Foundation grant supported the establishment of the Regional Nursing Centers Consortium (RNCC) by directors and staff from 13 Philadelphia-region nurse-managed centers to address common concerns and health policy issues. Finally, a series of grants from the Foundation in the late 1990s and early 2000s supported the development of software systems to collect data about demographic and health characteristics of clients served by the centers and services provided, and it purchased an electronic practice management and health record software system to be used in several of the centers.

CHALLENGES FACED BY NURSE-MANAGED CENTERS

In 2003, the Independence Foundation undertook a retrospective, qualitative study of 10 NMHCs it had funded during the prior 10 years, to identify past and ongoing challenges, and the strategies developed to address them (King, 2008). Although this report detailed a number of problems faced by the centers during that period, the major issue focused on how to become financially self-sustaining without compromising the mission of providing holistic comprehensive health care to underserved, indigent populations. A major threat to the financial sustainability of the NMHCs in Pennsylvania came from the 1994 Pennsylvania Health Choices legislation, which mandated all Medicaid recipients enroll in one of the state's Medicaid health maintenance organizations (HMOs) and, once enrolled, select a primary care provider who had been credentialed and approved by the respective HMO. Unfortunately, the initial legislation failed to include NMHCs as approved providers, partially due to lack of knowledge about NMHCs, as well as physician opposition. During the process of having this policy changed, the need for NMHCs to work together on such issues and to educate policymakers and others about NMHCs became clear, and led to the 1996 establishment of the RNCC, as noted above.

THE NATIONAL NURSING CENTERS CONSORTIUM

The RNCC, which rapidly grew from its initial 13 members in 1996 to 250 in 2008, and became the National Nursing Centers Consortium (NNCC) in 2002, has been the most important resource for the centers to address health policy issues. Through the cultivation of connections and collaboration at the federal, state, and regional levels, the NNCC has promoted the visibility of nurse-managed centers as important safety net providers, and has advocated for favorable reimbursement policies for the centers. It has provided technical assistance to centers to facilitate their applications to become credentialed by HMOs and to obtain Federally Qualified Health Center (FQHC) status, where feasible (see later section in this chapter). The NNCC also worked with centers in several states to obtain prescriptive privileges for NPs. With funding from the Independence Foundation, the NNCC implemented electronic data-collection systems in several of its member centers to collect health outcomes data to support its health policy advocacy efforts. These data-collection systems proved critical in the conduct of a Centers for Medicaid and Medicare-funded study that demonstrated that nurse-managed centers met the Institute of Medicine (IOM) definition of safety net providers, and that their adherence to selected Health Plan

Employer Data and Information Set (HEDIS) measures was similar to those of like providers (Hansen-Turton, Line, O'Connell, & Rothman, 2005).

NURSE-MANAGED HEALTH CENTERS IN THE 21st CENTURY

Role as Safety Net Providers

The definition of safety net providers developed by the Institute of Medicine (IOM) specifies: (a) that safety net providers, either by legal mandate or explicitly adopted mission, offer care to patients regardless of their ability to pay for those services; and (b) that a substantial share of safety net providers' patients are uninsured, Medicaid, and other vulnerable populations (IOM, 2004). The core safety net providers listed in the IOM summary include community health centers (CHCs), FQHCs, public hospitals, and local health departments. Missing from the list are NMHCs, despite their long history of providing low-income, medically underserved, vulnerable populations with high-quality health care services. Like CHCs, NMHCs are usually located in medically underserved areas in urban and rural communities, and in places such as public and Section 8 (federally subsidized) housing developments, schools, churches, community and recreation centers, and homeless and domestic violence shelters (Coleman & Hansen-Turton, 2003). Although it is clear that nurse-managed centers serve this population, they have not been officially recognized by the IOM as safety net providers.

Patients Served

When examining the characteristics of the clients served by NMHCs, it is clear that they meet the IOM definition of a safety net provider, because they serve a large percentage of uninsured clients, children, and individuals from minority racial or ethnic backgrounds. According to a national survey of NMHCs, 41% of the NMHC clients are African American, and 12% are Latino or Hispanic (National Nursing Centers Consortium, 2005a). More than a third of clients are children 18 years of age and younger (36%), and over half (51%) are adults between the ages of 19 and 64. Sixty-nine percent have completed high school and some of those have attended college (Hansen-Turton, 2005). Among those 18 and older, 54% report being unemployed, leaving less than half (46%) employed. A 2003 study of clients using Philadelphia-area NMHCs found that those who were employed, either full or part time, were less likely to have insurance than those who were unemployed (Hansen-Turton, Line, O'Connell, Rothman, & Lauby, 2004, p. 29). This finding is consistent with the Kaiser Family Foundation and the Health Research and Educational Trust 2006 survey (Henry J. Kaiser Family Foundation, 2006), and likely due to more of the unemployed being qualified for one of the Medicaid insurance products. Within the NMHCs, 46% of the patients are uninsured, and 37% are on Medicaid (NNCC, 2005a). Most NMHCs report that among their uninsured patients, the majority are unable to pay even a minimal fee for a health visit. And, their clients, largely from minority racial and ethnic backgrounds, more than half unemployed, and at least a third to a half uninsured, are among the nation's most vulnerable populations.

Importance in Addressing Health Disparities

As the data show, patients served by NMHCs are largely from vulnerable populations that are disproportionately affected by chronic illnesses, such as asthma, diabetes, and cardiovascular problems. A 2004 federally funded study of 11 Pennsylvania-based NMHCs found all of these illnesses to be very prevalent within their client population (Hansen-Turton, Line, O'Connell, & Rothman, 2005). Asthma-related diagnoses accounted for 32% of all pulmonary diagnoses, hypertension for 77% of all cardiovascular diagnoses, and diabetes and obesity 69% and 25%, respectively, of all metabolic diagnoses. A major focus of NMHCs is preventive health care and health promotion, aimed specifically at reducing health risks associated with chronic conditions like asthma, hypertension, diabetes, and obesity (Hansen-Turton, 2005). The other health services most often provided are immunizations, screenings, and well child, adolescent, and adult visits, which often include teaching about prevention or management of chronic illnesses (Hansen-Turton, 2005). This study's findings underscored the importance of NMHCs in addressing health disparities, both through management of existing illnesses and through the provision of preventative health care. The latter, along with the integration of behavioral health with primary care (common in many centers), is considered one of the most critical factors in eliminating health disparities (Hansen-Turton, 2005).

Staffing

According to data from the NNCC annual membership survey, staffing within NMHCs varies by the size of the center and the number of clients served. Nationally, APNs, including NPs, clinical specialists, and/or nurse midwives, comprise 43% of the nursing center workforce. Their work is supported by that of registered nurses (9%); therapists and social workers (6.5%); community outreach workers (4%); administrative support staff (12%); and health educators, students and others (25%); as well as physician collaborators for certified NPs' prescribing authority and/or for quality assurance and consultation (Hansen-Turton, 2005).

Role in Nursing Education

In the academic-based NMHCs, 25% of undergraduate nursing students and many of the advanced-practice students have clinical rotations in the health centers. Unlike Graduate Medical Education funds that provide payment to hospitals to offset physician training, these clinical rotations are not funded through service reimbursement systems. However, the centers receive indirect support through the in-kind education and practice efforts of nursing school faculty members. According to the American Association of Colleges of Nursing (AACN), "as front-line primary care and outpatient treatment become more dominant and hospitals focus more on acute care for the sickest patients, the demand for skilled nurse practitioners continues to climb. Despite this need, Medicare—the largest single source of federal funding for nursing education—currently does not support training for NPs and most other advanced practice nurses while, at the same time, continuing to subsidize hospital diploma programs that have been out of the mainstream of nursing education for decades" (AACN, 2000, p. 4).

Filling a Workforce Gap

There is a primary care physician shortage that is projected in the near future, and NPs and NMHCs are well positioned to fill this gap in primary care provision, as evidenced in this book. With now 4 decades of research, the evidence is clear that NPs provide care of comparable quality with physicians, and they have proven themselves as effective safety net providers, having served families with little or no health insurance for over 2 decades. When compared with like providers, nurse-managed centers have demonstrated higher rates of generic prescriptions and lower rates of hospitalizations than like providers, as well as parity in the rate of emergency room visits per 1000 members and use of appropriate medications for people with asthma. They see their members an average of 1.8 times more than other providers (NNCC, 2005b). Finally, NP salaries are 30–50% less than those of family practice physicians, thus lowering the cost of care. From a business perspective, it makes NPs a competitive alternative to family physicians, which helps position the profession as the future of primary health care.

CURRENT AND HISTORIC CHALLENGES TO FINANCIAL SUSTAINABILITY

Essential to the mission of NMHCs is providing holistic care to the underserved, which includes caring for the uninsured and providing health-enabling services, such as transportation to appointments, health education, outreach, and so on. The major challenge to the financial sustainability of NMHCs is that the level of reimbursement for services provided by third-party payers, usually Medicaid capitation in the case of nurse-managed centers, is not adequate to compensate for the amount of free care provided to uninsured clients, and currently does not cover the cost of enabling services. Recall that at least a third, but often as many as half, of the clients are uninsured and unable to pay even a minimal amount for their health care.

In the case of formally designated safety net providers, for example, the CHCs and FQHCs, the U.S. Congress has addressed the shortcomings of the managed care capitation system by creating a cost-based reimbursement system, entitled the prospective payment system (PPS). Under PPS, a provider is reimbursed for the entire cost of the services provided to Medicaid and Medicare patients, as long as the cost of these services does not exceed a predetermined amount set by state governments. For example, the average Medicaid-managed care capitation cost is $12 per month, compared with $135 per visit in a health center that has been successful in qualifying for PPS. Receiving PPS reimbursement is highly advantageous for safety net providers, because the higher level of reimbursement helps compensate for care for the uninsured. In the case of NMHCs, many were initially able to cover the cost of caring for the uninsured and medically underserved through start-up grants from the Bureau of Health Professions, Division of Nursing (DON) under Title VIII, but once that funding ended, they were challenged to compensate for uninsured care and looked for ways to receive a higher level of reimbursement. PPS was one potential, but difficult-to-obtain solution, without becoming an FQHC or an FQHC look-alike.

FEDERALLY QUALIFIED HEALTH CENTERS

An **FQHC** is a reimbursement designation referring to several health center programs funded under the Health Center Consolidation Act (Section 330 of the Public Health Service Act). They are nonprofit, community-based organizations that provide comprehensive primary care and preventive care, including oral, and mental health/substance-abuse services to persons of all ages, regardless of their ability to pay, and include several kinds of centers:

1. CHCs that serve a variety of Federally designated medically underserved area/populations (MUA or MUP).
2. Community Migrant Health Centers (CMHCs) that serve migrant and seasonal agricultural workers.
3. Health Care for the Homeless Programs that provide primary and preventive care and substance abuse services to homeless individuals and families.
4. Public Housing Primary Care Programs that serve residents of public housing and are located in or adjacent to the communities they serve.

Section 330 requirements mandate that FQHCs operate under a consumer Board of Directors' governance structure and function under the supervision of the Health Resources and Services Administration, which is part of the United States Department of Health and Human

Services. Although they provide services regardless of ability to pay, they do charge a fee according to a community-board-approved sliding-fee scale, based on patients' family income and size. In addition to PPS reimbursement, FQHCs receive additional financial benefits, free malpractice coverage under the Federal Tort Claims Act (FTCA), and sometimes an additional cash grant to subsidize care for the uninsured. In addition to FQHCs, the government also designates a category of health centers as "FQHC Look-Alikes." These health centers receive cost-based reimbursement for their Medicaid services, but do not receive malpractice coverage under FTCA or a cash grant (Taylor, 2004).

Obtaining FQHC Designation

Currently, the only way for nurse-managed primary care centers to receive PPS reimbursement is to become an FQHC. Unfortunately, centers operated by schools of nursing within private colleges and universities have been unable to apply for this designation, because they could not comply with the FQHC governance requirement that they be governed by a board, at least half of whom were consumers of the center, and that the board not be appointed by a single entity (e.g., the university). To meet the funding criteria for an HRSA Division of Nursing Special Projects grant, the center had to be established under the governance of the school of nursing, which was ultimately governed by the university. Thus, the institutional governance issue (ownership and control of the health center residing within the School of Nursing, and ultimately, the University Board of Trustees) historically prevented academic-based NMHCs from successfully applying for federal funding under the Consolidated Health Center Plan and Section 330, Community Health Center funding. Although most centers established community advisory boards for oversight purposes, these boards were not sufficient to meet legal governance requirements.

In spite of these challenges, 14 of the 150 NMHCs in the country are FQHCs. A few were established originally as health centers that served a homeless population or were a public housing primary care center and met other Section 330 requirements, enabling them to become federally qualified. Others became FQHCs through acquisition by existing FQHCs, through partnerships, or by developing contractual arrangements with existing FQHCs (King, 2008).

Congress has recognized the tremendous financial challenges NMHCs face, "encouraging the Health Resources and Services Administration to provide alternative means to secure cost-based (or PPS) reimbursement for nurse-managed health centers" (NNCC, 2005b, p. 5). However, to date, HRSA has not changed its policies. Consquently, a great number of these Division of Nursing-funded health centers have closed or risk closing, because they are not able to receive prospective payment for their Medicaid or Medicare populations to off-set their losses for serving a high uninsured population. Without a more permanent solution, such as a vehicle to obtain PPS or reimbursement at a level higher than traditional Medicaid managed care reimbursement, these health centers providers will likely close. In the Philadelphia area, for example, the four academic-based NMHCs faced with this predicament ultimately either transferred ownership of the health center's primary care services to a nurse-managed center that was an FQHC, or forged an affiliation agreement with an FQHC, in order to survive (King, 2008). Whereas such a strategy is not without numerous challenges, it has enabled all four centers to continue to grow and serve the needs of their communities.

THE FUTURE OF NURSE-MANAGED HEALTH CENTERS AND POLICY RECOMMENDATIONS

As of 2009, with a nation in an economic downturn, a health care system in crisis, and a new governmental administration, many changes in the health care service and reimbursement systems can be anticipated and hoped for. Although the United States has made several unsuccessful attempts to achieve universal coverage, the Institute of Medicine (2004) and many others believe that a major policy effort will be required at the federal level to ensure that everyone has access to health insurance. Although the current political climate may not be ripe for all of these recommendations, safety net providers, such as NMHCs, along with CHCs, could provide the basis for universal primary health care in the United States. If adequate funding were available to NMHCs, like their federally qualified CHC counterparts, both of these safety net providers would be financially secure and able to provide adequate health care coverage to vulnerable populations.

Despite NMHCs' effectiveness as safety net providers, they struggle financially, as the majority of them can not qualify to become an FQHC, the only avenue to PPS. Furthermore, in some regions of the country, managed care companies and third-party payers exclude NMHCs from their primary care provider panels, thus preventing them from receiving any reimbursement for care provided. In order for NMHCs to continue to provide primary health care services in underserved areas, the federal government must create mechanisms for NMHCs to become federally qualified, thereby enabling them to obtain PPS. In addition, managed care companies need to recognize NPs as primary care providers and contract with them, thereby placing them on equal financial footing with family physicians and with CHCs.

Interestingly, the U.S. Secretary of Health and Human Services, under existing Congressional authority, is in a position to grant waivers and give NMHCs PPS status. However, Secretaries have failed to act on this authority. Similarly, if the federal and state governments were to enforce existing antiprovider discrimination laws, and to take a stronger stance against Medicaid- and Medicare-managed care contractors who discriminate against NPs on the basis of licensure, NMHCs could obtain primary care contracts with third-party payers. Alternatively, passing a federal law mandating that states enforce the congressional intent of the Balanced Budget Act of 1997, requiring Medicaid-managed care companies to credential NPs as primary care providers, would also have a positive impact on these practices.

Now, more than ever, NMHCs are in a unique bargaining position to offer an alternative, cost-effective, safety net provider option for state governors to consider. Nevertheless, the future of the nurse-managed model of care still depends upon a place at decision-making tables to ensure that favorable health policies related to PPS and third-party reimbursement, funding mechanisms to pay for caring for the uninsured and underinsured, credentialing of NPs, and regulations regarding NP practice are enacted. Increasing the visibility of nurse-managed centers, cultivating relationships with influential governmental officials, monitoring forthcoming changes in the health care delivery system and being strategically prepared for them, mobilizing centers nationwide, and implementing strategies to strengthen the position of nurse-managed centers as mainstream health care providers will be vital. NMHCs have been compared with the hospice movement, which is now an integrated and well-funded service by Medicaid and Medicare, and judging from the latter movement's success, the future of nurse-managed centers looks very promising.

REFERENCES

American Association of Colleges of Nursing. (2000) *Nurse practitioners: The growing solution in health care delivery.* Retrieved July 30, 2009, from http://www.aacn.nche.edu/Media/Backgrounders/npfact.htm

Barger, S. E., Nugent, K. E., & Bridges, W. C. (1993). Schools with nursing centers: A 5 year follow-up study. *Journal of Professional Nursing, 9,* 7–13.

Bartlett, M. (2009). *The frontier nursing service: America's first rural nurse-midwife service and school.* Jefferson, NC: McFarland.

Boettcher, J. H. (1996). Nurse practice centers in academia: An emerging subsystem. *Journal of Nursing Education, 35,* 63–68.

Campbell, L. (2003). *Out of the briar patch: Diffusion and sustainability of nurse-managed practice.* Unpublished doctoral dissertation, University of Michigan, Ann Arbor.

Clear, J. B., Starbecker, M. M., & Kelly, D. W. (1999). Nursing centers and health promotion: A federal vantage point. *Family & Community Health, 21*(4), 1–14.

Coleman, S., & Hansen-Turton, T. (2003). Going national: National Nursing Centers Consortium. *Advance for Nurses, 11*(5), 14–18.

Glass, L. K. (1989). *The historical origins of nursing centers.* New York: National League for Nursing.

Hansen-Turton, T. (2005). The nurse-managed health center safety net: A policy solution to reducing health disparities. *Nursing Clinics of North America, 40,* 729–734.

Hansen-Turton, T., Line, L., O'Connell, M., & Rothman, N. (2005, Winter/Spring). NNCC releases a congressional commissioned evaluation report about nurse-managed centers. *National Nursing Centers' Consortium Update, 1,* 24–27.

Hansen-Turton, T., Line, L., O'Connell, M., Rothman, N., & Lauby, J. (2004, June). *The nursing center model of health care for the underserved.* Unpublished report submitted to the United States Health Care Financing Administration, Washington, DC.

Hansen-Turton, T., Ryan, S., Miller, K., Counts, M., & Nash, D. (2007). Convenient care clinics: The future of accessible health care. *Disease Management, 10*(2), 61–73.

Henry J. Kaiser Family Foundation. (2006). *Employer health benefits 2006 annual survey.* Retrieved July 30, 2009, from http://www.kff.org/insurance/7527/

Institute for Nursing Centers. (2004). *Aggregate survey report.* Okemos, MI: Author.

Institute of Medicine. (2004). *Insuring America's health: Principles and recommendations.* Washington, DC: National Academy Press.

King, E. S. (2005). *Nurse-managed health care funding initiative: Accomplishments, and current status.* Unpublished report, Independence Foundation, Philadelphia, PA.

King, E. S. (2008). A 10 year review of four academic nurse-managed centers: Challenges and survival strategies. *Journal of Professional Nursing, 24,* 14–20.

Matherlee, K. (1999). *The nursing center in concept and practice: Delivery and financing issues in serving vulnerable people.* (National Health Policy Forum Issue Brief No. 746).

National Nursing Centers Consortium [NNCC]. (2005a, March 18). *Congressional briefing*. Philadelphia: Author.

National Nursing Centers Consortium [NNCC]. (2005b). *Nurse-managed health centers*. Retrieved on July 30, 2009, from http://www.nncc.us/about/nmhc.html

Starbecker, M. M. (2000, September). *Historical perspective of Division of Nursing legislation*. Paper presented at the Health Services and Resources Administration, Division of Nursing, Nurse-Managed Centers Grantee meeting, Chevy Chase, MD.

Sullivan, E., Fields, B., Kelly, J., & Whelan, E. M. (1993). Nursing centers: The new arena for advanced nursing practice. In M. D. Mezey & D. O. McGivern (Eds.), *Nurses, nurse practitioners: Evolution to advanced practice* (pp. 251–264). New York: Springer Publishing Company.

Taylor, J. (2004, August 31). *The fundamentals of community health centers* (National Health Policy Forum background paper). Washington, DC: George Washington University.

U.S. Senate Appropriations Committee. (2005). *Senate Report 108-345* (p. 37).

Zachariah, R., & Lundeen, S. P. (1997). Research and practice in an academic community nursing center. *Image: Journal of Nursing Scholarship, 29*, 255–260.

14

The Pediatric Nurse Practitioner and the Child With Type 1 Diabetes: Partnership and Collaboration

TERRI H. LIPMAN

Nurse practitioners (NPs) play a vital role in the care of children and adolescents who live with diabetes mellitus. Because of their expertise in combining patient education with patient care, NPs provide diabetes management in the primary care setting, or as part of a multidisciplinary diabetes specialty team (Ward, 1998). Unlike the treatments for many chronic disorders, insulin doses for children vary widely and require frequent adjustment. NPs can legally prescribe diabetes medications, order diagnostic tests, and refer patients for consultations, unlike diabetes nurses who are not educated with advanced practice (Seley, Furst, Gray, Jornsay, & Wohl, 1999). The independence of NPs allows them to manage patient care using a telecommunication system, to provide access to diabetes care for children in a wide geographic area (Marrero et al., 1995), and provide coping-skills training for children and adolescents to improve metabolic control and quality of life (Grey, Boland, Davidson, Li, & Tamborlane, 2000).

Type 1 diabetes is the second most common chronic disease of childhood. It affects approximately 1 in 500 school-aged children (Lipman et al., 2006). Diabetes management is complex, and to be successfully managed requires collaboration among the health care team, the child, and the family. The goal of diabetes management is maintaining excellent metabolic control while allowing the child to live as normally as possible and to engage in age-appropriate activities. As diabetes care becomes more complex, education for the patient and family is increasingly necessary to provide the full spectrum of care. NPs provide care that is patient- and family-centered, and integrates the health, environment, culture, and socioeconomic needs of patients with diabetes. With the authority and autonomy to monitor, diagnose, and treat, NPs have a full scope of skills to ensure that children with diabetes have the best possible outcomes and quality of life.

The role of the NP includes counseling, education, and diabetes self-management training, with an emphasis on daily problem-solving skills (Fain, 2003). The pediatric NP in diabetes is a critical provider in the care of children with diabetes. Data have demonstrated improved diabetes outcomes for children followed in an NP-directed practice versus a physician-directed practice (Pishdad, Pishdad, & Pishdad, 2007), possibly because NPs are likely to practice evidence-based diabetes management (Ohman-Strikland et al., 2008). Several key areas of research guide the NP practice of children with diabetes.

THE DIABETES COMPLICATIONS AND CONTROL TRIAL

The findings of the Diabetes Complications and Control Trial (DCCT), a 9-year multicenter prospective study of 1500 patients with diabetes who were 13–39 years old at the start of the study, changed diabetes management. The patients were randomized into an intensive treatment group and a conventional therapy group. Intensive therapy was defined as a minimum of three insulin injections per day or the use of an insulin infusion pump. The researchers found that intensive therapy delayed the onset of retinopathy by 62%. Clinically significant neuropathy was reduced by 60%, and the development of clinical-grade albuminuria was reduced by 56% (The Diabetes Control and Complications Trial Research Group, 1993). It is crucial to note that the patients in the intensive therapy group were continuously involved in ongoing education and support in all aspects of diabetes management.

Because of the results of this study, tighter blood glucose control (i.e., glycosylated hemoglobin level $\geq 7\%$) is now the goal of diabetes management. The majority of children with diabetes are managed using multiple daily insulin injections or a continuous subcutaneous insulin infusion (CSII), known as an insulin pump, frequent blood glucose monitoring, carbohydrate counting, and a plan for activity. All of these components must be integrated to maintain near-normal blood glucose levels, and extensive education is involved. When children are cared for by NPs, the goal of diabetes education is to provide the family with the skills to empower them to manage the disease (Sullivan-Bolyai, Knafl, Deatrick, & Grey, 2003).

SCREENING FOR COMPLICATIONS AND COMORBIDITIES OF DIABETES

Type 1 diabetes is a disease with a number of complications and comorbidities. Diabetes complications include retinopathy, nephropathy, hypertension, hyperlipidemia, and neuropathy; the most common comorbidities are thyroid disease and celiac disease. A major issue for the NP is to both adhere to the guidelines of the American Diabetes Association for screening for the complications and comorbidities (American Diabetes Association, 2009) and adapt and integrate these guidelines for pediatric care (Montgomery & He, 2006). Current diabetes guidelines recommend regular screening for hyperlipidemia, retinopathy, celiac disease, thyroid disorders, microalbuminuria, and neuropathy in children and adolescents. In a study of family care practices, those practices employing NPs were more likely to measure lipid levels and urinary microalbumin levels (Ohman-Strikland et al., 2008).

Psychosocial and Developmental Issues

A role of the NP is to gear diabetes management to the developmental level of the child (Lipman et al., 1989). Developmental issues include sleep, dietary patterns, toileting, school matters, peer pressures, and, in adolescence, disordered eating, alcohol and drugs, and sexuality. Parents may have feelings of guilt related to the disease and its treatment, affecting discipline and limit-setting. Parents are often overprotective, which has an impact on decisions related to child care and sleepovers. Behavioral interventions to improve the coping skills of the child with diabetes improves metabolic control and quality of life (Grey, Boland, Davidson, Li, & Tamborlane, 2000), and family interventions may be helpful in reducing parent–child conflict about diabetes management and care. The pediatric NP is also focused on the successful transition of adolescents with diabetes from the children's health care service into the adult health care service (Fleming, Carter, & Gillebrand, 2002).

RACIAL DISPARITIES IN DIABETES
DIAGNOSIS, TREATMENT, AND OUTCOMES

African American and Hispanic children in the United States have the same or higher risk of developing diabetes as non-Hispanic White persons (Lipman, 1993; Lipman, Chang, & Murphy, 2002; Lipman et al., 2006). The enormous financial and social costs of childhood diabetes are likely to disproportionately affect minority families, because they are overrepresented among the poor in the United States (U.S. Census Bureau, 2009).

African American children with type 1 diabetes have poorer metabolic control (Auslander, Thompson, Dreitzer, White, & Santiago, 1997; Chalew et al., 2000; Delamater et al., 1999; Lipman et al., 2001).

Diabetes control in childhood has an impact on childhood mortality and sets the stage for outcomes in adults. Data from Chicago demonstrated a 9-fold increased risk of death for young African Americans with diabetes in Chicago, compared with non-Hispanic Whites with type 1 diabetes (Lipton, Good, Mikhailov, Freels, & Donoghue, 1999). In addition, there are racial differences in the goals and priorities of families of children with diabetes (Corbin, Ginsburg, Murphy, & Lipman, 2008; Ginsburg et al., 2005). Attention to these family issues must be integrated into the diabetes plan. The goal of the pediatric diabetes NP is to collaborate with all families to develop a plan of care that is culturally relevant and is based on the family's objectives.

SUMMARY: A MULTIDISCIPLINARY
APPROACH TO MANAGEMENT

Diabetes is a complex disorder requiring education, support, and collaboration from all members of the diabetes team, and is a unique disorder, in that the majority of management tasks and decisions occur in the home. Therefore, it is essential that the child and family be the center of the diabetes team. Self-care and a perception of family control over the disorder are hallmarks of successful diabetes management. Scheduling, meal plans, and interventions should be based on the activities, priorities, and culture of the family. The individualized approach is crucial.

Members of the diabetes team should include an advanced-practice nurse, a pediatric endocrinologist, dietician, social worker, psychologist, pediatrician, school nurse, and teacher. Frequent communication and periodic team meetings facilitate the sharing of information and the development of flexible management plans. The team must always be mindful that the family and the child are the experts in determining the child's short-term and long-term goals. The major goal of the other members of the diabetes team is to facilitate and support the actualization of the child's and family's goals.

REFERENCES

American Diabetes Association. (2009). Clinical practice recommendations. *Diabetes Care, 32*(Suppl. 1).

Auslander, W. F., Thompson, S., Dreitzer, D., White, N. H., & Santiago, J. V. (1997). Disparity in glycemic control and adherence between African-American and Caucasian youths with diabetes: Family and community contexts. *Diabetes Care, 20,* 1569–1575.

Chalew, S. A., Gomez, R., Butler, A., Hempe, J., Compton, T., Mercante, D., et al. (2000). Predictors of glycemic control in children with type 1 diabetes: The importance of race. *Journal of Diabetes and its Complications, 14*(2), 71–77.

Corbin, R., Ginsburg, K., Murphy, K. M., & Lipman, T. H. (2008, March). *The focus is on the family: Utilizing focus groups to assess perceptions of trust in diabetes treatment and outcomes.* Paper presented at the Annual Scientific Meeting of the Eastern Nursing Research Society, Philadelphia, PA.

Delamater, A. M., Shaw, K. H., Applegate, E. B., Pratt, I. A., Eidson, M., Lancelotta, G. X., et al. (1999). Risk for metabolic control problems in minority youth with diabetes. *Diabetes Care, 22*(5), 700–705.

The Diabetes Control and Complications Trial Research Group. (1993, September 30). The effect of intensive treatment of diabetes on the development and progression of long-term complications in insulin-dependent diabetes mellitus. *New England Journal of Medicine, 329*(14), 977–986.

Fain, J. A. (2003). It's time to recognize the importance of advanced practice care in diabetes. *Diabetes Education, 29*(4), 526.

Fleming, E., Carter, B., & Gillibrand, W. (2002). The transition of adolescents with diabetes from the children's health care service into the adult health care service: A review of the literature. *Journal of Clinical Nursing, 11*(5), 560–567.

Ginsburg, K. R., Howe, C. J., Jawad, A. F., Buzby, M., Tuttle, A., & Murphy, K. M. (2005). Parents' perceptions of factors that affect successful diabetes management for their children. *Pediatrics, 116,* 1095–1104.

Grey, M., Boland, E. A., Davidson, M., Li, J., & Tamborlane, W. V. (2000, July). Coping skills training for youth with diabetes mellitus has long-lasting effects on metabolic control and quality of life. *Journal of Pediatrics, 137*(1), 107–113.

Lipman, T. H. (1993). The epidemiology of Type I diabetes in children 0–14 years of age in Philadelphia. *Diabetes Care, 16,* 922–925.

Lipman, T. H., Chang, Y., & Murphy, K. M. (2002). The epidemiology of type 1 diabetes in children in Philadelphia 1990–1994: Evidence of an epidemic. *Diabetes Care, 25,* 1969–1975.

Lipman, T. H., DiFazio, D. A., Meers, R. A., & Thompson, R. L. (1989). A developmental approach to diabetes in children. Part I—Birth through preschool. *American Journal of Maternal Child Nursing, 14,* 255–259.

Lipman, T. H., Jawad, A., Murphy, K., Katz, L. L., Fuchs-Simon, J., Tuttle, A., et al. (2001). Incidence of type 1 diabetes in Philadelphia is higher in black than white children from 1995–2000: Epidemic or misclassification? *Diabetes, 50,* A39.

Lipman, T. H., Jawad, A., Murphy, K., Tuttle, A., Thompson, R., Radcliffe, S., et al. (2006). Incidence of type 1 diabetes in Philadelphia is higher in black than white children from 1995–1999: Epidemic or misclassification? *Diabetes Care, 29,* 2391–2395.

Lipton, R., Good, G., Mikhailov, T., Freels, S., & Donoghue, E. (1999). Ethnic differences in mortality from insulin-dependent diabetes mellitus among people less than 25 years of age. *Diabetes Care, 25,* 1969–1975.

Marrero, D. G., Vandagriff, J. L., Kronz, K., Fineberg, N. S., Golden, M. P., Gray, D., et al. (1995). Using telecommunication technology to manage children with diabetes: The computer-linked outpatient clinic (CLOC) study. *Diabetes Education, 21*(4), 313–319.

Montgomery, K., & He, W. (2006). Implementation of a clinical practice guideline for identification of microalbuminuria in the type 1 pediatric patient. *Journal of Pediatric Nursing, 21*(3), 235.

Ohman-Strickland, P. A., Orzano, J. A., Hudson, S. V., Solberg, I. L., DiCiccio-Bloom, B., O'Malley, D., et al. (2008). Quality of diabetes care in family medicine practices: Influence of nurse-practitioners and physician's assistants. *Annals of Family Medicine, 6,* 14–22.

Pishdad, G. R., Pishdad, R., & Pishdad, P. (2007). A nurse-managed diabetes care programme. *International Journal of Clinical Practice, 61*(9), 1492–1497.

Seley, J. J., Furst, P., Gray, T., Jornsay, D., & Wohl, N. R. (1999). The diabetes nurse 18.04actitioner: Promoting partnerships in care. *Diabetes Spectrum, 12*(2), 113–117.

Sullivan-Bolyai, S., Knafl, K., Deatrick, J., & Grey, M. (2003). Maternal management behaviors for young children with type 1 diabetes. *American Journal of Maternal Child Nursing, 28*(3), 160–166.

U.S. Census Bureau. *Historical poverty tables.* Retrieved May 20, 2009, from http://www.census.gov/hhes/www/poverty/histpov/hstpov2.html

Ward, J. F. (1998, June). Children and adolescents with diabetes mellitus. *Nurse Practitioner Forum, 9*(2), 94–97.

15 Adult Health and Gerontology Nurse Practitioner Care

MELISSA A. TAYLOR AND CHRISTINE BRADWAY

For over 10 years, students enrolled in the University of Pennsylvania School of Nursing's Adult Health Nurse Practitioner (AHNP) or Gerontology Nurse Practitioner (GNP) programs have had the option of following a dual-track curriculum model. This model was developed in the 1990s in response to requests from graduates, our understanding of expanding nurse practitioner (NP) roles and scope of practice, and growing interest of students applying to either the AHNP or GNP programs. Upon completion, dual-track graduates are eligible to sit for both of the current Adult and Gerontology NP national certification examinations (Cotter, Bradway, Cross, & Taylor, 2009). Our experiences with these students have been overwhelmingly positive. We continue to be in contact with many who have completed the dual-track curriculum, have closely followed their clinical practice experiences and careers, and have benefited from their continued engagement and collaboration to precept current University of Pennsylvania NP students. We believe these experiences will also serve us well and should be shared, particularly in light of the recently proposed advanced practice registered nurse (APRN) model (APRN Consensus Work Group & the National Council of State Boards of Nursing [NCSBN] APRN Advisory Committee, 2008). The exemplar case presented here highlights: (a) a brief review of features of the APRN model that specifically apply to adult and gerontology NPs; (b) an example from the first author's (MT) clinical practice; and (c) comments and recommendations for future education and evaluation of the adult–gerontology NP role.

FEATURES OF THE APRN ROLE SPECIFICALLY RELATED TO THE ADULT–GERONTOLOGY POPULATION FOCI

During the early to mid-1990s, the NCSBN APRN Committee (formerly APRN Advisory Board) developed a position paper on the regulation of advanced-nursing practice, and began work with APRN certifiers to make examinations more suitable for regulatory purposes. By the early 2000s, the NCSBN also initiated dialogue with other APRN stakeholder groups (APRN Consensus Work Group & the NCSBN APRN Advisory Committee, 2008). These discussions eventually led to collaborative work between educators, accreditors, certifiers, and licensers, and in 2008, dissemination of the *Consensus Model for APRN Regulation: Licensure, Accreditation, Certification & Education* (APRN Consensus Work Group & the NCSBN APRN Advisory Committee, 2008). This document details a newly developed regulatory model for APRN practice, education, certification, licensure, and accreditation. It includes four distinct APRN roles (certified NP [CNP], clinical nurse specialist [CNS], nurse anesthetist, nurse midwife) and nine areas of population foci, one of which is adult–gerontology (APRN Consensus Work Group & the NCSBN APRN Advisory Committee, 2008; Johnson, Dawson, & Brassard, 2010). According to this model, by December 31, 2015, all "graduates applying for APRN licensure must meet the stipulated licensure requirements" (Advanced Practice [APRN] Committee, 2008, p. 65). A key component of the model is that the Adult–Gerontology CNP or CNS will be prepared to care for young, middle-aged, older, and frail individuals; moreover, any APRNs in all of the four roles who provide care to adults "must be prepared to meet the growing needs of the older adult population" (APRN Consensus Work Group & the NCSBN APRN Advisory Committee, 2008, p. 9). The following example highlights the educational and clinical preparation of a current dually certified adult and gerontology NP, and how this role has been integrated into a typical internal medicine outpatient practice setting.

BACKGROUND OF ADULT AND GERONTOLOGY ROLES

A common clinical role for a dually prepared Adult–Gerontology Nurse Practitioner (AGNP) is providing care for patients in primary care practices with physicians who may specialize in either internal or family medicine, and in various geriatric settings (long-term-care facilities, assisted-living facilities, and continuing-care retirement communities [CCRCs]). One advantage of this role is the ability to manage and follow patients across systems at different levels of care. Because NPs are broadly trained across multiple settings, and in family theory and context, they use this knowledge along with their basic nursing experience to manage the care of the patient in the context of the family unit. Family-focused care enables the NP to provide, assess, and manage the individual patient in relationship to the patient's role as parent, child, or grandparent, and provide care that is developmentally sound. The following example is a typical clinical case that highlights the AGNP role in caring for a complex older adult and the family members over an extended period of time, and through a number of care-setting transitions.

Clinical Case of Ms. E.

Outpatient Visit

Ms. E. is an 86-year-old female who resides in the independent section of a CCRC. Being an NP dually certified in adult and gerontology care enables the provider to take care of several family members of different generations. For the last 2 years, Ms. E., her husband, daughter, and son-in-law have been followed by the same NP. The AGNP provides acute, chronic, and well visits for Ms. E.'s family members. Through these various patient encounters, the NP has become very familiar with this family, both as individual members and as a unit. The NP was also able to provide care for Ms. E. across several settings when Ms. E. experienced an illness, coordinate care with the family members who also were her patients, and intercede in a more streamlined manner than if she only saw the patient in one setting and did not know the patient within the context of her family. For example, she knew that Ms. E.'s daughter, Ms. C., helped Ms. E. and her husband with food shopping and errands. Ms. E.'s daughter was relatively healthy at 55 years of age, but recently had a biopsy of a breast cyst found on a routine mammography; the biopsy was negative. The NP was counseling Ms. C. about health promotion and the need for continued surveillance. Ms. E., who had multiple health problems, did not want to bother her daughter while she was concerned about her biopsy, tended to minimize some new symptoms that she was developing. The NP was aware of the mutual concern that the mother and daughter dyad had for one another, and was sensitive to both of their care needs and supported each of them through their currently evolving health needs. This case primarily focuses on the older Ms. E.'s care needs in the context of her family.

Ms. E.'s health history includes diagnoses of bipolar disorder, rheumatoid arthritis, hypothyroidism, hypertension, and osteoporosis. At a recent office visit, the AGNP examined her and found she was suffering from acute herpes zoster, with lesions extending down her right leg. The NP prescribed an oral antiviral agent for the patient, along with appropriate pain medications.

Home Visit

Over the course of a week, Ms. E. contacted the office multiple times requesting adjustments of her pain regimen. During a home visit, the AGNP identified that the zoster lesions were slowly resolving, yet Ms. E. continued to experience severe pain and had developed foot drop. Ms. E. refused any skilled therapy; however, she was agreeable to a home skilled nursing visit and physical therapy referral.

Hospitalization

Unfortunately, during the evening hours of the day of referral for home care, Ms. E. experienced a change in mental status and fell, sustaining a hip fracture. She was admitted to the local community hospital. Although all providers in the internal medicine practice (including the NP) are credentialed at this hospital, they do not make hospital rounds. Therefore, hospitalized patients are followed by a hospitalist service. Despite this, the NP was in constant contact with Ms. E.'s health care team and family throughout the hospital stay. In addition, she had a good relationship with the family, and was able to keep them informed and supported regarding Ms. E.'s care. Following hospitalization, Ms. E. was admitted to the long-term care section of the CCRC in which she resided for a skilled level of care. Her hospital discharge diagnoses were postherpetic neuralgia, foot drop, hip fracture, and urinary tract infection.

Skilled Care

One of the NP's collaborating physicians admitted Ms. E. to the skilled nursing facility (SNF). A few days later, the AGNP visited Ms. E. in the SNF for a follow-up visit. Since the NP has worked with Ms. E. in a variety of settings and with her family, she easily recognized that the patient's mental status and affect were quite different from her baseline. Ms. E. was very withdrawn and lacked interest in both eating and participating in therapies, both physical and occupational. The comprehensive NP visit included a review of her current chart, hospitalization records, and outpatient records. After reviewing the medical records and speaking with family, the AGNP determined that the patient's bipolar medications were significantly altered. She was no longer on the serotonin reuptake inhibitor (SSRI) that had stabilized her bipolar disorder for years. Instead, during her hospital stay, she was placed on a more current bipolar medication regimen. In collaboration with a geropsychiatrist, the NP slowly tapered off her present psychiatric medication regimen and restarted the previous SSRI.

Personal Care/Independent Living

After several weeks of skilled therapy, Ms. E. was discharged to her residential apartment in which 24-hour nursing care is available. She continued to receive extensive home physical therapy. With each week, she gained mental and physical strength. Eventually, she was able to discontinue personal assistance care and 24-hour nursing care. She now lives independently with her husband, and visits the internal medicine practice as an outpatient. Her daughter and son-in-law continue to be involved by providing transportation and shopping assistance, which is a function and role that they enjoy doing. Ms. E. continues to enjoy a stable health status, and has incorporated some new healthy lifestyles, such as walking exercise, recommended by the AGNP.

As an NP dually certified in adult health and gerontology, the NP is often able to follow patients and family members throughout various settings and stages of illness. Both certifications are beneficial to providing primary care for complicated patients of various age groups.

SUMMARY AND FUTURE RECOMMENDATIONS

From our experiences, and in light of recent recommendations (APRN Consensus Work Group & the NCSBN APRN Advisory Committee, 2008), we believe the future is bright for individuals educated, licensed, accredited, and certified in adult–gerontology population foci. As the United States and global population continues to age, we expect an even greater need for APRNs, including those who concentrate their practice on a variety of population foci (for example, the family/individual, women's health/gender-related, and psychiatric mental health APRNs), with an understanding of and expertise in adult health and gerontology. Competency recommendations are presently being developed by NP leaders in these areas, with a supportive grant from The John A. Hartford Foundation. In terms of education, many schools of nursing will need to revise current curricula and/or develop new programs to ensure that graduates are safe and competent in the concepts and skills regarding the adult–gerontology population. Moreover, alternate methods for identifying the appropriate number of clinical hours and mix of clinical experiences will also need to be evaluated and considered. For example, clinical evaluation tools for use in adult–gerontology CNP or other APRN roles need to be disseminated (Cotter, Bradway, Cross, & Talyor, 2009), revised, or developed. Finally, on a national level, certification, accreditation, licensure requirements, and examinations will need to be reviewed, and most likely revised or developed to accurately assess the knowledge base and skills of APRNs focusing on adult–gerontology populations.

REFERENCES

APRN Consensus Work Group & the National Council of State Boards of Nursing APRN Advisory Committee. (2008). *Consensus model for APRN regulation: Licensure, accreditation, certification & education.* Retrieved January 28, 2009, from www.ncsbn. org
Advanced Practice (APRN) Committee. (2008). *Report of advanced practice (APRN) committee.* Retrieved January 28, 2009, from www.ncsbn.org

Cotter, V. T., Bradway, C., Cross, D., & Taylor, M. (2009). Clinical evaluation tools for dual-track adult and gerontology nurse practitioner students. *Journal of the American Academy of Nurse Practitioners, 21*(12), 658–662.

Johnson, J., Dawson, E., & Brassard, A. (2010). Consensus model for APRN regulation: A new approach. In E. M. Sullivan-Marx, D. O. McGivern, J. A. Fairman, & S. A. Greenberg (Eds.), *Nurse practitioners: The evolution and future of advanced practice* (5th ed., pp. 125–142). New York: Springer Publishing Company.

16

Nurse Practitioner Contributions to HIV Care

CARL KIRTON

In 1980, HIV infection took the world by surprise: Here was a new disease, without any treatment, and suddenly the health care system was called upon to reengineer its delivery system to care for those affected by and caring for those with HIV disease. A new specialty role for the advanced-practice nurse emerged with the disease. The purpose of this chapter is to review the development of the role of the HIV/AIDS nurse practitioner (NP) in the context of the HIV epidemic. The current state of this field of specialization will be explored, along with a look toward the future.

HISTORICAL PERSPECTIVE

The first recognized cases of AIDS occurred in the United States in the early 1980s, when gay men in New York and California suddenly began to develop rare opportunistic infections and cancers that seemed stubbornly resistant to any treatment, and then swiftly took their lives. At this time, AIDS did not yet have a name, but it quickly became obvious that all the men were suffering from a common syndrome. The discovery of HIV, the human immunodeficiency virus, as the causative agent of this syndrome was made soon after (Bureau of Health Professions, Health Resources and Services Administration, U.S. Department of Health and Human Services, 2009).

HIV rapidly spread across the United States, fueled by international travel; unscreened blood transfusions; injection drug use, which became more prevalent in the 1970s; and the limited knowledge about the role that protected sexual activity plays in control of the spread of the virus. The 1980s was also a time of poor governmental response to this growing epidemic, and of fear and ignorance on the part of the health community, which resulted in the lack of a complete and comprehensive approach to the issues faced by individuals with HIV/AIDS. The AIDS epidemic took the health care community by surprise, and the fear of HIV infection created barbaric practices, archaic rituals, and an attempt to isolate those afflicted with this disease. Several moral issues confronted health care workers, such as duty to care for certain individuals or groups, the health care workers' right to refuse to care, and the growing risk of occupational exposure to this new virus. The AIDS epidemic represented a major challenge to the health care system, and required sweeping changes in health care practices.

Few health care systems were adequately prepared for the influx of patients with HIV disease. In New York City, the New York City Task Force on Single-Disease Hospitals was convened to consider the advantages and disadvantages of creating "AIDS hospitals" under the guise of "relieving overcrowding and to providing specialized care" (Rothman & Tynan, 1990). This notion was swiftly discarded when the committee reviewed the history of mental hospitals and tuberculosis sanitariums, in which patients and staff suffered from geographic and professional isolation (Rothman, 2007). The single-disease-hospital task force also recognized that patients with HIV required treatment by a wide range of specialists, including those in infectious diseases, pulmonary medicine, hematology, neurology, and oncology, "and that it would be almost impossible to assemble these resources" in new institutions (Rothman, 2007).

Some health care agencies responded to the HIV epidemic by congregating patients with HIV in units with dedicated staff who could respond quickly and who had interest in the evolving care paradigm of HIV practice. An advanced-practice clinician, Cliff Morrison, is credited with designing the first dedicated special care unit for people with HIV/AIDS at San Francisco General Hospital in 1983 (Helquist, Martin, &

Schietinger, 1999). This special unit, with integrated care and support services, became the "gold standard" for inpatient care, and was quickly duplicated across the country. On this unit, registered nurses (RNs) and clinical nurse specialists (CNSs) provided the care for its diverse and growing patient group. Many of the early advanced-practice clinicians were recruited from the oncology specialty practice, because of their expertise in managing the often-seen oncologic conditions early in the epidemic.

With the HIV epidemic rapidly expanding, states most burdened with a growing HIV population faced projected shortages of qualified clinicians to meet the growing provider needs, as well as the growing need to keep providers abreast of the expanding knowledge of this area of practice. The New York State Department of Health AIDS Institute (AI) responded by developing a 2-year fellowship program with clinical training and leadership development for physicians and NPs who could assume leadership roles in HIV-related direct care and program administration in New York State. In the early 1990s, schools of nursing throughout the country also responded by developing specialty tracks or minors in HIV/AIDS care within CNS or NP programs. Schools offering specialty nursing tracks included Hunter-Bellevue School of Nursing, Duke University, Columbia University, University of California, San Francisco, College of New Rochelle, and Massachusetts General Hospital Institute of Health Professions. Many of these programs continue today, and are instrumental in ensuring that a qualified pool of advanced-practice clinicians are prepared to care for the HIV population.

THE HIV/AIDS EPIDEMIC

The HIV/AIDS epidemic can best be characterized by two distinct eras: the period before the introduction of highly active antiretroviral therapies (HAART) (1980–1996) and the post-HAART era (1996–present). In the pre-HAART era, few effective therapies existed to effectively control viral replication and morbidity, and mortality from disease was high. During the pre-HAART period, the majority of HIV care was in acute care facilities using a dedicated unit or a scatter-bed approach to care. Hospitalization was necessary to diagnose and treat the various opportunistic infections seen at this time, and required consultation from infectious disease, pulmonary medicine, hematology, neurology, and oncology specialists.

Notwithstanding the model of care, NPs were often part of the team, and in many cases, were the direct care providers. Acute care NPs (ACNPs) required a skill set that consisted of pain management and palliative care, knowledge in the ordering and administration of chemotherapeutics and treatment of opportunistic infections, end-of-life care such as controlling symptoms, providing emotional support, dealing with financial and insurance issues, and assisting mothers with permanency planning for their children after their deaths.

Few programs of NP preparation had the expertise or the where-withal to keep pace with the rapidity or evolution of the advances that were being made in this field. The Association of Nurses in AIDS Care (ANAC) was formed in 1982 to promote the professional development of nurses involved in the delivery of health care to those infected or affected by HIV. Although not an NP-only organization, ANAC was quickly embraced by NPs who, at the time, had limited professional support and a need to network with other nurses across the country who were immersed in this new field of specialization. Recognizing that few schools of nursing had the expertise to educate HIV nurses, ANAC sponsored regional faculty development programs across the country, designed to keep faculty in schools of nursing abreast of the changes in the field of HIV/AIDS, and assisted programs with tools and techniques to integrate HIV content across programs.

With the introduction of HAART, better treatment combinations emerged that suppressed viral replication and provided significant improvements in the immunologic health of people infected with HIV. Suddenly, the paradigm of HIV as a chronic disease emerged, and care of the people with HIV shifted from the acute care to the ambulatory setting. As this new paradigm emerged, dedicated AIDS units across the country were dismantled as fewer and fewer HIV patients required hospitalization. Many of their disorders could be treated or managed on an outpatient basis. ACNPs either shifted to other acute care specialties or shifted their practice to the ambulatory setting. As the chronic-care era of HIV grew, patients were living longer, and, at the same time, the science of HIV grew more complex. Clinicians learned more about viral dynamics, viral resistance, new drug combinations, and new co-morbidities.

Early in the epidemic, the HIV/AIDS Nursing Certification Board provided a certification examination for RNs who worked in HIV/AIDS, and in 2001, recognized that advanced-practice clinicians also possessed unique knowledge and expertise that could be tested and verified. The first advanced-practice examination was given in November 2003, and successful candidates use the credential AACRN, the acronym for Advanced AIDS-Certified Registered Nurse. Candidates for examination are RNs with advanced educational preparation (master's degree or higher) who function in advanced-practice roles, such as a CNS or NP, and demonstrate advanced knowledge, skill, and expertise in the practice of HIV/AIDS nursing (Relf, Berger, Crespo-Fierro, Mallinson, & Miller-Hardwick, 2004).

NPs can also demonstrate their HIV/AIDS expertise through credentialing by the American Academy of HIV Medicine (AAHIVM). AAHIVM is an independent organization with a diverse membership of HIV providers that includes advanced-practice clinicians. AAHIVM credentialing has been available since 2001 to both members and nonmembers of AAHIVM. Successful candidates are designated as an "HIV specialist," and approximately 10% of its members are NPs (Grossman, 2006). It is important to note that AAHIVM examination is one way to achieve the specialist credential. Some states have defined an HIV specialist by examination or by the number of hours of care or the number of patients in a caseload. An HIV specialist demonstrates competency in HIV, and is able to engage in the key activities listed in Exhibit 16.1.

QUALITY OF NP CARE IN HIV PRACTICE

More than 40 years of research has established that NPs provide high-quality, cost-effective, and personalized care. The body of evidence regarding the quality of NP practice supports that it is at least equivalent to that of physician care, and is discussed in this text. In a recent study comparing the quality of HIV care provided by advanced-practice clinicians with that of physicians (Wilson, Landon, & Hirschhorn, 2005), researchers found NP and physician assistant (PA) performance on eight quality measures of HIV care to be similar to or better than physicians, even after controlling for patient and HIV clinic characteristics. Under certain circumstances, these NPs and PAs provide HIV

Exhibit 16.1

EXPECTATIONS OF AN HIV SPECIALIST

An HIV specialist should have an understanding of and familiarity with the following areas:

- **Latest information about HIV disease and treatments.** Advances in antiretroviral therapy continue to make HIV a dynamic field. Data regarding new drugs and their combinations continue to emerge, changing standards of practice. Familiarity with these new drugs, their side effects, including treatment-related lipid disorders, and interactions with other drugs is a feature of basic HIV care.

- **State-of-the-art diagnostic techniques,** including quantitative viral measures and resistance testing.

- **Immune system monitoring.**

- **Strategies to promote treatment adherence,** including methods to elicit information about adherence from patients, techniques to measure adherence in clinical practice, and referral sources for adherence support services.

- **Management of opportunistic infections and diseases.** Basic familiarity with the clinical presentation and proper diagnostic approach to opportunistic diseases, and a strong grasp of the therapeutic strategies to manage them, are an essential part of basic HIV care.

- **Management of HIV-infected patients suffering from commonly associated comorbid conditions,** including tuberculosis, hepatitis B and C, and syphilis.

- **Access and referral to clinical trials.**

- **Postexposure prophylaxis protocols and infection control issues.**

- **Guidelines for prophylaxis to prevent vertical transmission and systems for referral to obstetrical providers with experience in management of HIV-infected pregnant women.**

- **Care coordination.** Proper referral to other providers for specialty care (e.g., oral, ophthalmologic, obstetrics, gynecology, dermatology, nutrition, drug treatment).

- **Patient education,** including risk reduction/harm reduction counseling.

- **Preconceptional counseling for women of childbearing age,** including knowledge of contraceptive methods and ways to prepare for a healthy pregnancy.

Exhibit 16.1 *(continued)*

EXPECTATIONS OF AN HIV SPECIALIST

EXPECTATIONS OF AN HIV SPECIALIST IN PEDIATRICS

The HIV specialist in pediatrics should collaborate with the mother's HIV specialist and obstetrical care provider to obtain maternal history prior to and during delivery.
In addition to the expectations of the medical specialist, an HIV specialist in pediatrics should have an understanding of:

- **Factors associated with perinatal HIV transmission,** including the impact of maternal viral load, antiretroviral therapy, mode of delivery, mode of feeding (breastfeeding versus bottle feeding), and **interventions to reduce transmission.**

- **Diagnostic testing schedule for the HIV-exposed infant,** including interpretation of HIV tests in the newborn, appropriate diagnostic tests, and recommended testing schedules.

- **The diagnosis, treatment, and prophylaxis of infections in HIV-infected and HIV-exposed infants, children, and adolescents.**

- **Immune system monitoring,** including an understanding of the normal range of CD4 counts in children at different ages.

- **Antiretroviral treatment of HIV-infected infants, children, and adolescents,** including timing of initiation, the pharmacokinetics of particular antiretroviral agents, appropriate antiretroviral combinations, adverse effects of medications, and adverse interactions of medications.

- **Regulatory requirements,** including those regarding expedited and newborn testing for newborns, and reporting and partner notification for adolescents.

- **Immunization schedules for HIV-infected infants and children,** as well as for non-infected infants and children living in homes with HIV-infected person(s).

- **Mental health, psychosocial, and educational needs of HIV-infected children and their families,** including those related to disclosure of the infection, loss of family members, sexual responsibility, and educational difficulties.

- **Adherence monitoring and support,** including barriers to adherence specific to children and adolescents of different ages and developmental levels, and approaches to overcome such barriers.

Note: Retrieved January 28, 2010, from http://www.hivguidelines.org/admin/Files/policy/hiv-spec-pol/HIV%20Specialist%20Report.pdf care similar to that of physician HIV specialists and infectious disease physicians, and better care than generalist physicians who are not HIV experts.

THE FUTURE OF HIV ADVANCED PRACTICE

Each year, approximately 50,000 individuals in the United States are infected with HIV, and it is estimated that approximately 1.2 million people are living with HIV/AIDS (Hall et al., 2008). Today, the care of the patient goes beyond the provision of a complex antiretroviral regimen and management of opportunistic infections; it includes the management of contemporary HIV comorbidities, such as hepatitis C, substance use, and cardiovascular, renal, and liver disease. Preconception care, once thought to be irrelevant in HIV care, is now a key part of the care of women of childbearing age. As people live longer with HIV, meeting the needs of older HIV adults is another emerging branch of HIV care. Ensuring the expansion of the HIV workforce to meet these, as well as other facets of HIV care, will be a significant challenge in the future. The American Academy of HIV Medicine has estimated that more than 32% of today's HIV clinicians will retire and stop providing care for HIV patients over the next 10 years (Gatty, 2009; Schouten & Sosman, 2009). The Bureau of Health Professions, Health Resources and Services Administration (HRSA) has launched an initiative to determine the capacity of the HIV primary care workforce, regionally and nationally; the focus will be on physicians, PAs, NPs, nurses, pharmacists, and dentists (Bureau of Health Professions, Health Resources and Services Administration, 2009). To address the needs of the declining HIV workforce, the Bureau of Health Professions plans to conduct a study that will address a number of issues, including discerning whether shortages in clinical personnel are HIV-specific or part of the larger primary care shortage; whether capacity and recruitment challenges are primarily urban, rural, or both; and whether there are distinct regional variations in HIV workforce patterns. Without a stable and qualified workforce, at a minimum, access to life-saving therapies will be severely restricted.

SUMMARY

Since the start of the HIV epidemic, NPs have been a part of the workforce responding to the evolving epidemic. HIV care that is of high quality, accessible to all in need, and provided by experienced practitioners is a shared goal of patients, providers, and policymakers. Empirical evidence exists that the care provided by NPs is equivalent to physicians in specialty practice, and in some cases, exceeds that of the generalist physician. Predicted shortages of qualified NPs to care for a growing elderly HIV population will be a significant challenge to HIV care in the future.

REFERENCES

Bureau of Health Professions, Health Resources and Services Administration, U.S. Department of Health and Human Services. (2009). Kaposi's sarcoma and pneumocystis pneumonia among homosexual men—New York City and California. *Morbidity and Mortality Weekly Report, 30*, 305–308. Retrieved April 5, 2009, from http://www.healthworkforceinfo.org/

Gatty, R. (2009). New AAHIVM survey warns of looming workforce shortages in HIV medicine. *HIV Specialist, 1*(1), 8–15.

Grossman, H. (2006). Addressing the need for HIV specialist: The AAHIVM perspective. *AIDS Reader, 16*, 479–486.

Hall, H. I., Ruiguang, S., Rhodes, P., Prejean, J., An, Q., Lee, L. et al. (2008). Estimation of HIV incidence in the United States. *Journal of the American Medical Association, 300*, 520–529.

Helquist, M., Martin, J. P., & Schietinger, H. K. (1999). *The AIDS epidemic in San Francisco: The response of the nursing profession, 1981–1984* (Vol. 1). Berkeley, CA: University of California.

Relf, M., Berger, B., Crespo-Fierro, M., Mallinson, R., & Miller-Hardwick, C. (2004). The value of certification in HIV/AIDS nursing. *Journal of Association of Nurses in AIDS Care, 15*(1), 60–64.

Rothman, D. J. (2007). The single disease hospital: Why tuberculosis justifies a departure that AIDS does not. *Journal of Law, Medicine & Ethics, 21*, 296–302.

Rothman, D. J., & Tynan, E. A. (1990). Advantages and disadvantages of special hospitals for patients with HIV infection: A report by the New York City Task Force on single-disease hospitals. *New England Journal of Medicine, 323*(11), 764–768.

Schouten, J., & Sosman, J. (2009). Who will care for them? Workforce shortages in primary care spills over to HIV medicine. *HIV Specialist, 1*(1), 6–7.

Wilson, I., Landon, B., & Hirschhorn, L. (2005). Quality of HIV care provided by nurse practitioners, physician assistants, and physicians. *Annals of Internal Medicine, 143*, 729–736.

17

Roles of Nurse Practitioners in the U.S. Department of Veterans Affairs

KAREN R. ROBINSON

Nurse practitioner (NP) roles, over the last several decades, have changed significantly as a result of altering patient needs and expectations, pressures related to reimbursement and managed care, a shift in the care delivery from hospital to community and home settings, a growth of patient advocacy, and changing attitudes about the role (Keane & Becker, 2004). The U.S. Department of Veterans Affairs (VA) employs the largest group of NPs in the country, and offers numerous opportunities for health care in multiple clinical settings and specialties. Because of the enormity of the VA and complexity of health care, it challenges NPs to develop their roles so they can meet the comprehensive needs of the veteran population. This chapter will detail how NPs in the VA have taken advantage of opportunities by using their critical thinking abilities and becoming creative in further advancing their roles. Additionally, challenges will be made to this group to provide leadership in the future that promotes health system effectiveness and optimal patient outcomes.

BACKGROUND

The VA, like other health care systems that recognized that NPs provide compassionate and competent care, first appointed them as primary

Table 17.1

THE DEPARTMENT OF VETERANS AFFAIRS DATA

Number of VA Employees	278,566
Number of Registered Nurses	43,533
Number of Nurse Practitioners	3,344
Number of VA Medical Centers	153
Number of Ambulatory Care and Community-Based	909
Outpatient Clinics	
Number of VA Nursing Homes	135
Number of VA Vet Centers	232
Number of VA Home Care Programs	108
Number of VA Residential Rehabilitation Treatment	45
Programs	
Projected U.S. Veterans Population	23 million
Projected U.S. Female Veterans Population	1.8 million
Number of Veterans treated in the VA Health Care System during FY 2008 (October 1, 2007–September 30, 2008)	5.5 million

Note: From http://www1.va.gov/opa/fact/vafacts.asp

providers of patient care in 1973. Headed by the Secretary of Veterans Affairs, the VA is the second largest of the 15 Cabinet departments, and operates nationwide programs for health care, financial assistance, and burial benefits. From 54 hospitals in 1930, when created by Executive Order 5398, the VA's health care system now has 153 hospitals, with at least 1 in each state, Puerto Rico, and the District of Columbia (Table 17.1). The VA health care facilities provide a broad spectrum of medical, surgical, and rehabilitative care (U.S. Department of Veterans Affairs, 2008a).

The VA has experienced considerable growth in the medical system workload over the past few years. The number of patients treated increased by 29%, from 4.2 million in 2001 to 5.5 million in 2008. By the end of fiscal year 2008, the VA's outpatient clinics registered over 60 million visits, and inpatient facilities treated 773,600 patients (U.S. Department of Veterans Affairs, 2008a).

Of the approximately 23 million veterans, the median age is 60 years, 7.5% are female, and Vietnam-era veterans represent the single largest period-of-service component, with Gulf War-era veterans second (*VA Organizational Briefing Book*, 2008). Major illnesses of these individuals include pulmonary disease, coronary artery disease, congestive heart failure, cancer, pneumonia, diabetes, substance abuse, and mental illness.

There are 3,344 NPs employed in the VA system representing 7.7% of the total RN workforce (U.S. Department of Veterans Affairs, 2008b). As the VA has responded to United States sector health issues such as professional shortages, increased technology, and interprofessional team care, innovation for NP roles within the VA have expanded. NPs are now employed in primary care, home, and acute settings, as well as in subspecialty and administrative areas. In these roles, NPs deliver essential and preventive care, providing patient and family education, and coordination of care. They provide specific services, such as obtaining medical histories and performing physical examinations. They are able to diagnose and treat many health problems. Others deliver employee health care at the VA and other work sites or care for special groups of patients with HIV infection, multiple sclerosis, and cancer (Robinson & Petzel, 2003; U.S. Department of Veterans Affairs, n.d.). An area of growing need is women's health care, as the number of women veterans has increased and they are increasingly eligible for service-connected benefits (U.S. Department of Veterans Affairs, 2008a). Many of the VA's women veterans' health coordinators are NPs. They provide annual gynecological examinations and follow-up medical procedures and coordination of services with other VA services.

The majority of NPs in the VA have a master's degree (approximately 97%), a national advanced clinical certification, and a license as an NP. The VA does continue to employ some NPs who were educated through other training programs and are not master's-prepared (approximately 3%). These individuals may have a more limited scope of practice (Under Secretary for Health, 1997, 1999). NPs have prescriptive authority to prescribe pharmacologic and nonpharmacologic treatments.

In 1996, the VA was transformed from an inpatient-based system into an outpatient-based primary care health network, doubling the need for VA nonphysician providers (U.S. Department of Veterans Affairs, 2008d). NPs certainly became key figures to this new care scheme, and were critical to the success of this organizational transformation, as evidenced by their progression from 43 NP positions in 1973 to approximately 1400 in 1997, and more were needed. At the same time, the VA Headquarters' Nursing Strategic Healthcare Group (NSHG) was aware of the shortage of NPs nationwide. VA facilities across the country were reporting difficulties in hiring NPs, and reported local programs had lengthy admission waiting lists. VA nurse executives were also reporting that some clinical nurse specialists (CNSs) were displaced from their inpatient practice. Based on all of these facts, the NSHG determined that an approach for increasing the number of NPs in the VA would be to educate existing CNSs as NPs through a postmaster's certificate program. Because the nurses were located across the country, a distance learning program seemed to be the way to proceed. The VA partnered with the Uniformed Services University of the Health Sciences Graduate School of Nursing (USU GSN). A total of 70 nurses from VA facilities across the United States, Puerto Rico, and the Virgin Islands graduated from the program (Beason, 2005).

The Advanced Practice Nurse Advisory Group (APNAG) was established to serve in an advisory capacity to the VA National Nursing Executive Council (NNEC). The mission of the APNAG is to provide a national focal point for information relating to issues pertinent to advanced-practice nurses (APNs) and their practice in VA facilities and clinics. Issues may involve licensure, use, roles, scope of practice, recruitment and retention, workload capture, and prescriptive authority.

EXAMPLES OF VA NURSE PRACTITIONERS' ROLES

With the support of VA leaders and innovation by VA NPs to address needs in the VA and work in collaborative teams, a variety of NP roles have evolved in the VA over the last 36 years. Some of the more specialized roles that have developed over time are in areas such as acute care, gastroenterology, interventional radiology, surgery, nephrology, neurosurgery, pain management, palliative care, and quality management. The following examples are intended to provide the readers more detailed information about some of the roles of NPs in the VA and how patient outcomes are achieved.

Compensation and Pension Examination Program

The VA is comprised of the Veterans Benefits, Veterans Health, and National Cemetery Administrations, which have important linkages in terms of providing veteran services. One such linkage is related to veterans' applications for compensation and pension (C&P) for injuries or medical conditions incurred or aggravated during active military service (U.S. Department of Veterans Affairs, 2008a).

A major factor in determining a veteran's C&P status is a clinical or disability examination, which can be conducted at most VA medical centers. Results of this examination are critical indicators of a veteran's health and burial benefits. The process is initiated when the veteran submits a claim for a condition to the Regional Office. The Regional Office would then request an examination relevant to the particular claim. Examinations are necessarily quite detailed and wide-ranging to assess and document a veteran's condition. Examiners must render assessments, in legally mandated language, regarding the claim and potential benefit. Upon completion, they are reviewed internally and returned to the Regional Office, whereby adjudicators assign percentages to the disability. At the Tucson, Arizona, VA Medical Center, seven APNs and two physicians, certified as Disability Examiners, provide these examinations to veterans. The group completes about 400 examinations per month, and achieves an audit average score of 94%, as compared with the national average of 90% (D. Rhoads, personal communication, December 23, 2008).

Complementary and Alternative Medicine Integrative Health Program

Similar to the U.S. population, veterans have been seeking a new approach to care of chronic illness that emphasizes holistic methods, prevention of disease, and wellness, as well the treatment of disease. Integrative health is a holistic model that brings together conventional allopathic health care with modalities and therapies that are under the classification of complementary and alternative medicine (CAM) (National Center for Complementary and Alternative Medicine [NCCAM], 2005).

Initial surveys on the use of CAM indicated over one-third of respondents reported that they had used at least one CAM therapy during the past year (Eisenberg et al., 1993). In a follow-up study, it was reported that there was a 25% increase in CAM use, from 33.8% in 1990 to 42.1% in 1997 (Eisenberg et al., 1998). CAM therapies were most frequently used for chronic conditions, such as back problems, anxiety, depression, and headaches.

An NP at the VA Medical Center in Salt Lake City, Utah, developed the Integrative Health Clinic and Program (IHCP) for veterans with chronic non-malignant pain and stress. The goal of the IHCP was to improve health-related quality of life (QOL) and lower pain-related psychopathology, such as depression and anxiety. The clinic provides holistic, nonpharmacological, mind–body and research-based CAM therapies within a conventional VA health care system. The IHCP therapies and classes include acupuncture, aquatic bodywork, choose-to-heal mind–body skills classes, herbal/supplement/drug interaction counseling, medical hypnosis, meditation, qigong, tobacco cessation, weight management classes, and yoga. In addition, the Native American sweat lodge, drumming ceremonies, and a healing garden fall under the umbrella of IHCP (Smeeding, 2009).

The NP at the Salt Lake City VA, as part of her requirements for the PhD in health promotion program, conducted an IHCP outcome study (Smeeding, 2009). The study results indicated that the Integrative Health program was effective in lowering depression and anxiety and improving health-related QOL in those with non-spinal-cord-related pain (joint pain, headache, and fibromyalgia), as compared with the spinal-cord-related pain group (back pain and neck pain). The spinal cord pain group had improvements in the health-related QOL category of bodily pain. The results suggested the nonpharmacological IHCP is an effective program for veterans with chronic non-malignant pain (Smeeding, 2009).

Gerontology/Extended Care Centers

Grzeczkowski and Knapp (1988) highlight one health corporation's definition of a gerontological NP as "a health provider, caring for patients who, by utilizing her/his nursing skills and knowledge of physical assessment and disease processes can reliably evaluate a patient's problems, formulate and execute a coherent plan for their management, in cooperation with a physician, but taking into consideration all the social and nursing aspects of the patient's problems" (p. 64C). Furthermore, they discussed a 6-month study conducted in a 120-bed facility that showed significant benefits to elderly patients after employment of a gerontological NP. Benefits included reduction of drug use, urinary tract and respiratory infections, indwelling catheter usage, and pressure-related skin breakdown. Positive outcomes, in terms of increases in discharges to home settings and patient/family satisfaction, were also reported.

Many VA gerontology NPs are employed in extended care centers that offer patient services such as skilled nursing care, rehabilitation therapies, reconditioning, radiation therapy, complex medical management, wound care, prosthetic training, management of geropsychiatric conditions, respite services, end-of-life care, spinal cord injury care, and comprehensive general geriatric evaluation and management. In these settings, NPs manage chronic diseases, as well as diagnose and treat acute diseases, with a focus on the holistic approach to meet the medical, social, and functional needs of older patients. In addition, NP activities include admission screening; history and physical examinations; prescribing medications, treatments, and procedures; program development; patient and staff education; local, state, and national leadership in committees related to nursing practice; preceptorship for graduate NP students; and research. Prescribing and admitting privileges can be included in their scope of practice (C. DePew, personal communication, January 16, 2009).

In many VA settings, gerontology NPs lead the interdisciplinary health care team, with the team collaboratively managing the veterans' care. The health care team consists of NPs, physicians, nurses, chaplains, dieticians, psychiatrists, and pharmacists, as well as recreational, physical, and occupational therapists. The role of NPs can be easily linked to the various members of the team, thereby providing them the advantage of connecting with each discipline and assuming the leadership position of the team (Smith, Vezina, & Samost, 2009). NPs possess the clinical expertise, knowledge, and abilities to be able to facilitate the team to maximize independent functioning, promote health, and enhance QOL for chronically ill, older veterans.

Home-Based Primary Care

The Eastern Colorado Health Care System Home-Based Primary Care Program is based at the Denver VA Medical Center. This program targets frail, chronically ill, older veterans who not only have frequent urgent and emergency care visits, but also prolonged hospital and rehabilitation stays and inadequate home support (North, Kehm, Bent, & Hartman,

2008). The interdisciplinary team offers evaluation, treatment, and supportive services provided by NPs, dietitians, occupational therapists, medical social services, and pharmacists. NPs on the team, functioning in the role of the patient's primary care provider, make home visits for evaluation and management purposes, as well as oversee coordination of care and follow-through of the care plan.

Interested in determining whether or not the program was making a difference, the team conducted a longitudinal study to assess the effects of an NP-directed home-based primary care program in regard to meeting standard performance measures, reducing hospitalizations and emergency department visits, and cost-effectiveness in managing a complex, elderly veteran population (North, Kehm, Bent, & Hartman, 2008). Inclusion criteria for use data included all patients who had been enrolled in the program for at least 12 months, and had received care at the Denver VA at least 12 months prior to enrollment in the home-based primary care program.

The group reported that the number of hospitalizations, emergency department visits, and "no show" appointments for 104 veterans receiving home-based primary care were all significantly lower ($p < 0.01$) as compared with use by the same group for 1 year before home-based primary care enrollment (North, Kehm, Bent, & Hartman, 2008). Most impressive was the 84% reduction that occurred in the number of hospitalizations. The number of emergency department visits and "no show" visits were each reduced by 48% and 46%, respectively. Total cost savings were over $1 million, with hospitalization reductions accounting for 98% of the cost saving.

Informatics

After spending several years developing a program called Veterans Health Information Systems and Technology Architecture (VistA), medical professionals within the VA in the late 1990s were able to electronically enter histories, physicals, and progress notes directly into a patient's medical record. With the advancement in this technology, the VA quickly became a leader in further developing the electronic medical record to ensure that critical patient information is not stored in a paper file somewhere, but is readily accessible to all providers who may see a veteran, and appropriately protects medical privacy. They implemented additional systems such as provider electronic order entry and clinical practice guidelines to further avoid medical mistakes, reduce costs, and improve care. "Clinical Reminders" became a mechanism for providers to use to ensure that health screenings would be completed according to the clinical practice guidelines.

An NP at the Dubuque, Iowa, VA Outpatient Clinic is employed as an Informatics Liaison working with clinical application coordinators and others to write clinical reminders that make sense to other NPs and physicians. She also educates new providers on how to use the computerized medical record, and demonstrates practical approaches to documentation (S. Timmerman, personal communication, January 16, 2009).

Interventional Radiology

Because interventional radiology has become a common adjunct in vascular access care, NPs are now practicing in this area. This is the case in the Vascular Interventional Radiology Department at the Samuel S. Stratton VA Medical Center in Albany, New York. When a dedicated vascular access NP began to perform PICC line insertion and use real-time ultrasound, the rate of PICC catheter-related blood stream infections dropped from six to nine per year to zero. Improvements were also made in monitoring and the care of the inserted PICC line, dressing changes, and staff education. These actions resulted in improved quality of care, decreased length of stay, and a cost avoidance of $315,000 to the facility in 2007 (M. Biscossi, personal communication, December 23, 2008).

Nurse Manager/Nurse Practitioner

NPs need to be managed by NPs who can bridge the clinical and administrative areas. Many of them can be viewed as successful nurse leaders who are visionary activists who believe in getting involved. They are investors in the organization and its goals, and serve as integrators and interpreters of its major functions. Nurses in leadership positions can influence and motivate others (Baillie, Trygstad, & Cordoni, 1989). Grzeczkowski and Knapp (1988), in the case of gerontology NPs, firmly believe that they possess the necessary clinical skills and managerial abilities needed to assume nursing administrative roles such as directors of nursing in long-term care settings. Henderson (1996), a geriatric NP, describes her role as director of health services with specific administrative functions of defining the specific health services offered, developing appropriate policies and procedures, hiring staff, and monitoring financial aspects of the program.

Fain, Asselin, and McCurry (2008) propose that advanced-practice clinicians educated at the doctoral level would be prepared to develop practice innovations, assume leadership positions in education, executive, and clinical settings, collaborate with interdisciplinary teams to improve health care outcomes, and act as a change agents to effect health care policy. These are all important attributes of a successful nurse leader/administrator.

In 2007, the VA Medical Center in St. Louis, Missouri, created the position of Nurse Manager/NP. In this leadership role, the individual not only manages a full panel of primary care patients, but is also responsible for ensuring that established standards of nursing practice and standards of care are maintained, initiates and participates in interdisciplinary efforts at the clinic, service, and medical center levels, and maintains a Quality Improvement/Performance Improvement program at the unit level. The nurse manager/NP ensures staff meets performance measure requirements and serves as a consultant when developing or updating collaborative practice agreements (P. Becker-Weilitz, personal communication, January 2, 2009).

A challenge of being in a dual role is attempting to manage a panel of patients while at the same time staying current with the administrative duties. However, this clinician/manager still finds opportunities to assist "the new ones [to] grow and mature and the seasoned ones [to] realize some of their goals and dreams" (P. Becker-Weilitz, personal communication, January 2, 2009).

Primary Care

An NP working in a primary care setting at the VA Medical Center in Columbia, Missouri, recognized that a majority of the elderly, male patients in her panel had joint and muscle problems (D. Salisbury, personal communication, January 6, 2009). Traditionally, these patients would get a physical examination, diagnostic testing such as X-rays and magnetic resonance imaging scans, a trial of conservative treatments such as nonsteroidal antiinflammatory medication, and physical therapy. In some cases, they would be referred to specialty services. If conservative therapies failed, they would then be referred to orthopedic service. However, it was noted that the Orthopedic Department was extremely busy and it would take 2–3 months before a patient could be seen in their clinic. The NP's collaborating physician performed his own musculoskeletal procedures, so she approached him about the idea of developing an NP-managed primary care procedure clinic to perform these procedures. She received approval to proceed, learned how to do the injections, and developed a clinic protocol. Procedures performed in this clinic include shoulder, knee, elbow, carpal tunnel, trigger finger, and trochanter bursa kenalog injections. Her services have now expanded to the inpatient units. She sees 30 patients per month, and just has clinic 1 afternoon per week (D. Salisbury, personal communication, January 7, 2009). In terms of outcomes, the NP reports that this is a temporary pain-relief modality for a number of chronic conditions.

In 2007, the VA in Minneapolis, Minnesota, developed a Primary Care Access clinic, consisting of two components; Primary Care Same Day and New Patient Access. The team consists of two physicians, one NP, one registered nurse, one licensed practical nurse, and one medical support assistant. The clinic is located across from the urgent care and emergency room in the hospital, within a primary care clinic. When a patient presents to the Emergency Department/Urgent Care, triage is initiated and the appropriate level of care is determined. The patient with nonurgent needs is sent to the Primary Care Same Day clinic to be seen by a primary care physician or NP. Veterans may also use these services by calling the primary care call center to make an appointment, or by just walking in to the clinic (A. Toth, personal communication, January 7, 2009). The other component, the New Patient Access clinic, was developed to ensure all veterans have a primary care provider; thereby ensuring continuity of care and appropriate follow-up. In this clinic, a complete history and physical examination is completed, appropriate referrals made, medications prescribed, and a care plan developed; therefore, a primary provider is established and the veteran is enrolled in the VA system. Since the implementation of this program in 2007, Emergency Department visits have significantly decreased by approximately 90 visits per month, and there has been an increase in patient satisfaction reports related to wait times and overall quality of care.

Psychiatric Care

Major changes in the health care delivery system have supported the increased use of psychiatric nurses in advanced-practice roles. As a result of managed care approaches, access to third-party payment, and federally funded programs, NPs are responding to the increasing need for mental health services for those individuals with substance abuse, posttraumatic stress disorder (PTSD), and acute and chronically ill mental health diagnoses. The VA is experiencing the same increasing need of veterans for these mental health services, as evidenced by various research studies conducted in VA facilities (Chermack et al., 2008; Laffaye, Cavella, Drescher, & Rosen, 2008; Magruder et al., 2004; Schnurr & Lunney, 2008).

One example of a VA research study, by Magruder and colleagues (2004), was conducted in an attempt to estimate the prevalence of PTSD in VA primary care clinics. Results revealed PTSD symptom levels were significantly related to age (younger veterans had more severe symptoms), employment status (disabled persons had higher symptom levels), and war zone experience. Veterans with high PTSD symptoms exhibited worse functional status across both physical and mental health domains.

Schnurr and Lunney (2008), in an attempt to address the knowledge gap of gender differences in QOL among individuals with PTSD, randomized two groups of veterans treated in VA settings. One group consisted of male Vietnam veterans who received group therapy, and the other group was composed of females from all eras who received individual psychotherapy. Results revealed overall QOL was poor in men and women, and in general, they did not differ in QOL or in how PTSD was associated with QOL. The investigators concluded that QOL should receive increased attention in clinical efforts to assist those veterans with PTSD; certainly in an area where NPs have the capability and expertise to significantly improve patient outcomes.

Substance abuse remains a leading cause of premature and preventable illness, disability, and death among Americans, including veterans. Chychula and Sciamanna (2002), two NPs with the Behavioral Health

Service at the Philadelphia VA, recognized that individuals struggling with substance abuse are more likely to present or return to a primary care provider who is not an addiction specialist, but yet these individuals may be in a stage of readiness to change their behavior. In an effort to assist the primary care provider, Chychula and Sciamanna (2002) detailed motivation interventions that can encourage a patient to enter treatment for substance abuse, as well as how to recognize post-abstinence symptoms that are present after acute withdrawal symptoms. These interventions can serve as a bridge to support the individual's decisions to move from a world of substance abuse to a lifestyle free from alcohol and drug use.

VA medical centers across the country have NPs who are able to deliver primary mental health care services to veterans. Their clinical practice focuses on a wide range of activities, including involvement in completing health assessments and examinations, conducting health screening and evaluations, designing and conducting mental illness preventative interventions, and conducting individual and group psychotherapy, as well as formulating, implementing, and evaluating outcome-based treatment plans.

FUTURE OF NURSE PRACTITIONERS IN THE VETERANS ADMINISTRATION

NPs were first appointed to the VA as primary providers of patient care in 1973. Just as the health care environment has become more complex, so has the role of NPs. They no longer just work in primary care, but have expanded their roles to include almost every aspect of health care. What does the future hold for this group of VA health care professionals?

All indicators point to continued growth in the number of veterans being treated at the VA. For example, in fiscal year 2009, it is estimated that the VA will treat approximately 5.8 million veterans. Of this number, about 3.9 million veterans are the VA's highest priority patients, including veterans returning from service in Operation Iraqi Freedom (OIF) and Operation Enduring Freedom (OEF), veterans with service-connected disabilities, those with lower incomes, and veterans with special health care needs. The VA will treat about 333,000 OIF/OEF veterans in 2009, a 14% increase over 2008. Resources for mental health care will reach $3.9 billion in 2009, a 9% increase, which will assist in strengthening efforts to ensure the VA provides equitable access throughout the nation for veterans with mental health disorders (U.S. Department of Veterans Affairs, 2008c). With the veteran population aging and having multiple medical problems, as well as soldiers returning home with severe injuries, one VA NP predicts the continued expansion of home-based primary care programs with NPs as key team members (R. Rowe, personal communication, August 20, 2008).

Guadagnino (2008) argues that the supply of NPs, let alone doctorate-prepared NPs for leadership positions, is projected to fall short of the demand for their services in the future. Specialty practices including oncology, endocrinology, cardiology, and transplant surgery have a growing need of NPs to manage the patients' primary care and chronic health needs. There continues to be a growing shortage of primary care physicians; therefore, it is certainly inevitable that more primary care patients will be seen by NPs.

There are NPs in the VA who are either currently enrolled in doctorate programs or already have a Doctorate in Nursing Practice (DNP). One individual, who plans to complete a program this year, hopes to use her skills in a way that will impact policy changes to better incorporate evidence-based practice in mental health nursing (J. Holdren, personal communication, August 27, 2008). Others who have a DNP are conducting research, such as one NP at the Salt Lake City VA who studied the outcomes of a CAM integrative health program (S. Smeeding, personal communication, January 7, 2009). Another DNP in the VA developed a method to target Vietnam veterans with Agent Orange presumptive cancer conditions using the computer; thereby improving the compensation and benefit process time frame (S. Burkart-Jayez, personal communication, August 21, 2008). In the Philadelphia VA Medical Center, APNs with PhDs are conducting primary research in brain injury, sleep, and psychosocial support for oncology patients.

The future for NPs in the VA looks bright. They are a creative and innovative group of health care professionals who are continually looking for ways to improve their practice and delivery of care to the veteran. Their roles are continuing to evolve, and this author predicts, by 2015, NPs will be involved in every aspect of primary and specialty care that is offered by the VA. Additionally, although more NPs will have a PhD or DNP, the majority of the group will continue to practice with a master's degree in nursing. NPs, whether PhD or DNP, will provide expertise in research, leadership, health policy, evidence-based practice, and clinical content; therefore, they will not only continue their clinical practice, but will be able to assume leadership positions in developing practice innovations and in improving the VA's health care system as it increasingly becomes more complex.

REFERENCES

Baillie, V. K., Trygstad, L., & Cordoni, T. I. (1989). *Effective nursing leadership: A practical guide.* Rockville, MD: Aspen.

Beason, C. F. (2005). Lessons learned: A successful distance learning collaborative between the Department of Veterans Affairs and the Department of Defense. *Military Medicine, 170,* 395–399.

Chermack, S. T., Zivan, K., Valenstein, M., Ilgen, M., Austin, K. L., Wryobeck, J., et al. (2008). The prevalence and predictors of mental health treatment services in a national sample of depressed veterans. *Medical Care, 46,* 813–820.

Chychula, N. M., & Sciamanna, C. (2002). Help substance abusers attain and sustain abstinence. *Nurse Practitioner, 27*(11), 30–47.

Eisenberg, D. M., Davis, R. B., Ettner, S. L., Appel, S., Wilkey, S., Van Rompay, M., et al. (1998). Trends in alternative medicine use in the United States, 1990–1997: Results of a follow-up national survey. *Journal of the American Medical Association, 280,* 1569–1575.

Eisenberg, D. M., Kessler, R. C., Foster, C., Norlock, F. E., Calkins, D. R., & Delbanco, R. L. (1993). Unconventional medicine in the United States: Prevalence, costs, and patterns of use. *New England Journal of Medicine, 328,* 246–252.

Fain, J. A., Asselin, M., & McCurry, M. (2008). The DNP…Why now? *Nursing Management, 39*(7), 34–37.

Grzeczkowski, M., & Knapp, M. (1988). The gerontological nurse practitioner as director of nursing in the long-term care facility. *Nursing Management, 19*(4), 64B–64F.

Guadagnino, C. (2008). *Growing role of nurse practitioners.* Retrieved February 3, 2010, from http://www.physiciansnews.com/cover/508.html

Henderson, M. L. (1996). Elder care: One geriatric nurse practitioner's experience in a continuing care retirement community. In J. V. Hickey, R. M. Ouimette, & S. L. Venegoni (Eds.), *Advanced practice nursing: Changing roles and clinical applications* (pp. 298–305). Philadelphia: Lippincott.

Keane, A., & Becker, D. (2004). Emerging roles of the advanced practice nurse. In L. A. Joel (Ed.), *Advanced practice nursing: Essentials for role development* (pp. 31–57). Philadelphia: F.A. Davis.

Laffaye, C., Cavella, S., Drescher, K., & Rosen, C. (2008). Relationships among PTSD symptoms, social support, and support source in veterans with chronic PTSD. *Journal of Traumatic Stress, 21,* 394–401.

Magruder, K. M., Frueh, B. C., Knapp, R. G., Johnson, M. R., Vaughan, J. A., Carson, T. C., et al. (2004). PTSD symptoms, demographic characteristics, and functional status among veterans treated in VA primary care clinics. *Journal of Traumatic Stress, 17,* 293–301.

National Center for Complementary and Alternative Medicine (NCCAM). (2005). *The use of complementary and alternative medicine in the United States.* Retrieved February 3, 2010, from http://nccam.nih.gov/news/camsurvey_fs1.htm#list

North, L., Kehm, L., Bent, K., & Hartman, T. (2008). Can home-based primary care cut costs? *Nurse Practitioner, 33*(7), 39–44.

Robinson, K. R., & Petzel, R. (2003). Roles of nurse practitioners in the U.S. Department of Veterans Affairs. In M. D. Mezey, D. O. McGivern, & E. M. Sullivan-Marx (Eds.), *Nurse practitioners: Evolution of advanced practice* (4th ed., pp. 284–302). New York: Springer Publishing Company.

Schnurr, P. P., & Lunney, C. A. (2008). Exploration of gender differences in how quality of life relates to posttraumatic stress disorder in male and female veterans. *Journal of Rehabilitation Research & Development, 45,* 383–394.

Smeeding, S. J. (2009). *Outcome evaluation of the Integrative Health Clinic at the Veterans Affairs Salt Lake City healthcare system.* Unpublished doctoral dissertation, University of Utah, Salt Lake City, UT.

Smith, T. D., Vezina, M. L., & Samost, M. E. (2009). Mediated roles: Working through other people. In L. Joel (Ed.), *Advanced practice nursing: Essentials for role development* (2nd ed., pp. 211–229). Philadelphia: F. A. Davis.

Under Secretary for Health. (1997, July 7). *Information letter: Utilization of nurse practitioners and clinical nurse specialists.* Washington, DC: Department of Veterans Affairs.

Under Secretary for Health. (1999, February 24). *Information letter: Utilization of nurse practitioners and clinical nurse specialists.* Washington, DC: Department of Veterans Affairs.

U.S. Department of Veterans Affairs. (2008a). *Facts about the Department of Veterans Affairs.* Retrieved February 3, 2010, from http://www.va.gov/opa/fact/vafacts.asp

U. S. Department of Veterans Affairs. (2008b). *Office of Nursing Services Annual Report 2008.* Washington, DC: Author Retrieved on March 3, 2010, from http://www

U.S. Department of Veterans Affairs. (2008c). *FY 09 VA budget request highlights.* Retrieved February 3, 2010, from http://www1.va.gov/opa/pressrel/pressrelease.cfm?id=1448

U. S. Department of Veterans Affairs. (2008d, April). *VA nursing—A profession and a passion.* Washington, DC: Author.1.va.gov/NURSING/docs/2008_ONSannualRpt.pdf.

U.S. Department of Veterans Affairs. (n.d.). *VA careers.* Retrieved February 3, 2010, from http://www.vacareers.va.gov

VA Organizational Briefing Book. (May 2008). *Overview of the Department of Veterans Affairs.* Retrieved February 3, 2010, from http://www.va.gov/ofcadmin/docs/vaorgbb.pdf

Ethical Issues in Advanced-Practice Nursing

CONNIE M. ULRICH AND MINDY B. ZEITZER

INTRODUCTION

By all accounts, the U.S. health care system needs to be radically restructured (Ulrich & Grady, 2009). The statistics are troubling; it is expected that health care will consume nearly 20% of the gross domestic product (GDP) by 2017, and cost more than $4.3 trillion. With an estimated 47 million citizens uninsured and an additional 25 million underinsured, it is not surprising that the majority of Americans feel like systematic change is needed (How, Shih, Lau, & Schoen, 2008; Jecker, 2008; Schoen, Collins, Kriss, & Doty, 2008). Frustrations are common, as problems include disparities in access, quality, and outcomes of care. Additionally, nearly one in five Americans is medically disenfranchised—those without an established medical or health care home due to primary care physician shortages. The confluence of an aging, chronically ill society, physician and nurse shortages, and constrained economic resources amidst the U.S. fiscal crisis will present significant ethical challenges in the delivery of care. Advanced-practice nurses (APNs)* will be no exception, as they, too, will tackle professional,

---

*For the purpose of this chapter, the terms *advanced-practice nurse* (APN) and *nurse practitioner* (NP) are used interchangeably as per the literature reviewed and cited.

239

ethical, societal, and regulatory challenges in meeting the needs of their patients and must be prepared to appropriately address them. The purpose of this chapter is to address the ethical issues nurse practitioners (NPs), as one group of APNs, face as they address the emerging, emergent, and preventative health care needs of the public.

As fittingly defined by Hanson and Hamric (2003), "[a]dvanced nursing practice is the application of an expanded range of practical, theoretical, and research-based therapeutics to phenomena experienced by patients within a specialized clinical area of the larger discipline of nursing" (p. 205). In 2004, nearly a quarter-million nurses were prepared at the advanced-practice level, and it is expected that their growth will continue in response to significant health care labor shortages and societal needs. As such, they will confront many ethical problems as they continue to define their autonomous role(s) within collaborative models of practice, establish their moral and professional leadership, and work toward prescriptive and reimbursement equity.

ETHICAL ISSUES IN ADVANCED PRACTICE

The advanced-practice role in nursing is one of historical, clinical, and moral relevance. And, although political and regulatory barriers still exist, many states now legitimately recognize NPs and do not confine patient choice. As is true for their physician colleagues, ethical issues and problems appear to arise from the profession's primary obligation and commitment to the health and welfare of their patients, as outlined in nursing's extant national and international Codes of Ethical Conduct (American Nurses Association, 2001; International Council of Nurses, 2006). Specifically, APNs are called to be moral leaders—those whose patient advocacy goals are respectful, beneficent, and just; and who work toward equity within the health care system, as well as address thorny ethical issues that have an impact on both research and practice, and promote dignified and humane care for the public's good (American Nurses Association, 2001). Thus, it seems easy to justify why Grace (2008) claims that "any obstruction to what is seen, in the clinical judgment of the APN, as needed care for a patient is an ethical issue" (p. 135). Of course, the ethical issues are many, and therefore, it is first important to define and distinguish the types of ethical issues and problems APNs encounter and any subsequent untoward distress that might ensue.

Any situation that presents itself with moral or ethical challenges represents an ethical issue (Purtillo, 2005). Today, this might represent fundamental ethical questions on topics related to the use of genetic markers to predict disease states, the role of cognitive neuroscience and its relationship to behavioral characteristics, conflicts of interest, quality end-of-life care, recruitment and retention of human subjects, allocating finite resources, and a host of other novel and up-and-coming health care technologies used to advance both clinical care and research outcomes. An *ethical problem* exists when core moral values and duties are threatened, and requires the APN to reflect on what he or she believes to be morally right or wrong in a particular situation. In his groundbreaking work on ethical issues in nursing practice precisely 25 years ago, philosopher Andrew Jameton (1984) identified three different types of moral/ethical problems that are particularly important for today's advanced practitioner: moral uncertainty, moral dilemma, and moral distress. Although data are limited to better understand the depth of ethical problems in advanced practice, given what we do know, it seems plausible that APNs experience all three types of problems.

First, APNs experience *moral uncertainty* when they find themselves in particular situations in which the ethically correct action is not necessarily clear. In one study, Ulrich and colleagues (2006b) found that 25% of advanced practitioners (i.e., NPs and physician assistants [PAs]) felt isolated in making ethical decisions and wanted more ethics education to assist them in their decision making. Second, there are times in clinical practice when an APN can justify two or more morally accepted courses of action but both cannot be followed; hence, the APN experiences a *moral dilemma*. For example, suppose the APN is confronted with a patient who is at risk for Huntington's disease, meaning he/she has a parent or first-degree relative who has been diagnosed with this specific type of genetic neurological disorder. Huntington's disease is both progressive and debilitating; patients suffer with physical, psychological, and cognitive dysfunction. The APN is responsible for discussing the risks and benefits of genetic testing with the patient, which may include the loss of health insurance, loss of employment, and a change in disability status. The patient must then decide whether the benefits and burdens of genetic testing are acceptable and whether he or she is willing to risk these losses or forgo discovering his or her true risk of developing the disease.

Once a positive result is found, the result is an indelible mark on the patient's medical and insurance record. The NP is fully aware of the difficult choices that must be made, and is torn by doing what is perceived as "right" for the patient in a health care system that seems "unfair." The NP advises the patient to pay for the genetic testing with cash, use a false name, and records the visits in such a way that the patient is protected. To protect the patient in case of a positive result, the NP also recommends obtaining life insurance, private disability insurance, and long-term care insurance. The NP has a duty to do what is right for the patient, but feels as though she has to manipulate the system in order to do so and questions whether her actions are ethically defensible. Thus, in this scenario, the NP is doing right but also wrong. Indeed, it is the duty of professionals to take actions to protect their patients. But deceiving the system to do so is ethically troubling. On the other hand, working within established policies and procedural reimbursement guidelines may leave the NP feeling as though he/she did not do "good" enough in providing necessary care.

Finally, *moral distress* has received much attention in the nursing literature, and several studies discuss its impact on patient quality of care and nurse-related outcomes (Corley, 1995; Corley, Elswick, Gorman, & Clor, 2001; Hamric & Blackhall, 2007). When nurses are constrained to follow a course of action that they believe to be unethical, they may experience distress. These constraints certainly vary, but can include such things as time pressures, patient demands, resource limitations, and authoritative powers within organizational structures. Bell and Breslin (2008) argue that moral distress occurs "as a result of being forced to act in a manner that contravenes personal and professional values." (p. 94) For example, in a recent study examining the ethical conflicts associated with managed care, 23% of advanced practitioners felt that it was sometimes necessary to ignore their own clinical judgment and follow the mandates of insurance companies, and three-quarters reported ethical concerns (Ulrich et al., 2006a, 2006b). This type of distress can lead to feelings of powerlessness, anger, anxiety, frustration, and fatigue. Additionally, one of four nurses has indicated a desire to leave her/his position.

ETHICAL ISSUES IN PRIMARY CARE

NPs encounter a multitude of ethical issues in their clinical practice, and often struggle with divided loyalties between their historical fiduciary ethic to the patient and their contractual obligations to meet the "bottom line" and efficiency goals of the organization (Johnson, 2005; Ulrich, Soeken, & Miller, 2003; Ulrich et al., 2006b). Unfortunately, few studies specifically address the types of ethical issues NPs encounter, and most of these studies have been conducted with NPs in primary care (see Table 18.1).

In fact, Ulrich and colleagues (2006b) reported that more than half of primary care NPs and PAs experienced issues with managed care policies that threatened the availability (67.4%) and quality (58.7%) of the care they provided. NPs grapple with having to bend the rules or manipulate the system in order to do what is right for their patients (Laabs, 2005). Ulrich and Grady (2009) note that, "Even when the provider does the best he or she can, it may not feel good enough" (p. 6). In Laabs's (2005) study of moral problems encountered by NPs in primary care, 49% of NPs experienced distress related to ethical issues. Of these, 26% were somewhat distressed, 15% were moderately distressed, and 8% were highly distressed. NPs appeared to be highly distressed about situations related to clinical decisions by others and patients unable to pay for services. Moreover, when NPs felt their integrity had been compromised, they experienced self-doubt, regret, outrage, and frustration. They often reconciled their compromised integrity by avoiding situations that caused distress, and rationalized or convinced themselves that they did everything they could for a patient and, therefore, were not to blame for any negative outcomes. NPs also showed compensating behavior, where they accepted blame but attempted to find methods to compensate for their failures (e.g., lowering their expectations) (Laabs, 2007).

ETHICAL ISSUES IN ACUTE AND CHRONIC CARE

Ethical issues for NPs in acute and chronic care are uncharted territory, as a paucity of literature exists to better understand the most salient issues that have an impact on their ability to provide ethical nursing care.

Table 18.1

ETHICAL ISSUES IN ADVANCED-PRACTICE NURSING CATEGORIZED BY GUIDING ETHICAL PRINCIPLES AND VALUES

Beneficence   **Moral Agency Concerns**

- Balancing agency role and concern over becoming agents for the health plan rather than patient advocates
- Protecting the rights of patients
- Manipulating the system or bending the rules to provide needed care
- Managed care policies/procedures that threaten the quality of care
- Genetic testing (i.e., protecting the patient from negative consequences)

Supportive Practice Concerns

- Use of ethics resources (i.e., ethics consults called in too late to be helpful)
- Transitional concerns (i.e., lack of DNR orders for outside the hospital transfers)

Respect for Persons   **Informed Consent**

- Patient not informed
- Failure of providers to educate their patients
- Advanced directives and/or surrogates not honoring patient's advance directives
- Confidentiality
- Patient refuses treatment
- Patient withholds information
- Misunderstanding of patients and families

Patient–Provider Relationships

- Discriminatory treatment of patients
- Prejudice of others toward care of the poor and minorities
- Conflict of parent and minor regarding termination of pregnancy
- Inappropriate patient requests

Justice   **Distributive Justice Issues**

- Lack of access to health care on local and global levels
- Providing expensive health care to undocumented patients
- Allocation of costly resources
- NP care not available to all (i.e., other groups limiting NP practice)
- Insurance not paying for necessary services
- Insurance drug formularies that excessively restrict medication
- Patient abuse of insurance such as Medicaid for minor complaints
- Need to tailor patient care based on what insurance company will pay for
- Managed care policies/procedures that threaten availability of care
- Patient unable to pay

Table 18.1 *(continued)*

ETHICAL ISSUES IN ADVANCED-PRACTICE NURSING CATEGORIZED BY GUIDING ETHICAL PRINCIPLES AND VALUES

Personal/ Professional Integrity	**Patient Care Concerns**
	■ Balancing professional role as patient advocate with costs associated with providing care
	■ Patient care needs being overridden by business decisions
	■ Child/parent/practitioner relationship

Practice-Related Concerns

- Misrepresentation of medical assistants as RNs
- Refilling medications for other providers when NP disagrees with plan of care
- Physician signing off NP notes without reading them
- Competition between MDs and NPs for patients
- Physician finding ways to get more money from Medicare
- Clinical decisions by others
- Physician collaboration/conflict in nurse–physician relationships
- Pressure to prescribe
- Pressure to see patients
- Incentives for productivity offered by managed care
- Impaired physician
- Disagree with plan of care
- Compromised personal values and ethics
- Conflicts of interest

Table is not exhaustive: (Butz, Redman, Fry, & Kolodner, 1998; Fontana, 2008; Hannigan, 2006; Johnson, 2005; Laabs, 2005; Ulrich et al., 2003, 2006).

We do know, however, that issues of informed consent for treatment and research, privacy and confidentiality, conflicts surrounding end-of-life and palliative care, decisional capacity, requests for assisted suicide, access to care, role-boundary blurring, and other facets of caregiving seem to cut across both acute and chronic care domains.

Although little research has investigated the ethical issues for NPs in the acute care setting, hospital-based physicians experience a unique set of issues that differ from those who work in a clinic setting (Rajput & Bekes, 2002). This is often true because of the "need for rapid decision making, often based on incomplete information and without a prior patient–physician relationship, and difficulty in establishing trust" (Rajput & Bekes, 2002, p. 870). Physicians, like NPs, are often confronted with issues of informed consent and are required to help determine the decision-making capacity of the patient (Pantilat & Lo, 2005). This is of particular concern when patients lack decision-making capacity or their decision-making capacity is in question. Furthermore, with hospitalized patients, advanced directives become quite pertinent. Health care providers are often faced with questions related to patients' wishes about cardiopulmonary resuscitation, mechanical ventilation, intensive care, and artificial nutrition and hydration, as well as surrogate decision making and withdrawing care or withholding treatment (Pantilat & Lo, 2005). NPs in primary care are in a prime position to assist patients and families in completing advanced directives and making these decisions; however, when patients are hospitalized, these decisions are often made quickly and under physical and emotional stress, placing the patient, the family, and the NP in a precarious situation, resulting in an advanced directive that may not reflect the patient's true wishes (Schlenk, 1997).

For NPs working in acute care, role-boundary blurring is a recurrent issue. Unfortunately, NPs perceived this "blurring" as an affront to their professional nursing identity because of its potential to medicalize their role, encroach on medical territory, and devalue the unique contributions they bring to patient care and the health care system (Cummings, Fraser, & Tarlier, 2003; Tye & Ross, 2000). Many of the NP's duties are similar to those of his or her physician counterparts (e.g., diagnosing, treating, and prescribing); when there are misunderstandings associated with the NP role among colleagues, it is easy to experience pressures to conform to the "medical way" of thinking and treating patients. Not having clear role descriptions further contributes to the blurring, which fosters frustration among NPs and their colleagues (Cummings et al., 2003; Tye & Ross, 2000). It also places them in awkward situations, as the staff/team have varying expectations of what it is the NP should be doing (Cummings et al., 2003; Tye & Ross, 2000). Ultimately, this boundary blurring creates a negative work environment (Cummings et al., 2003; Tye & Ross, 2000), strains collegial relationships, and compromises patient care by precluding the advanced NP from fulfilling the role for which he/she was educated.

Hospital-based NPs are typically surrounded by a team of colleagues treating the patient. The NP is often caught between meeting the expectations of these colleagues—nurses, physicians, residents, and other health care team members—while caring for the patient, and fulfilling his or her additional role obligations (i.e., educational programming and research activities) (Cummings et al., 2003). Being caught in this middle position can be tenuous and lead to moral distress, frustration, and burnout (Cummings et al., 2003), and affect the way the NP is able to deal with challenging situations. NPs and clinical nurse specialists have also pin-pointed lack of resources, staff shortages, work overload, and lack of autonomy, leading to inability to perform appropriate job duties as additional issues causing distress (Jones, 2005). However, "there is an alternative view of the in-the-middle position, which is that it presents numerous opportunities" (Hamric, 2001, p. 255). Because NPs are surrounded by multiple colleagues within the hospital, they are in an optimal position to seek guidance and consultation from many parties when they are confronted with ethical challenges. They do, however, need to "be able to tolerate uncertainty, and maintain their own integrity while respecting the opinions of others" (Pantilat & Lo, 2005, p. 127).

ETHICAL ISSUES IN COLLABORATIVE PRACTICE

Health care providers are increasingly seeing patients with chronic conditions and complex needs in all medical venues—acute care, outpatient and ambulatory care, nurse-managed community clinics, and long-term care. For example, it is not unusual to coordinate and provide care for the patient with heart failure who also has sleep disturbances and depression, or the patient with diabetes who is also obese and has hypercholesterolemia and coronary artery disease (Anonymous, 2009a). "Good chronic care will require care teams, which will, in turn, require workforce development" (Anonymous, 2009b, p. 63). NPs are a critical part of the health care team for complex patients. Other team members may include physicians, social workers, and rehabilitation therapists. These team members work within an organizational and political system to facilitate optimal patient care outcomes. Thus, interacting with other health care professionals is a key component of the daily activities of NPs. Collaboration has been defined by various authors, but Gardner (2005) described it in this way:

> Collaboration is both a process and an outcome in which shared interest or conflict that cannot be addressed by any single individual is addressed

by key stakeholders. A key stakeholder is any party directly influenced by the actions others take to solve a complex problem. The collaborative process involves a synthesis of different perspectives to better understand complex problems. A collaborative outcome is the development of integrative solutions that go beyond an individual vision to a productive resolution that could not be accomplished by any single person or organization. ("What is Collaboration?" Section 4)

The benefits of collaborative practice exist for both patients and providers. These include, but are not limited to, improved quality of care, patient outcomes, and communication, as well as personal satisfaction, shared responsibility, and mutual respect (Charlton, Dearing, Berry, & Johnson, 2008; Flanagan, 1998; Greene, 2001). Collaborative relationships, however, are not without value conflicts, particularly NPs' relationships with their physician colleagues and the diverse knowledge and skill set that each professional group brings to practice (Laabs, 2005; Ulrich et al., 2006a). In fact, Laabs (2005) found that 72% of primary care NPs experienced ethical issues with physician collaboration. Much of these ethical issues stemmed from disagreement with an established plan of care and clinical decisions that had been made by others. Moreover, NPs experienced distress when they found that patients had not been educated by providers, were asked to refill prescriptions for other providers when they disagreed with the plan of care, encountered an impaired physician, perceived limited supervisory oversight (e.g., physician sign-off on documentation written by an NP without reading it), and faced professional competition for patients (Laabs, 2005).

Reimbursement is another salient ethical issue in collaborative practice, because of state-specific legislation outlining practitioners' scope of practice, as well as the number of Americans who are uninsured and underinsured seeking care. Many NPs report ethical angst when their collaborating physicians attempt to find ways to obtain financial gain from health insurance programs, such as Medicare (Laabs, 2005). When NPs encounter a colleague committing fraud, whistle blowing generates a great amount of discomfort, as he/she risks retaliation and disdain from coworkers, as well as a tarnished reputation and damaged collegial relationships (Hannigan, 2006). Judgmental differences between physicians and NPs in how to best achieve reimbursement goals can create emotional conflict among providers. In a study by Ulrich and colleagues

(2006a), however, the majority of NPs and PAs (79%) believed that physicians value their unique perspective; therefore, conflict should not be sidestepped, as the voice of each party is important to the process. "If we keep the focus of collaborative efforts on mutual goals of patient good, then collaborative relationships are likely to be effective in achieving these goals" (Grace, 2008, p. 150).

STRATEGIES TO IMPROVE ETHICAL DECISION MAKING

Although NPs face a multitude of ethical issues and dilemmas, formal education on ethics or ethical decision making is not included in many advanced-practice training programs. Interestingly, Fontana (2008) interviewed NPs from various specialties, and discovered that many experienced ethical issues in prescribing pain medications to chronically ill patients. NPs were concerned about protecting themselves from potential scrutiny from the Drug Enforcement Agency and prescribing adequate pain control to ensure the beneficent care of the patients. One respondent in this study commented that, "If you have someone on a narcotic long term, it gets people's attention even if it is justified, so I feel like I am under the microscope when I prescribe those drugs" (p. 33). In fact, many respondents altered their prescribing practices to reduce their perceived risk. The NPs, however, described these prescribing decisions as clinical, rather than ethical, and failed to identify the conflict between protecting themselves and prescribing adequately for the patient (Fontana, 2008). This study in particular points to the need for increased ethics education in advanced practice.

Ethics education is an important first step that helps build the foundation for NPs to recognize and address ethical issues in their practice, and develop the critical skills needed to analyze these situations. However, additional measures need to be taken, as well. First, research is critical if we want to discover the specific types of issues NPs encounter so we can create an ethics curriculum that supports initiatives to address their unique concerns. Second, NPs need to engage in open dialogue with health care team members, as well as have open access to ethics resources, if available. Additionally, NPs need to voice their ethical concerns without fear of reprisal. Being able to identify and address ethical issues is part of their responsibility, and without the appropriate education and avenues to address these issues, they are left unprepared to face these realities. Therefore, in order for NPs to fulfill their ethical responsibility, they need to be better educated in ethics and made aware of the avenues available to them.

ETHICAL DECISION-MAKING MODELS

Ethical decision-making models exist to provide guidance on ethical dilemmas and serve as a framework from which NPs can delineate troublesome issues. These models can range from simple to quite complex. However, because NPs are often busy, it is crucial that they are able to call upon a model that will efficiently help them make a decision related to the problem(s) they are experiencing. Ethical decisions are often not made in isolation, but rather in partnership with an interdisciplinary team, the patient, and/or the patient's family. The following steps can be used to assist in the decisional process: First, all ethical decisions must begin with identifying the facts of the particular case under review. Thus, as in any basic patient assessment, it would be important to know the patient's medical diagnosis, prognosis, history of illness, and whether the problem is acute, chronic, or emergent. And, what is the ethical problem? For example, does the patient have the mental capacity to make autonomous decisions and is he/she legally competent? If not, is there a surrogate who can make decisions on behalf of the patient and are the patient's expressed treatment or research preferences known? Second, the NP must further determine the nature and dimensions of the problem by evaluating who is involved and who might be affected. Also, what are the benefits and risks to the patient and family members, and has informed consent been provided? This evaluation may also include determining which core bioethical principles are at stake: respect for autonomy, beneficence, nonmaleficence, and justice. Third, NPs in conjunction and after consultation with colleagues must identify possible solutions or courses of action considering professional code of ethics and nursing organizational groups, state practice guidelines, professional values and beliefs, the patient's values and beliefs, and other legal and regulatory bodies. If available, ethics committees can be helpful in supporting ethical deliberations, providing a critical analysis of the issue(s) and potential courses of action. The provider should then evaluate each possible course of action; in doing so, consequences to all parties must be considered—that is, to the patient, the family, the provider, and any other external parties. Finally, the NP needs to choose and implement the course of action and reevaluate the situation.

CONCLUSIONS

As the nursing and physician shortages continue to grow and the numbers of uninsured and underinsured patients multiply, the need for accessible and cost-efficient quality patient care increases. To fill this need, the number of NPs providing care will also need to increase. NPs are educated to be leaders in their respective field of inquiry and in the communities to which they serve. However, they too will face mounting ethical challenges as the demands of patient care become more complex, and resources remain tight in the current U.S. fiscal climate. Preparing NPs to assume leadership roles will require graduate preparation for the ethical issues they most likely will encounter, and the avenues to which they can turn for help and support. "More substantive thinking is needed to help advanced practitioners address the realistic ethical challenges of providing care, ethically negotiate their options, and feel supported in acting on their reasoned moral convictions" (Ulrich & Grady, 2009, p. 7). NPs are competent, dedicated providers who are essential to sustaining the public's health. Thus, every effort must be made to educate, recruit, and retain qualified NPs who can shape policies that reflect patient-centered care and improve the quality of our health care delivery system.

REFERENCES

American Nurses Association. (2001). *Code of ethics for nurses with interpretive statements*. Retrieved January 30, 2009, from http://nursingworld.org/ethics/code/protected_nwcoe813.htm
Anonymous. (2009a). Prologue: The scope of the problem. *Health Affairs*, 28(1), 14.
Anonymous. (2009b). Reorganizing chronic care delivery. *Health Affairs*, 28(1), 63.
Bell, J., & Breslin, J. M. (2008). Healthcare provider moral distress as a leadership challenge. *JONAS: Healthcare, Law, Ethics, & Regulation*, 10(4), 94–97.
Butz, A., Redman, B. K., Fry, S. T., & Kolodner, K. (1998). Ethical conflicts experienced by certified pediatric nurse practitioners in ambulatory settings. *Journal of Pediatric Health Care*, 12(4), 183–190.
Charlton, C. R., Dearing, K. S., Berry, J. A., & Johnson, M. J. (2008). Nurse practitioners' communication styles and their impact on patient outcomes: An integrated literature review. *Journal of the American Academy of Nurse Practitioners*, 20(7), 382–388.

Corley, M. C. (1995). Moral distress of critical care nurses. *American Journal of Critical Care, 4*(4), 280–285.

Corley, M. C., Elswick, R. K., Gorman, M., & Clor, T. (2001). Development and evaluation of the moral distress scale. *Journal of Advanced Nursing, 33*(2), 250–256.

Cummings, G. G., Fraser, K., & Tarlier, D. S. (2003). Implementing advanced nurse practitioner roles in acute care: An evaluation of organizational change. *Journal of Nursing Administration, 33*(3), 139–145.

Flanagan, L. (1998). Family physicians and nurse practitioners—A perfect team. *Family Practice Management, 5*(6), 60–63.

Fontana, J. S. (2008). The social and political forces affecting prescribing practices for chronic pain. *Journal of Professional Nursing, 24*(1), 30–35.

Gardner, D. (2005). Ten lessons in collaboration. *Online Journal of Issues in Nursing, 10*. Retrieved January 26, 2009, from www.nursingworld.org/MainMenuCategories/ANAMarketplace/ANAPeriodicals/OJIN/TableofContents/Volume102005/No1Jan05/tpc26_116008.aspx

Grace, P. J. (2008). *Nursing ethics and professional responsibility in advanced practice.* Sudbury, MA: Jones & Bartlett.

Greene, J. (2001). Growing ranks: Benefits of collaboration with nurse practitioners. *American Medical News.* Retrieved January 26, 2009, from http://proxy.library.u-penn.edu:2651/amednews/2001/03/12/prsa0312. htm

Hamric, A. B. (2001). Reflections on being in the middle. *Nursing Outlook, 48*, 254–257.

Hamric, A. B., & Blackhall, L. J. (2007). Nurse-physician perspective on the care of dying patients in intensive care units: Collaboration, moral distress, and ethical climate. *Critical Care Nurse, 35*(2), 422–429.

Hannigan, N. S. (2006). Blowing the whistle on healthcare fraud: Should I? *Journal of the American Academy of Nurse Practitioners, 18*(11), 512–517.

Hanson, C. M., & Hamric, A. B. (2003). Reflections on the continuing evolution of advanced practice nursing. *Nursing Outlook, 51*(5), 203–211.

How, S. K. H., Shih, A., Lau, J., & Schoen, C. (2008). *Public views on U.S. health system organization: A call for new directions.* Retrieved December 19, 2008, from http://www.commonwealthfund.org

International Council of Nurses. (2006). *The ICN code of ethics for nurses.* Retrieved January 30, 2009, from http://www.icn.ch/icncode.pdf

Jameton, A. (1984). *Nursing practice: The ethical issues.* Englewood, NJ: Prentice-Hall.

Jecker, N. S. (2008). A broader view of justice. *American Journal of Bioethics, 8*(10), 2–10.

Johnson, R. (2005). Shifting patterns of practice: Nurse practitioners in a managed care environment. *Research and Theory for Nursing Practice: An International Journal, 19*(4), 323–340.

Jones, M. L. (2005). Role development and effective practice in specialist and advanced practice roles in acute hospital settings: Systematic review and meta-analysis. *Journal of Advanced Nursing, 49*(2), 191–209.

Laabs, C. A. (2005). Moral problems and distress among nurse practitioners in primary care. *Journal of the American Academy of Nurse Practitioners, 17*(2), 76–84.

Laabs, C. A. (2007). Primary care nurse practitioners' integrity when faced with moral conflict. *Nursing Ethics, 14*(6), 795–809.

Pantilat, S. Z., & Lo, B. (2005). Ethical issues in the hospitalized patient. In R. M. Wachter, L. Goldman, & H. Hollander (Eds.), *Hospital medicine* (2nd ed.). Philadelphia: Lippincott Williams & Wilkins.

Purtillo, R. (2005). *Ethical dimensions in the health professions* (4th ed.). Philadelphia: Saunders Elsevier.

Rajput, V., & Bekes, C. E. (2002). Ethical issues in hospital medicine. *Medical Clinics of North America, 86*(4), 869–886.

Schlenk, J. S. (1997). Advanced directives: Role of the nurse practitioner. *Journal of the American Academy of Nurse Practitioners, 9*(7), 317–321.

Schoen, C., Collins, S. R., Kriss, J. L., & Doty, M. M. (2008). How many are underinsured? Trends among U.S. adults, 2004–2007. *Health Affairs, 27*(4), w298–w309.

Tye, C. C., & Ross, F. M. (2000). Blurring boundaries: Professional perspectives of the emergency nurse practitioner role in a major accident and emergency department. *Journal of Advanced Nursing, 31*(5), 1089–1096.

Ulrich, C., & Grady, C. (2009). Doing "good" with limited resources: Is it good enough in the provision of quality clinical care? *Clinical Scholars Review, 2*(1), 5–7.

Ulrich, C. M., Danis, M., Ratcliffe, S. J., Garrett-Mayer, E., Koziol, D., Soeken, K. L., et al. (2006a). *Ethical issues in nurse practitioners and physician assistants.* Unpublished raw data.

Ulrich, C. M., Danis, M., Ratcliffe, S. J., Garrett-Mayer, E., Koziol, D., Soeken, K. L., et al. (2006b). Ethical conflict in nurse practitioners and physician assistants in managed care. *Nursing Research, 55*(6), 391–401.

Ulrich, C. M., Soeken, K. L., & Miller, N. (2003). Ethical conflict associated with managed care: Views of nurse practitioners. *Nursing Research, 52*(3), 168–175.

Business and Payment Structures for Nurse Practitioners

There is probably no more daunting, complicated, or essential area of information for nurse practitioners (NPs) than the mastery of reimbursement, models of care, and federal and state regulation. Little information or inclination in undergraduate education or subsequent generalist practice prepares NP students or beginning practitioners for this major component of their practice. The emphases to this point have been on clinical competence, caring, and patient satisfaction, not the external business and regulatory dynamics.

Few nurse experts are more prepared in these topics than the authors whose work is assembled in this section. Sullivan-Marx, recognized for her contribution to various formal advisory groups on payment and ability to present these topics in an understandable fashion, sets the groundwork for the following chapters on managed care, nurse-managed community-based care, and quality and safety components of the practice model.

NPs as part of multidisciplinary or single-discipline practices have to develop a strong understanding of the business model, risks and opportunities, and responsibility for understanding shifting regulations. Miller describes the architecture of managed care, how payment is structured, and the need for credentialing in order to gain provider status. Nurses and NPs' assumptions about practice are often obstacles to skillful negotiation with managed care organizations. Miller details the key aspects of such contracting and credentialing, and emphasizes the importance of the effectiveness of NPs' messages to consumers, who, when well informed, will request these services.

NPs have two dichotomous goals: to become fully integrated into the mainstream reimbursement system, and to continue their key role in meeting the needs of patients, particularly the under- and uninsured, as safety net providers. Ritter expertly lays out the obstacles to payment for the system of nurse-managed health centers, including managed care organizations' policies. The resolution of these issues and obstacles by the National Nursing Centers Consortium is a classic case study of organizational efforts to create broad supportive networks and better-informed practitioners to meet both of these goals.

Quality drives finance in the best of worlds. Being attuned to meeting quality care is, therefore, essential for best practice and for solid financial foundations. Quality care and improvement as part of NP practice is thoroughly discussed by Fiandt and Pohl, who note the critical need for practitioner leadership in quality improvement (QI) efforts considered essential to reforming health care delivery. NPs must be able to incorporate organized strategies for QI into their practices. As the authors indicate, planning in this area is key to practice improvement and development of much-needed databases to show the effectiveness and efficacy of NP practice models, which, in turn, stabilizes finances.

These chapters provide a significant explanation of the practice landscape, with an emphasis on the need to understand what the business model, regulations that shape reimbursement, and the other responsibilities and opportunities outside of the core clinical demands on NPs.

19 Business, Policy, and Politics: Success Factors for Nurse Practitioner Practice

EILEEN M. SULLIVAN-MARX

For many years, I have been lecturing on the issues of how nurse practitioners (NP) and other advanced-practice nurses (APNs) can be reimbursed by private third-party payers, Medicare, Medicaid, or garner private-payer funds. The process of health care finance and how health professionals are paid is so convoluted that it was often difficult to answer questions posed by members of an audience or class. Many times the initial answer to, "How do I get paid for what I do, or how do I bill for my services as an NP?" was, "It depends." Usually, this was not a well-received reply, particularly in those years of uncertainty just before and after the Balanced Budget Act of 1997, which granted Medicare reimbursement to NPs and certified nurse specialists (CNSs) in all geographic areas and settings.

To answer questions about payment, it began to dawn on me that when it comes to knowing how to get paid for what we do as NPs, there are three contextual factors in play: business, policy, and politics. Understanding each can bring clarity to tough situations and expedite change. The interplay of business, policy, and politics is key for NPs who provide care with funds from federal or state sources, and whose authority and independent scope of practice is frequently challenged.

257

Table 19.1

COLLINS' KEY FRAMEWORK

1. First the who, then the what
2. Confront the brutal facts
3. The hedgehog concept
4. A culture of discipline
5. Technology accelerators
6. Keep the flywheel turning

Note: Adapted from Collins (2001).

Success in practice and businesses is critical for NPs to sustain and grow their contribution to society's needs for health care.

In his book, *Good to Great* (2001), Collins makes the point that many companies or organizations are good, but being good may actually stand in the way of becoming a great company. For NPs who are employed in or run a good health care practice, and want to achieve greatness, they need to understand the factors that move their practices toward greatness, factors that are often either business, policy, or political in nature. In this chapter, I will use Collins' framework (see Table 19.1) to discuss NPs and their practices as a force that has reached a "good" status in the Unites States, but still needs to achieve greatness, and what business, policy, and political steps we need to take to get there as individual NPs and as organizations. In the next section, I will present key concepts that Collins recommends for NP practices to achieve greatness.

FIRST THE WHO, THEN THE WHAT

NPs came on the health care scene in 1965, and thus, became the "who" to meet primary health care provider gaps, along with physician assistants and the growing specialty of family medicine. Over the years, NPs have moved forward from nurses who assessed children's health in rural areas to a plethora of certifications and specialties. In a sense, NPs were the "who" that then created the "what" in health care. How did this happen? Collins (2001) identified that greatness in business companies is linked with attracting the right people and "getting the wrong people off the bus" (Collins, 2001, p. 44), and, in turn, ensuring that the right people are in the right position. To use Collins' metaphor, get the right people on the bus in the right seats, and the wrong people off the bus after checking that there is not a seat for them, and then decide "where to drive the bus" (Collins, 2001, p. 63). For the NP movement, NPs have consistently been identified as the right people to be in seats when innovative and new approaches are developed in health care. As a result of innovation, NP specializations have flourished. However, at this juncture, NP specialties have so proliferated that there is a growing interest for state boards of nursing to standardize advanced-practice roles nationally. Professional nursing specialty organizations would create certification that would allow for flexibility in practice (Johnson, Dawson, & Brassard, 2010).

In health care, NP businesses often develop when a group of like-minded practitioners get together and launch a practice. Getting the right persons together and continuing to refine the right mix of expertise in a practice as it moves forward is key to achieving excellence. This will involve finding ways to recruit and keep the best people, and move others who may not fit to other projects or out of the organization altogether. Human resource workers and advice from career planners can help to develop skills in this area. The processes may take time, and require constant attention and rigor. Collins' advises three practices for people decisions that work:

When in doubt, don't hire.

When you know you need to make a people change, act.

Put your best people on your biggest opportunities, not your biggest problems. (p. 63)

The Family Practice & Counseling Network (FPCN) in Philadelphia founded by Donna Torrisi, MSN, CRNP, is one of the most successful and nationally excellent NP community partnership practices in the United States. I asked Donna Torrisi to comment on the concepts of finding the right people, keeping them in the right positions, and moving forward as she has over the years as Executive Director of FPCN (Family Practice & Counseling Network, n.d.-a). Ms. Torrisi considers "First the Who, then the What" to be the most important component of Collins' framework. Finding the right people takes time, she notes, hiring is only the beginning. Then, make sure that they are meeting your expectations. "Listen to your gut, if you know something is not right, take care of it immediately, which may mean ending your relationship with the person." Take time to find the right person; the right people are out there but it can take many months to find them. "Don't settle, and feel like you know them well before hiring them," says Ms. Torrisi. Most people are the right person because of their interpersonal skills, more than their competencies or technical skills. "When the right people are in place, everyone benefits, and you can retain good staff to lead to great things," says Ms. Torrisi (D. Torrisi, personal communication, February 2, 2009).

CONFRONT THE BRUTAL FACTS

Knowing difficult facts that threaten a business and confronting these facts with action does not always occur. According to Collins (2001), businesses may know the facts that are threatening their organization in a current situation, but stay with the status quo to avoid further risk leading to lost opportunities. Truth telling and hearing the truth to learn how best to understand what needs to be addressed in an organization or company, and then taking steps to engage and debate issues, are critical. Open-ended questions by leaders who want to hear the truth in an atmosphere in which truth is valued will enable forward movement. Leaders must maintain the paradoxical position of confidence and faith that success will be ultimately achieved, while simultaneously facing reality, whatever that may entail.

The University of Pennsylvania School of Nursing established the Penn Nursing Network in 1999 to grow and own nursing practices to support its academic mission, integrating faculty responsibility for research, teaching, and practice (Evans & Lang, 2004). One of the most successful practices from a faculty and community perspective was a community nurse-managed practice, called the Health Annex. This practice, initially funded by a Health Resources and Services Administration (HRSA) grant, provided behavioral health, women's health, and primary health care in an underserved area of Southwest Philadelphia. The faculty practice was successful in several regards. There was strong connection with the community, a nursing database was used for clinical records, several faculty practiced at the site, research studies were initiated, and Penn nursing students were an active part of the practice. In

2003, however, the practice had to confront brutal facts in business, policy, and political contexts. From a policy perspective, families and individuals who used the service were either uninsured or covered by newly emerging capitated Medicaid plans. The Health Annex was a participant in one of the Medicaid plans, but not in all, and so was losing money providing primary and behavioral health services for the uninsured patients. The Health Annex needed to become a Federally Qualified Health Center (FQHC) to receive funding that would cover these much-needed services. However, because the Health Annex was owned by the University of Pennsylvania School of Nursing, which has its own 501c3, and FQHCs need to operate under their own 501c3, ownership by the University was an impediment for the Health Annex to become an FQHC. Politically, there was great support from the community, local legislative representatives, and the City of Philadelphia. For the Health Annex to become an FQHC and serve the community, it needed to become a stand-alone practice no longer owned by the School of Nursing. The faculty and the School of Nursing had to confront this brutal fact. In 2004, the School of Nursing transferred ownership of the Health Annex to FPCN, a nurse-managed community practice that developed the practice as an FQHC, grew the practice, and expanded it in 2007 to an established shopping area with community support. The Health Annex continues as a strong model of community partnership nursing practice, offering behavioral, and now, dental health services (The Family Practice & Counseling Network, n.d.-b).

The Health Annex and the School of Nursing retain a relationship for education and community service. The Penn Associate Dean for Practice & Community Affairs sits on the advisory board, Penn NP students have clinical rotations at the site, and Health Annex NPs are appointed as clinical preceptors or associates to the School of Nursing faculty. The School of Nursing gained several advantages with separation, such as sustaining and growing the nurse-managed practice when brutal facts were confronted. However, the tradeoff was also significant, as the School of Nursing lost faculty practices that had the potential to grow nursing science in an embedded practice.

THREE CIRCLES OF THE HEDGEHOG CONCEPT

Why a hedgehog? Collins (2001) uses the metaphor of a hedgehog to demonstrate the importance of simplification. A hedgehog curls into a ball when attacked and displays spikes that ward off any enemy. It is a simple, yet completely effective, strategy that the hedgehog is best at, obviously passionate about, and receives benefit by surviving the attack. In business, understanding three simple questions and how they intersect will provide businesses and NPs with an elegant way to focus practice and succeed:

What are you deeply passionate about?

What can you be best in the world at?

What are your economic drivers (p. 96)?

I have asked audiences of NPs and other health professions to think about these questions, particularly when they are more worried about the economic drivers than the other two questions. The intersection of the three concepts is key to finding greatness. Collins's work in *Good to Great for Social Sectors* states that in a nonprofit world, economic drivers could also be considered to be resources or goals that drive a project (Collins, 2005). For example, a particular family NP (FNP) may be best at counseling new mothers and passionate about women's health care. But the practitioner may not be able to be reimbursed for these services from third-party payers or get paid at rates that would support a business. To stay with the passion, the FNP may look for different economic drivers, such as writing a grant, opening a boutique service and foregoing reimbursement, or contracting with an insurer to facilitate payment to special needs populations. However, when there is no passion but there are economic drivers, a business may not succeed. One such example may be a primary care practice that is approached by a hospital or company to provide health assessments for corporate executives for a contracted fee. If there is no person who has a passion for this work or who is particularly good at or interested in corporate executive health, the business is at risk, perhaps because quality care would not be met or retention of staff would be problematic. From the perspective of Collins' (2001) model, the business would not achieve greatness because all three forces of the hedgehog concept were not in place.

At the University of Pennsylvania School of Nursing, we have started and owned several businesses. Some have continued, but others ended, either because of losing the persons with the passion to do the work, or because we no longer were "best at" a particular venture, or because there was a loss of the economic driver for the business. The clinical practice that has been retained the longest is the Living Independently For Elders (LIFE) Program. This program is a Program of All-Inclusive Care for Elders (PACE) model of care for older adults in the community who are otherwise eligible for nursing home care. We have successfully grown this program, which provides daily for 370 + older persons 24/7 in the community who are frail, with comorbidities, and from lower socioeconomic backgrounds. In 10 years, we have provided care to over 650 older adults in the community immediately adjacent to the University, supporting the mission of the University to serve the community. It is a site of excellence in care using a nurse-managed and interdisciplinary care model with excellent outcomes, including low hospitalization rates, low hospital length of stay, low emergency department visits, high satisfaction, and reduced cost by providing care at 85% the cost of nursing home care for comparable patients (Commonwealth of Pennsylvania Department of Public Welfare, 2007).

This practice represents all three areas of the hedgehog concept; it represents a passion of the SON faculty to provide best practice, discover new knowledge through research, and educate our students in the best models of care. At Penn, we had an excellent capacity of gerontological nurses, including faculty, alumni, and students to support the practice, something that we are "best at." The economic drivers are obtained through mainstream third-party sources and highly endorsed by the Commonwealth of Pennsylvania's (2003) Office of Long Term Living.

Academic nursing practices need to adhere to the hedgehog principle of knowing what you are best at, staying with your passion, and using economic drivers. We aligned our passion for nursing models of care with being best at geriatric nursing, and had strong economic drivers from third-party payers, the community, and the university to successfully grow the practice and reach excellence. One year after we aligned the three concepts, the practice grew by 70%. Moreover, following this growth, we were aligned with the University's mission for community and civic engagement. Success led to recognition in national and regional awards and public media attention. In addition to the primary mission to provide excellent care, we also achieved our goals to educate over 100 students annually, participate in on-going research, and provide public service through such community outreach as a health program on a local radio station. Fiscally, we are able to contribute to the School of Nursing's revenues, enabling the dean to create Investment for the Future funds for staff tuition and faculty research pilot funds.

CULTURE OF DISCIPLINE

After understanding and identifying the three areas of the hedgehog concept, a culture of discipline of freedom and responsibility must be instituted in an organization. Employees must have the freedom to be responsible for their work, and systems must be in place to support their work. According to Collins (2001), several issues that are particularly relevant for NPs who are struggling with conflicts between business, policy, and political issues are as follows:

1. Opportunities for growth are more likely when staying within the three concepts, in other words, What is your passion? What are you best at? What are your economic drivers?
2. Overly bureaucratic cultures arise to compensate for incompetence and lack of discipline.
3. Budgets should be used to decide which activities best fit in the Hedgehog Concept.
4. "Stop doing" lists are more important than "to do" lists (pp. 142–143).

Often in NP businesses, clinical practice, or organizational work, heavily laden policies are developed to address gaps in political or legislative arenas. Policies can get in the way of moving ahead, because overbearing policies will limit freedom and entrepreneurial spirit. As the NP movement became larger and more mainstreamed in U.S. health care, some of the initial creativity for NPs to practice was curtailed as policies were developed state-by-state without national coordination. NPs are now addressing the Hedgehog Concepts nationally to develop policies for certification and specialization that will create a culture of discipline for the nursing profession and enable political action and businesses to flourish (Johnson, Dawson, & Brassard, 2010).

As the Director for the Center for Nurse Entrepreneurship at the University of Rochester School of Nursing, Patricia Chiverton, PhD, RN, FAAN, worked with nurse faculty and the Medical Center to identify nurse businesses that focused on health promotion and wellness. When an opportunity surfaced for the School of Nursing to purchase and operate a travel health practice at the University, the nurse faculty applied the culture of discipline by identifying that health promotion and wellness was a good fit for the School's priorities, and they would not veer into illness management practices (P. Chiverton, personal communication, February 6, 2009; University of Rochester Center for Nursing Entrepreneurship, n.d.). By staying within the goals of health promotion, they were able to work with Passport Health, a national company, to establish a center in the School of Nursing and grow one center into two others, and ultimately cover an eight-county region. The success of the business has enabled students in primary care to have clinical experiences in this area and has facilitated research activities (Passport Health, n.d.).

TECHNOLOGY ACCELERATORS

Electronic health record systems, online claims billing, telehealth communication, home monitoring devices, and other technologies are currently influencing how health care is delivered, paid for, and evaluated. Investment in technologies by an NP practice needs to be considered as to the influences of business, policy, and politics. Policy may mandate or strongly incentivize online claims billing; however, a business decision regarding electronic records would need to take into consideration the resources and investment capital needed. Business decisions to move ahead may involve risk, but also political benefits. Electronic health records help identify NP work, and link it with specific outcomes used to demonstrate in a political arena the difference NP practice can make among consumers. Although this technology has propelled NPs forward, inclusion of NPs as providers in insurer policies and electronic data bases limits the full potential of NP practice (Hansen-Turton, Ritter, & Torgan, 2008).

Collins (2001) emphasizes that it is not technology alone that makes a great organization but the use of technology after the other steps—the right people who confront the brutal facts, establish the Hedgehog Concept and a culture of discipline—are in place. Technology can be critical to accelerate a business. Convenience or retail care clinics, such as the Minute Clinic (n.d.-a), are a good example of using technology to promote NP practice. NPs have always been very good at short-term acute care, engaging patients and families quickly, prioritizing health problems, providing specific care, and satisfying patients (Brown & Grimes, 1995; Mehrotra, Wang, Lave, Adams, & McGlynn, 2008). In retail clinics, NPs have communication access as soon as a potential client sees the electronic kiosk in the retail business, signs in electronically, and is given information about the immediate availability of the NP, general information regarding his or her problem, and has his or her insurance or payment verified on site to expedite the visit process.

Cheryl McDonald, MSN, CRNP, Regional Director of the Philadelphia area Minute Clinics (n.d.-b) states that the technology of service, online support, electronic information, and rapidly meeting care needs "breaks down barriers to access to care" (C. MacDonald, personal communication, February 6, 2009). From the kiosk sign-in that links customers with a national data base, to the link with insurance eligibility, to a national electronic medical record, NPs can accurately expedite a customer's needs. In these clinics, NPs are doing what they do best successfully through the technology drivers.

KEEP THE FLYWHEEL TURNING

Collins (2001) notes that momentum in great organizations is like a flywheel that is difficult to get moving, but once moving, will fly on its own weight. To achieve this moment, Collins (2001) makes several points that are relevant to NPs:

1. Good to great transformations in organizations or businesses seems to be a gradual cumulative process more than a dramatic sudden leap forward.
2. Buildup and breakthrough are consistent patterns as organizations move ahead.
3. The magnitude of a good-to-great transformation is apparent only after it occurs and organizations look back; there was no specific event, marketing technique, or acquisition that made it happen. It was day-to-day application of the right actions and conditions for a long-term goal (pp. 186–187).

Madeline Wiley, MSN, ARNP, and Robert Smithing, MSN, ARNP, are FNPs who have operated primary care businesses since 1983 in the suburban Philadelphia and Seattle areas. To keep the flywheel turning over the years, they have created a strong network and outreach effort. This outreach serves to not only create markets for their businesses, but also to address political and policy issues that support their business. As independent entrepreneurs, they consider themselves the right people to launch an NP primary care practice. Then they confronted the brutal facts of state policy that was not supportive of NPs in Pennsylvania, and established what they were best at, passionate about, and what drove them economically. They also used the internet and other technology services to accelerate their NP primary care practice and keep the flywheel turning in their current practice, including NP Central, a resource for patients and NPs (NP Central, n.d.). We have an "independent streak," says Madeline Wiley.

These NP entrepreneurs have succeeded because they have consistently adhered to what they were best at—primary health care, and what they were passionate about—NPs as independent primary care providers in suburban settings. Wiley and Smithing used economic drivers to adjust their business models to maintain their passion and what they were best at. They keep the flywheel turning by using discipline with insurance contracts. To keep the flywheel turning over the years, they have created a strong network and outreach effort. This outreach serves to not only create markets for their businesses, but also to address political and policy issues that support their business. They moved from Pennsylvania to Washington in 1984 for a more supportive NP practice state-policy environment. As independent entrepreneurs, they considered themselves to be the right people to launch an independent NP primary care practice.

They do not identify any one moment when they broke through to success, but they clearly articulate that they took the right actions for conditions during their 25 years of success. Ms. Wiley notes that one critically important factor occurred when they sold their second practice to a company and remained employees of the practice, keeping their active patients. In this contract, they inserted language that they could buy back charts at any time, as long as they were not a competitor to the owner of the company. When the company that bought them decided to divest primary care from their company, Ms. Wiley and Mr. Smithing were able to buy back their patient charts and continue their practice essentially uninterrupted (M. Wiley & R. Smithing, personal communication, February 14, 2009). Their current practice, Family Health Care of Kent, uses the byline "Caring, Competent, and Convenient Healthcare," and provides NP family health care (Family Care of Kent, n.d.).

CONCLUSIONS

NP businesses have grown, but not yet flourished, in U.S. health care. Understanding the context of business, policy, and political issues is critical for NP practices to create and grow. The flexibility and multiplicity of NP skills and talents are a tremendous resource to addressing access and quality health services. Using Collins' (2001) model is a very useful tool for good NP health care practices to achieve greatness. Success of NP practices will resonate with policymakers and politicians as a great resource for solutions to the health care crisis in the United States. Globally, APNs can use lessons learned from NP practices in the United States and Collins' method to create innovations in health care in their respective countries.

REFERENCES

Brown, S. A., & Grimes, D. E. (1995). A meta-analysis of nurse practitioner and nurse midwives in primary care. *Nursing Research, 44*, 332–339.

Collins, J. (2001). *Good to great.* New York: HarperCollins.

Collins, J. (2005). *Good to great and the social sectors: Why business thinking is not the answer* [Monograph]. Retrieved on January 24, 2009, from http://www.jimcollins. com/books/g2g-ss.html

Commonwealth of Pennsylvania. (2003). Department of Public Welfare. *Report to Office of Long Term Care.*

Commonwealth of Pennsylvania. (2007). Department of Public Welfare, Office of Long Term Living.

Evans, L. K., & Lang, N. M. (2004). *Academic nursing practice: Helping to shape the future of health care.* New York: Springer Publishing Company.

Family Care of Kent. (n.d.) Retrieved February 12, 2009, from http://www.familycare ofkent.com/

The Family Practice & Counseling Network. (n.d.-a). Retrieved February 18, 2009, from http://www.fpcn.us/index.cfm?id=20870&fuseaction=browse&pageid=1

The Family Practice & Counseling Network. (n.d.-b). Retrieved February 18, 2009, from http://www.fpcn.us/index.cfm?id=34216&fuseaction=browse&pageid=29

Hansen-Turton, T., Ritter, A., & Torgan, R. (2008). Insurers' contracting policies on nurse practitioners as primary care providers: Two years later. *Policy, Politics, & Nursing Practice, 9*, 241–248.

Johnson, J., Dawson, E., & Brassard, A. (2010). Consensus model for APRN regulation: A new approach. In. E. M. Sullivan-Marx, D. O. McGivern, J. A. Fairman, & S. A. Greenberg (Eds.), *Nurse practitioners: The evolution and future of advanced practice* (5th ed., pp. 125–142). New York: Springer Publishing Company.

Mehrotra, A., Wang, M. C., Lave, J. R., Adams, J. L., & McGlynn, E. A., (2008). Use and costs of care in retail clinics versus traditional care sites. *Health Affairs*, 27, 1283–1292.

Minute Clinic. (n.d.-a). Retrieved February 12, 2009, from http://www.minuteclinic.com/en/USA/

Minute Clinic. (n.d.-b). Retrieved February 12, 2009, from www.minuteclinic.com/en/USA/PA/Clinics.aspx

NP Central. (n.d.). Retrieved February 12, 2009, from http://www.npcentral.net

Passport Health. (n.d.). Retrieved February 12, 2009, from http://www.passporthealthusa.com/rochester/locations.html

University of Rochester Center for Nursing Entrepreneurship. (n.d.) Retrieved July 31, 2009, from http://www.son.rochester.edu/CNE/

20 Systems of Payment for Advanced-Practice Nurses

EILEEN M. SULLIVAN-MARX AND DAVID KEEPNEWS

In an era of rapid fluctuation in the business and financing of health care, all health care professionals must have skills enabling them to take advantage of practice opportunities, and also to overcome challenges to their practices. Both as autonomous providers of health care and members of interdisciplinary teams, nurse practitioners (NPs) and other advanced-practice nurses (APNs) make significant contributions in all sectors of health care delivery. In 1997 Congress passed the Balanced Budget Act, which included provisions recognizing NPs and clinical nurse specialists (CNSs) as providers of professional services under Medicare, effective 1998. Thus, all categories of APNs are now recognized by Medicare as providers of professional services. This status has brought responsibilities for APNs to develop new skills to meet growing demands in practice administration, accurate billing and documentation, and contract negotiation. The purpose of this chapter is to provide the context in which payment policies have and are developing and to provide an overview of current health care payment structures for APNs.

BACKGROUND ON ADVANCED-PRACTICE NURSES

By gaining direct Medicare reimbursement status in 1998, APNs became part of mainstream health care payment. Achieving this status helped to further establish APNs as legitimate independent providers of primary and specialty care. Subsequently, new advanced nursing practices in in-home primary care, acute care, mental health care, and gerontological care have emerged, among others. However, despite abundant research demonstrating the quality and efficacy of APNs, barriers remain that impede use of APNs in mainstream health care delivery, and that stifle development of innovative care models (Lugo, O'Grady, Hodnicki, & Hanson, 2007; Medicare Payment Advisory Commission, 2002; Sekschenski, Sansom, Bazell, Salmon, & Mullan, 1994).

Society, however, has struggled with the recognition of the APN's authority in the health care environment (Baer, 1993). Payment is one method used by society to overtly recognize a professional group's authority to practice. Barriers to payment for APNs, therefore, often reflect a struggle over professional issues, such as scope of practice, prescriptive authority, educational preparation, professional certification, and economic competition (Lugo et al., 2007). Consequently, legislative and policy initiatives for reimbursement of NPs developed in a piecemeal fashion, and often vary from state to state (Abood & Keepnews, 2000; Pearson, 2009). APNs need to be aware that practice and payment are intertwined, requiring on-going vigilance by nurses and nursing organizations to maintain and expand nursing's contribution to health care delivery.

Regardless of existing barriers to payment, many changes in health care present opportunities for NPs and other APNs, including primary care, acute care, specialty care, home care, long-term care, and rural areas (Bakerjian, 2008; Becker, Kaplow, Muenzen, & Hartigan, 2006; Kane, Flood, Keckhaver, Bershadsky, & Lum, 2002; Kaplan, Brown, Andrilla, & Hart, 2009). Attention to the economic forces at work in health care and development of business skills are crucial if APNs are to take full advantage of opportunities.

PAYMENT MECHANISMS FOR ADVANCED-PRACTICE NURSES

Although many APNs continue to develop independent nurse-managed businesses, most commonly, APNs are employees of a health care professional group or health system and receive salaries and benefits from their employer. Salaries are based on revenues generated by APNs, as well as on the value that they bring to a practice setting in terms of revenue, access, cost savings, and/or quality. Reimbursement or payment for services provided by APNs occurs through several mechanisms. In managed care plans, APNs may receive payment as an identified provider for a panel of patients. APNs who are not identified as the primary provider of care, but are employed by a professional practice group, receive payment through their employer's managed care arrangement. For example, if an APN is an employee in an independent practice association (IPA) that has a contract with a managed care plan for capitated payment for a group of patients or has an established fee schedule with a managed care plan, APN services are covered as part of the professional group's contract.

In the Medicare Part B payment structure, APNs can receive payment for their services in either of two ways. First, APNs can directly bill for their services and receive direct reimbursement at 85% of the prevailing physician rate (65% for certified nurse midwives (CNMs). Second, services provided by APNs may be billed "incident to" physician services at 100% of the physician rate. "Incident to" billing has specific requirements and, for NPs, is only applicable to non-hospital settings, and even then, when the physician is available on site. APN services may also be reflected in Medicare Part A payment to hospitals, skilled nursing facilities, and home care and hospice agencies. Further, each state determines billing requirements for APNs for the Medicaid program and private payer (Medicare Payment Advisory Commission, 2002). In the following sections, each of these reimbursement systems and mechanisms will be discussed in greater detail.

MANAGED CARE

Consumers and Managed Care

APNs must understand the dynamics of financial, clinical, and administrative agendas in managed care to present themselves as cost-efficient providers of quality care (see chapter 21 in this book). They must recognize, moreover, that managed care is driven by enrollment contracts with employers and, to a lesser extent, consumers. In an environment in which consumers and managed care organizations (MCOs) are less aware of the contributions of APNs or view the APN as an uncommon entity who happens to work with a physician, APNs will have difficulty presenting themselves as a marketable alternative to physicians, and may be more successful arguing for their role in value-added services that ultimately benefit employers, consumers, and managed care. In environments in which the APN role is well known by consumers and there is a physician shortage or limitation in access to care, APNs can be successful in marketing themselves as a legitimate provider of primary or specialty health services.

Role of Advanced-Practice Nurses in Managed Care

Changes in both health care financing and restructuring of delivery systems over the last decade have limited "solo" practice arrangements and emphasized employment and contractual arrangements for most professional providers. Managed care includes many models that integrate elements of health care delivery and payment (see chapter 21 in this book). Managed care models are structured so that financial risk and responsibility for patient outcomes range across a continuum. Clinician providers who remain independent practitioners and contract with managed care payers assume a moderate financial risk (Abood & Keepnews, 2000; Buppert, 2008).

APNs who have been successful in negotiating contracts with MCOs have done so with careful preparation, particularly when they identify a need that they can fill with a specific group of patients/enrollees. Strategies for success include meeting with managed care administrators, partnering with other health professionals and health systems, using political support and legal advice, and persisting in the face of denial (Buppert, 2008).

Financial Arrangements for Advanced-Practice Nurses

Issues that APNs must address in negotiating with MCOs, health systems, or professional practice groups include:

- Contract between the APN and employer and payer
- Risk sharing
- Clinical privileges
- Malpractice insurance

- Percentage of payment to collaborating physician
- Participation in bonus payment plans.

MEDICARE

Background

Medicare provides basic health insurance to Americans over the age of 65, and those persons who are disabled, or have end-stage renal disease (approximately 38 million Americans). According to the Medicare Payment Advisory Committee (MedPAC), "Of the $1.9 trillion spent on personal health care in the United States in 2007, Medicare accounted for 22 percent or $409 billion" (Medicare Payment Advisory Commission, 2009, p. 5). Medicare accounts for 3% of the U.S. gross domestic product (GDP) (Medicare Payment Advisory Commission, 2009).

Medicare consists of four parts. Part A (Hospital Insurance) covers inpatient hospital services, skilled nursing facility services, home health agency services, and hospice care. Medicare Part B (Supplemental Medical Insurance) covers services of professional providers. Medicare Part C is more commonly referred to as Medicare Advantage; it is a program through which Medicare beneficiaries can choose to receive their Part A and Part B (and often their Part D) services through a private health plan, most often a managed care plan. Medicare Part D is the Medicare prescription drug program.

Part A is provided to Medicare beneficiaries as an entitlement program funded through a federal payroll tax paid by employers and employees. Part B is a voluntary program funded by a combination of general tax revenues and a premium paid by participating Medicare beneficiaries. Nursing services provided in a hospital system, skilled nursing facility, home health agency, and hospice are covered under Medicare Part A. Medicare Part B covers services of professional providers, including physicians, podiatrists, NPs, CNSs, CNMs, certified registered nurse anesthetists, physician assistants, chiropractors, clinical psychologists, social workers, physical and occupational therapists, nutritionists, and speech language audiologists. Medicare Part B also covers laboratory services, outpatient hospital care, and some home health care and supplies (Medicare Payment Advisory Commission, 2001).

In 1983, federal efforts to address growth in Medicare Part A inpatient hospital expenditures led to the development of a prospective payment system (PPS) based on diagnosis-related groups (DRGs). Starting in 1998, PPS systems have been implemented for skilled nursing facilities, home health agencies, and outpatient hospital services.

Federal payment reforms to control rapidly escalating costs of physician services in Medicare Part B began with policy review under the Physician Payment Review Commission (PPRC) in the 1980s. Recommendations from the PPRC in 1989 led to provisions in Public Law 101-239, the Omnibus Budget Reconciliation Act of 1989 (OBRA-89), that established the Medicare Fee Schedule (MFS), which sets fees based on resources used. The MFS is based on a resource-based relative value scale (RBRVS), a methodology developed by health economists and adopted for use in the MFS by P.L. 101-239 (Hsiao, Braun, Yntema, & Becker, 1988). Prior to 1989, physician payment was based on "usual and customary and reasonable" fees determined by regional Medicare carriers.

Medicare Fee Schedule

In the MFS, fee-for-service (FFS) payment for services provided by health professionals is based on the resource costs used to provide the service. Each service is classified according to the Current Procedural Terminology (CPT) coding system developed by the American Medical Association (AMA) in 1966 and updated annually (AMA, 2009a). There are over 7000 CPT codes, of which the most common are the Evaluation and Management Services, such as an office or outpatient visits for a new patient (99201-99205), ranging from low (1) to high (5) in both complexity and time (AMA, 2009a). To establish the allowable payments for a service, the Center for Medicare and Medicaid Services (CMS) develops a fee schedule for each CPT code using RBRVS methodology, and based on recommendations from the AMA Relative Value Update Committee (RUC), professional organizations, carriers, and the public. The fee is established by accounting for the relative work value of the service, practice cost, and professional liability insurance, each adjusted for geographic location, and using a dollar conversion factor. In addition, the RBRVS is used by managed care systems to set fee schedules, measure clinician productivity, and analyze value of services provided. Although

Medicare has increasingly expanded participation for beneficiaries in Medicare Advantage programs, capitated payment, and managed care plans, FFS plans (in which the provider of the service is directly reimbursed) continue to be a common payment mechanism in Medicare, particularly in rural areas and for the sickest beneficiaries. However, although there has been a decline in the number of beneficiaries in FFS Medicare, Medicare spending per FFS beneficiary increased between 2000–2008 (Medicare Payment Advisory Commission, 2009). The costliest group of beneficiaries in 2006 represented 43% of all FFS Medicare spending; these are individuals with multiple chronic conditions, those who use inpatient hospital services, and those in the last year of life (Medicare Payment Advisory Commission, 2009).

CURRENT PROCEDURAL TERMINOLOGY AND OTHER BILLING CODING SYSTEMS

The American Medical Association (AMA) established the CPT coding system in 1966 following the inception of Medicare, in order to classify physician procedures. CPT codes are established and updated annually by the AMA CPT Editorial Panel. The CPT Editorial Panel is comprised of representatives of the AMA, medical specialty societies, payers, and health professionals (AMA, 2002b). Since 1993, the American Nurses Association (ANA) has had a representative on the CPT Advisory Committee and Health Care Professional Advisory Committee (CPT HCPAC) to the CPT Editorial Panel, and has been directly involved in the process of CPT code development and revision.

Services are also billable to Medicare and other payers by using the Health Care Common Procedural Coding System (HCPCS), which includes CPT codes, some codes from the International Classification of Diseases System-Clinical Modfication (ICD-CM), and other health care codes developed to describe technology and supportive care services. HCPCS codes are generally supportive services and supplies, but may have relative work values associated when applicable, such as physician (or practitioner) review of an electrocardiogram with interpretation (G007) (Abood & Keepnews, 2000). ICD-CM codes are largely diagnostic codes, but may include some procedures; they do not have assigned relative work values for Medicare purposes. These classification systems were developed for reimbursement of physician services, but have been used for all providers (e.g., psychologists, physical therapists) who may provide billable services.

RESOURCE-BASED RELATIVE VALUE SCALE PROCESS

Following Congress' mandate for Medicare to pay physician services based on an RBRVS, the CMS (then known as the Health Care Financing Administration [HCFA]), along with the American Medical Association and other medical specialty societies, established a process to develop relative work values for each CPT code in 1990. AMA established the Relative Value Update Committee (RUC), composed of representatives of AMA and medical specialty societies, to survey clinicians regarding the value of the work, to review the results of surveys, and to make recommendations to HCFA (now CMS). In 1993, organizations that represent other health care professionals who bill Medicare, including the ANA, were added to the RUC process. Requests for new or adjusted relative work values for CPT codes are initially addressed through the AMA's Relative Value Update process. Professional specialty societies or groups, the CPT Editorial Panel, or CMS may identify the need for relative work value changes. Evidence to establish or alter relative work values are developed by surveys of practicing clinicians, who rate the value of work for a specific CPT code in comparison with a related CPT code using magnitude estimation methodology. Relative work values are scaled estimates of the work involved for a specific code that take into account: (a) time, (b) technical skill and physical effort, (c) mental effort and judgment, and (d) psychological stress associated with patient risk (AMA, 2004a). Specialty societies or professional organizations present findings from surveys and their recommendations to either the AMA's RUC or the HCPAC. The HCPAC generally reviews relative work values for services provided by health professionals other than physicians, for example, physical therapy services. Recommendations from the RUC and HCPAC committees are forwarded to CMS. Relative values for the work, practice expense, and professional liability components of a CPT-coded service are totaled and multiplied by a conversion factor to determine the allowable Medicare charge for each CPT-coded service. Final recommendations for the MFS are published by CMS in the *Federal Register*, following a public comment period.

The ANA has a representative to the AMA CPT Editorial Panel and RUC process. ANA has a voting seat on the HCPAC that makes relative work value recommendations for health professional services to CMS. ANA also has a voting seat on the Practice Expense Subcommittee of the RUC, which in 2000, was charged with making recommendations for relative values for the practice expense component of the MFS. This committee established relative practice expense values for CPT-coded services. The greatest component of practice expense is salaries for nursing and medical assistant personnel.

Since 1995, when the first mandated review of RBRVS values took place, APNs have been directly involved in the development of relative work values for primary care services, home visit codes, care plan oversight, psychiatric mental health services, and specialty codes in critical care, surgical procedures, and continence management. Through the ANA and other nursing organizations, NPs and APNs have completed surveys to develop relative work values for evaluation and management services, and were coalition participants with primary care and mental health professionals to develop new and accurate relative work values for evaluation and management codes, including home visits (Sullivan-Marx & Maislin, 2000).

DIRECT REIMBURSEMENT FOR ADVANCED-PRACTICE NURSES UNDER MEDICARE PART B

Amendments to the Social Security Act passed by Congress and signed by President Clinton as part of The Balanced Budget Act (BBA) of 1997 (Public Law 105-33) gave direct Medicare reimbursement (at 85% of the physician rate) to NPs and CNSs. Prior to 1997, incremental legislative and policy changes over 15 years were in place, allowing NPs to bill for Medicare services in rural areas and nursing facilities, and allowing CNSs to bill in rural areas at 85% of the prevailing physician rate. The BBA of 1997 broadened the opportunities for billing by: (a) removing geographic area limits and (b) removing limits on direct billing by setting. Billing for NPs and CNSs at the lower rate of 85% of the prevailing physician rate had been in place prior to the BBA of 1997, and was not changed by this legislation.

When directly billing Medicare Part B, NPs and CNSs are required to be "working in collaboration with a physician" (Social Security Act,

Sec. 1861). Medicare law defines collaboration as "a process in which a nurse practitioner (or clinical nurse specialist) works with a physician to deliver health care services within the scope of the practitioner's professional expertise, with medical direction and appropriate supervision as provided for in jointly developed guidelines or other mechanisms as defined by the law of the State in which the services are performed." Collaboration with a physician is required for services reimbursed by Medicare, even if this is not required by the state in which the service was rendered.

Reimbursement to NPs and CNSs is available "only if no facility or other provider charges or is paid any amounts with respect to the furnishing of such services" (Social Security Act, Sec. 1861). The intent of this provision is to ensure that Medicare pays only once for a particular service provided by an NP or CNS. In order to ensure correct billing procedure, NPs and CNSs need to be absolutely clear about the source of their salaries to avoid billing Medicare Part B for services that are included in a facility's Part A payment. For the same reason, NPs and CNSs should also be sure not to bill Medicare directly for services billed by a physician as "incident to" services. In addition to these provisions, APNs must accept assignment from Medicare, meaning that APNs cannot bill Medicare beneficiaries for amounts greater than Medicare allowable charges for the service provided.

HOSPITAL SERVICES

In 2002, CMS issued instructions stating that NPs, CNSs, CNMs, or physician assistants may bill for evaluation and management services shared with a physician for hospital inpatient, outpatient, or emergency room services provided on the same day, as long as the physician had a face-to-face visit with the patient on that day. The NP, CNS, CNM, or PA and physician must be part of the same group practice (Medicare Carriers Manual Section 15501 [B]).

To clarify and allow direct billing of NPs and CNSs in hospital inpatient and outpatient settings, CMS issued a policy change in 2007, stating that, "direct billing and payment for the professional services of NPs and CNSs furnished to hospital patients (inpatients and outpatients) must be made to the NP or the CNS. However, if NPs or CNSs reassign payment to the hospital for their professional services to hospital patients, payment must be made to the hospital for these services at 85% of the physician fee schedule" (U.S. Department of Health and Human Services, 2007).

Pertinent to mostly acute care NPs, Medicare issued critical care billing clarifications in 2008. When NPs adhere to scope of practice and licensure requirements and meet the specifications for providing time-based critical care services, they can bill for their services and receive payment directly. Time spent in delivering critical care services must be at the bedside or in the immediate vicinity. Shared billing does not apply when billing critical care services as an NP, however, because adjusted rules allow for modifiers and other codes for billing when multiple providers are involved in care of critically ill patients (U.S. Department of Health and Human Services, 2008).

"INCIDENT TO" BILLING UNDER MEDICARE PART B

Prior to the BBA of 1997, NPs could bill Medicare as physician employees under guidelines for services that were furnished "incident to" physician services. The BBA of 1997 did not remove the ability for NPs to bill Medicare using "incident to" mechanisms. Billing "incident to" in a physician's office setting reimburses the physician practice at 100% of the prevailing physician rate, but requires adherence to strict guidelines and is not applicable in the hospital setting. The Medicare Part B guidelines for incident to billing are:

> Incident to services must be provided by employees of a physician under the physician's direct supervision. In addition, the physician must be in the office suite while the service is being provided and be immediately available to provide assistance and direction. The physician also must have provided direct, personal professional services to initiate the course of treatment and must furnish subsequent services at a frequency consistent with active management of the course of treatment. Incident to billing is not allowed for the first visit for a new patient or for subsequent visits that present a new problem. In these cases, physicians must personally examine patients to bill for services at the physician rate; otherwise, services are billed at the nonphysician practitioner rate. (Medicare Payment Advisory Commission, 2002, p. 7)

MEDICAID

Medicaid is a federally mandated program that pays for health care services to low-income families with dependent children, the low-income aged, and disabled persons. Medicaid is administered by the states, pursuant to guidelines established by the federal government, and is financed jointly by the federal and state governments. Prior to 1989, reimbursement of APNs varied according to individual state policy and legislation. To increase access to primary care services for low-income families and children, the U.S. Congress included a provision in the Omnibus Budget Reconciliation Act of 1989 requiring Medicaid payment for certified pediatric and family NPs, regardless of whether they are supervised by or associated with physicians or other health care providers. Since 1989, some states have opted to reimburse more broadly than required by federal law, allowing Medicaid payment for all NPs and at least some CNSs. Payment varies from 70–100% of the prevailing physician rate. Twenty-one states reimburse APNs at 100% of the physician rate (Buppert, 2008).

Medicaid programs have increasingly turned to managed care arrangements, including primary care case manager (PCCM) programs, in order to control use and contain costs. In many instances, MCOs providing Medicaid services have failed to include APNs as primary care providers. Thus, although all states cover NP and CNM services in FFS Medicaid, access to APN services is often limited if they are blocked from serving as primary care providers in Medicaid-managed care programs. Nursing organizations have sought changes in federal Medicaid law that would ensure that NPs may be primary care providers in Medicaid-managed care plans.

MEDICARE ADVANTAGE

More than 10 million Medicare beneficiaries receive their Part A and Part B services through private health plans that participate in the Medicare Advantage program. Most of these beneficiaries also receive their Part D (prescription drug) benefits through their Medicare Advantage plan. Medicare Advantage plans are paid on a capitated basis by Medicare. Many plans also charge beneficiaries an additional premium. The payment formula for Medicare Advantage plans has been the focus of some controversy. As of 2009, Medicare Advantage plans cost more, on average, than "traditional" FFS Medicare. Some efforts to reduce or contain Medicare costs have included proposals to reduce payments to Medicare Advantage plans. As of this writing, these proposals have been unsuccessful.

PROGRAM FOR ALL-INCLUSIVE CARE FOR THE ELDERLY

The philosophy of the Program for All-Inclusive Care for the Elderly (PACE) model is to maintain older adults in the community with minimal disruption of their lives. The PACE model is based on the successful On Lok program in San Francisco that provides a comprehensive, multidisciplinary, community-based program for older adults in their homes with capitated Medicare and Medicaid funding. Initially, originally a Medicare waiver program, PACE models are now a standard Medicare program, and are currently part of Medicare Advantage programs (U.S. Department of Health & Human Services, 1999). Services provided include primary and specialty care, adult day care, home care, nursing, social work, rehabilitative services, prescription drugs, and coordination of hospital and nursing home care by PACE staff. APNs can provide specialty, as well as primary, care medical services. The University of Pennsylvania School of Nursing received approval as a PACE site for its Living Independently for Elders (LIFE) Program in 1998, and has grown today to serve 385 frail older adults in West Philadelphia, using a nurse-managed and interdisciplinary model achieving lower rates of preventable hospitalization, emergency department visits, and nursing home use than any other PACE model in Pennsylvania (Evans & Lang, 2004).

OTHER FEDERAL PROGRAMS

Federally Qualified Health Centers

In 1992, Federally Qualified Health Centers (FQHCs) were established to provide health promotion and preventive services and access to primary care services for Medicare beneficiaries (U.S. Department of Health and Human Services, 1992). FQHCs originated from community health centers and migrant health centers established under the Public Health Service, and include any facility receiving funding from the Public Health Service Act or meeting requirements to receive a grant from this act. Clinics or facilities that meet these requirements, but do not receive a public health service grant, are called FQHC "look-alikes." Services covered in these health centers include health promotion activities usually not covered in the Medicare program, such as annual physical examinations, health screening and diagnostic tests, immunizations, and preventive health education (U.S. Department of Health and Human Services, 1992). Services of "individual practitioners who may be employed in FQHCs, including…nurse practitioners, nurse midwives…- may be covered under Medicare Part B" (*Federal Register*, 1992, p. 24965). NPs working in FQHCs, therefore, cannot also submit billing for Medicare Part B services directly (U.S. Department of Health and Human Services, 1992).

Military Health Insurance

TRICARE, a health insurance program operated by the Department of Defense, provides coverage to active duty military personnel, their families, and retired military personnel. TRICARE includes three options—TRICARE Prime (a health maintenance organization-type option), TRICARE Extra (a preferred provider organization [PPO] -type option), and TRICARE Standard (an FFS option). TRICARE Standard is the former Civilian Health and Medical Program of the Uniformed Services (CHAMPUS) program.

All three options include some coverage of NP services. Under TRICARE Prime, NPs may serve as primary care managers (PCMs). NPs may also serve as preferred providers under TRICARE Extra. As a FFS program, TRICARE Standard offers the widest choice of providers. Like CHAMPUS, its predecessor, TRICARE Standard provides for payment of services by NPs (as well as psychiatric CNSs). It does not require referral or supervision by a physician.

Federal Employee Health Benefit Plan

Federal employees can voluntarily receive health insurance through the Federal Employees Health Benefit Plan (FEHBP). Two laws have mandated FEHBP coverage of services for nurses. First, in 1985, Congress mandated reimbursement to all nonphysician providers, including registered nurses, for services provided under this plan.

In 1990, Public Law 101-509 mandated direct payment to NPs, psychiatric CNSs, and CNMs for services provided to federal employees participating in this plan. Collaboration or supervision by any other health care provider is not required.

TRADITIONAL "INDEMNITY PLAN" REIMBURSEMENT

Coverage of APN services by private indemnity plans is regulated at the state level. In the last 30-plus years, NPs and other APNs have been successful in establishing state legislation supporting reimbursement for their services. State insurance laws address components of health care coverage that include insurers affected (nonprofit and commercial or for-profit), providers affected, or reimbursable services. State laws will vary by type of insurer and whether the benefit to be covered for APN services is mandatory or a mandatory option. In a mandatory "option" regulation, consumers of health care must request to have APN services included in their coverage; although in legislation for mandatory coverage, APN services must be included in coverage. Rates of reimbursement vary, and may be a percentage of the prevailing physician rate (Buppert, 2008; Pearson, 2002).

ISSUES WITH ADVANCED-PRACTICE NURSES AND PAYMENT

Medicare

One of the earliest attempts to ascertain the extent of use of CPT billing codes by otherwise "invisible" nurse specialists found that use of codes ranged from family NPs who provided 233 CPT codes, to school nurses who performed 58 codes (Griffith & Robinson, 1993). In 1996, Medicare payment to NPs under the MFS was limited to services that were provided by NPs whose services could be billed to Medicare, in other words, those who practiced in rural areas or in skilled nursing facilities. Thus, the most frequently billed codes by NPs prior to the Balanced Budget Act of 1997 were nursing facility visits. Home visits (Medicare

Part B provider services to patients in their homes) were the least frequently represented, because NPs could not bill Medicare for these services, except in rural areas.

Payment to APNs through "incident to" billing appears in Medicare Claims Data as physician-provided, rendering APN services invisible in the federal data bases. With direct Medicare billing, APNs can now track services that are billed in federal data bases, and also track revenue that they have generated in a practice, but only those that are billed under the APN's name and provider number. With shared service billing in hospitals and billing to group practices, the Medicare activity of NPs remains largely invisible. Thus, as NPs continue to set up systems for billing under their own provider identifier rather than under a physician identifier, their contribution to Medicare services will become clearer.

Professional nursing organizations have established information services and "hotlines" for questions about correct billing procedures. Gaps in published material on APN billing have been closed as new texts have been written, and general billing texts now include material on billing for APN services. Information regarding organizations for APNs can be accessed at Web sites that are provided in chapter 28 in this book. Questions that APNs should be able to answer in their practices include:

1. What specific CPT code is used for the specific services provided?
2. What documentation in the patient's record is required for the service that is billed?
3. When is the service provided a billable service? Or is the service already included in payment by another source, such as Medicare Part A?
4. What resources do I need so that my services are accurately and legally billed?

Fraud and abuse by health care providers has been the subject of increasing activity by both federal and state governments over the past several years. Government agencies have devoted increasing resources to investigation and enforcement, and recent federal legislation has increased both the breadth of practices that may be considered illegal, as well as the potential penalties for violations.

Most NPs are ethical, honest practitioners. Unfortunately, this is not sufficient protection. NPs need to have a working familiarity with reimbursement laws and with what they are expected to do to avoid legal or regulatory violations.

Some of the more common examples of activities that may be considered fraud or abuse include: billing for services that were not actually furnished to the patient; misrepresenting a patient's diagnosis in order to justify or increase payment; misrepresenting the services as being medically necessary; billing for services in excess of those needed by the patient; billing for services that were not furnished as billed (for instance, by "upcoding" to a more expensive service); and billing for services that are not covered. Among its provisions, the federal Health Insurance Portability and Accountability Act (HIPAA) of 1996 (P.L. 104-191) introduced broad penalties for defrauding, or attempting to defraud, virtually any health plan, whether federal, state, or private. HIPAA also prohibits making knowing and willful false statements in connection with the delivery or payment of health care services. It provides for criminal penalties, including fines and prison sentences, for violation of these provisions.

HIPAA also broadened the standards under which civil penalties against providers may be imposed. A provider may be liable for submitting a claim that she knows *or should know* is false. A provider may be held accountable for claims submitted in her/his name (for instance, by a billing service). Ignorance of improper billing practices by a billing service or office personnel may not be a sufficient response to allegations of fraud and abuse. If a bill reflects services that were not delivered, or if it includes services billed at a higher level than actually delivered, it is generally not an adequate response to allegations of fraudulent billing. This is one reason why NPs and other clinicians should be aware of what is billed under their names and provider numbers.

The Medicare and Medicaid Patient Protection Act of 1987 (42 U.S.C. §1320a-7b[a]) identifies six types of conduct that may be considered felonies, and may result in fines of up to $25,000 and/or up to 5 years' imprisonment. Among the prohibited activities is a broadly described one: *knowingly and willfully making or causing to be made any false statement or representation of a material fact in any application for any benefit* under the Medicare or Medicaid program. This not only prohibits billing for services that were not provided, it also prohibits other false statements with regard to billing, and conduct related to such false statements.

The Federal Anti-Kickback Statute (42 U.S.C. §1320a-7b[b]) prohibits knowingly and willfully offering, paying, soliciting, or receiving
anything of value in order to induce furnishing of services under
Medicare, Medicaid, or other state health care programs. Violating this
law is a felony that is punishable by fines of up to $25,000, imprison-
ment of up to 5 years, and exclusion from Medicare, Medicaid, and
other federal health care programs. The antikickback law applies to
referrals (for instance, an NP paying another provider for each patient
referred to the NP). But it may also apply to other arrangements, such
as discounts, rebates, or other reductions in fees. The Office of Inspector
General (OIG) of the U.S. Department of Health and Human Services
maintains a list of "safe harbors"—arrangements that will not be considered a violation of the antikickback law. This list is updated periodically
through the federal rule-making process, and is contained in the Code
of Federal Regulations at 42 CFR §1001.952.

The federal False Claims Act (31 U.S.C. § 3729) is a major source
of federal fraud and abuse activity. It imposes civil liability on anyone
who submits a false or fraudulent claim paid by the government. Its
reach is not limited to health care services; in fact, it was first enacted
during the Civil War to address fraud by military contractors. 1986
amendments strengthened the law, and made it clear that it applied
to false claims submitted to the Medicare and Medicaid programs. An
important feature of the False Claims Act is the fact that it allows a
private individual—known as a "qui tam relator" (or, more informally,
a whistleblower)—to bring suit in federal court on behalf of the government. If the allegations are proven in court, or result in an out-of-
court settlement, the qui tam relator can collect a share of the recovered
damages (ranging between 15 and 30%).

Self-referral is another important area of federal enforcement activity. Federal laws (known as Stark I and II) establish limits on a physician's ability to refer patients to clinical laboratories and several other
health services in which the physician (or an immediate family member) has a financial interest. The intent of these laws is to avoid referrals
made for economic self-interest rather than actual patient need. As
written, the laws are specific to physicians; they do not address referrals
by NPs. But NPs should be aware of these laws. The laws express a
clear policy against referring patients based on the provider's self-
interest, and it is certainly possible that the laws may be amended at
some point in the future to address self-referral by providers other
than physicians. More immediately relevant, referrals made by an NP

may invoke the Stark laws if the physician "controls or influences" the referral. The question of whether an NP is acting independently or under a physician's "control or influence" is answered by examining the specific facts and circumstances surrounding the referral.

POTENTIAL PAYMENT AND INSURANCE REFORMS RELEVANT TO ADVANCED-PRACTICE NURSING PRACTICE

Regardless of the political context and time, reforms in health coverage and health care delivery will be ongoing processes. To be able to proactively plan and respond to changes in payment systems and structures, NPs need to remain informed and to work closely with professional organizations to ensure that NPs have continued ability to be a part of mainstream U.S. health care. Outside of the United States, nurses should work with emerging payment systems in their respective countries, as well.

In the United States, facets of the health reform for change include infrastructure, organization of health care delivery, provider payment incentives, patient activation, quality of care, and population health. Payment reform generally is categorized in the areas of: (a) redesigning or adjusting fees for service payments, (b) developing payment incentives based on performance, and (c) bundling or global/comprehensive payments (Guterman, Davis, Schoenbaum, & Shih, 2009; Mechanic & Altman, 2009; Wilensky, 2009). In consideration of potential changes, NPs may see adjustments for payment relative to their services in the following categories.

Readjustment of Fee for Service

As described earlier, NPs and organized nursing have been involved in refining FFS payment through activities to establish relative work values for payment. Because NPs commonly work in teams, NPs will need to make sure that NP work is defined in any attempts to realign payment in an FFS payment for professional services.

Provider Payment Incentives

Also known as "Pay for Performance," provider payment incentives simply reward providers for achieving specific outcomes. Incentives for providers to reach quality are increasingly being implemented, as both providers of care and payers recognize that incentivizing efforts to produce outcomes through payment can be an effective means to increase quality (Guterman, Davis, Schoenbaum, & Shih, 2009; Mechanic & Altman, 2009). NPs are actively involved in reform efforts, but would benefit from greater engagement with other stakeholders and policy experts. Such engagement is being organized through the American Academy of Nursing and other consumer organizations, such as the Robert Wood Johnson Foundation and the AARP (see chapter 4 in this book).

In Pennsylvania, the Chronic Care Commission, which has several NPs and nurse leaders as members, has implemented a pilot study incentivizing primary care providers to reach outcomes for care of persons with diabetes and asthma based on measurable outcomes, such as HgA1c and reduction in emergency department visits. Nurse-managed clinics, and primary care practices that employ NPs, are included in the pilot study program currently underway. Findings from such pilot programs will inform policymakers, providers, and consumers about the critical need to achieve outcomes through coordination of care, health education, and use of electronic individual health data.

Chronic Care Management

The need to address cost of care of patients with multiple chronic conditions is paramount in the United States (Berenson et al., 2008; Medicare Payment Advisory Commission, 2009). As part of chronic care management, NPs are members of teams or direct primary care providers responsible for a panel of patients. In addition, nurse-managed centers often achieve quality outcomes. There is no prohibitive reason for NPs not to be included in any chronic care payment model; indeed, research related to long-term care outcomes demonstrates that NPs are prominent in translational work demonstrating improvements in chronic care (see chapter 7 in this book). However, nurses and NPs continue to be invisible in payment models, described as nonphysician providers or staff to manage and coordinate care, such as in the movement to establish the medical home model (Fisher, 2008). The medical home model developed as a method to care for children with disabilities, and as such, has strong ties with pediatricians. To identify that NPs have relevance in the medical home concept, the American Academy of Pediatrics issued a joint statement in April 2009 (Tayloe, 2009) indicating support for NPs to be involved in medical home movement, but not to "direct" medical homes. NPs who have independent practices certainly could direct medical home concepts, and do so in nurse-managed centers (MacStravic, 2006; Torrisi & Hansen-Turton, 2005).

Transitional Care Model

The Transitional Care Model (TCM) is a demonstrated care model in which APNs provide care management through telephone calls and home visits, and care coordination with physicians and nurses to reduce re-hospitalization and emergency department visits following hospitalization for hospitalized older adults, as well as those with heart failure (Naylor et al., 2004). TCM has drawn considerable interest as a successful, efficient model for improving care. As health reform looms in the United States, NPs may find some opportunities for payment in this model of care.

SUMMARY AND CONCLUSIONS

Thirty-five years ago, APNs were considered pioneers in health care delivery models, forging a place for themselves in primary care and specialty care. Today, inclusion of APNs in health care systems is increasingly standard practice. Consistent growth in numbers and use of NPs has led to the inclusion of APNs in mainstream health care payment structures. Both business and governmental models of practice have recognized the advantages of including APNs in systems of care for cost savings and quality outcomes. APNs, however, have had a steep learning curve to acquire the requisite business skills and knowledge of reimbursement relevant to their practices. Current emphasis in linking financial responsibility with provision of quality care, and the need to address care of underserved, uninsured, and specialized patient groups, has made it inevitable that APNs take an active part in policy and business in order to continue as essential and viable providers of care. Globally, NPs and policymakers have begun to implement scope of practice within payment for care, mostly in situations in which NPs are providing services to underserved patients or are part of hospital budgets. As NPs continue to develop across the world, lessons learned from the United States regarding how to mainstream NP practice into payment for services will be crucial.

REFERENCES

Abood, S., & Keepnews, D. (2000). *Understanding payment for advanced practice nursing services.* (Volume One: Medicare reimbursement.) Washington, DC: American Nurses Publishing.

American Medical Association. (2002a). *Medicare RBRVS: The physician's guide.* Chicago: Author.

American Medical Association. (2002b). *Physician's current procedural terminology.* Chicago: Author.

Annas, G. J. (1997). Patients' rights in managed care: Exit, voice, and choice. *New England Journal of Medicine, 337*(3), 210–215.

Baer, E. D. (1993). Philosophical and historical bases of primary care nursing. In M. D. Mezey & D. O. McGivern (Eds.), *Nurses, nurse practitioners: Evolution to advanced practice* (pp. 102–116). New York: Springer Publishing Company.

Bakerjian, D. (2008). Care of nursing home residents by advanced practice nurses. *Research in Gerontological Nursing, 1,* 177–185.

Becker, D., Kaplow, R., Muenzen, P. M., & Hartigan, C. (2006). Activities performed by acute and critical care advanced practice nurses. *American Journal of Critical Care, 15,* 130–148.

Berenson, R. A., Hammons, T., Gans, D. N., Zuckerman, S., Merrell, K., Underwood, W. S., et al. (2008). A house is not a home: Keeping patients at the center of practice redesign. *Health Affairs, 27,* 1219–1230.

Buppert, C. (2008). *Nurse practitioner's business practice and legal guide* (3rd ed.). Boston: Jones and Bartlett.

Fisher, E. S. (2008). Building a medical neighborhood for the medical home. *New England Journal of Medicine, 359,* 1202–1205.

Griffith, H. M., & Robinson, K. R. (1993). Current procedural terminology (CPT) coded services provided by nurse specialists. *Image: Journal of Nursing Scholarship, 25,* 178–186.

Guterman, S., Davis, K., Schoenbaum, & Shih, A. (2009). Using Medicare payment policy to transform the health system: A framework for improving performance. *Health Affairs, 28*(2), w238–w250.

Henry, S. B., Holzemer, W. L., Randell, C., Hsieh, S.-F., & Miller, T. J. (1997). Comparison of nursing interventions classification and current procedural terminology codes for categorizing nursing activities. *Image: Journal of Nursing Scholarship, 29,* 133–138.

Hooker, R. S., & McCaig, L. F. (2001). Use of physician assistants and nurse practitioners in primary care, 1995–1999. *Health Affairs, 20,* 231–238.

Hsiao, W. C., Braun, P., Yntema, D., & Becker, E. R. (1988). Estimating physicians' work for a resource-based relative value scale. *New England Journal of Medicine, 319,* 835–841.

Kane, R. L., Flood, S., Keckhaver, G., Bershadsky, B., & Lum, Y. S. (2002). Nursing home residents covered by Medicare risk contracts: Early findings from the EverCare evaluation project. *Journal of the American Geriatrics Society, 50,* 719–727.

Kaplan, L., Brown, M.-A., Andrilla, C. H., & Hart, L. G. (2009). Rural-urban practice patterns of nurse practitioners in Washington state. *Journal for Nurse Practitioners, 5,* 169–175.

Lang, N. M., Sullivan-Marx, E. M., & Jenkins, M. (1996). Advanced practice nurses and success of organized delivery systems. *American Journal of Managed Care, 2,* 129–135.

Lugo, N. R., O'Grady, E. T., Hodnicki, D. R., & Hanson, C. M. (2007). Ranking state NP regulation: Practice environment and consumer healthcare choice. *American Journal for Nurse Practitioners, 11*(4), 8–24.

MacStravic, S. (2006). Medical versus health homes for patients. *Journal of Nurse Practitioners, 2,* 206–208.

Medicare Payment Advisory Commission. (2001, December). *Report to the Congress: Reducing Medicare complexity and regulatory burden.* 1–48.

Medicare Payment Advisory Commission. (2002, June). *Report to the Congress: Medicare payment to advanced practice nurses and physician assistants.* 1–27.

Medicare Payment Advisory Commission. (2009, June). *A data book: Healthcare spending and the Medicare program.*

Morgan, R. O., Virnig, B. A., DeVito, C. A., & Persily, N. A. (1997). The Medicare-HMO revolving door: The healthy go in and the sick go out. *New England Journal of Medicine, 337,* 169–175.

Naylor, M., Brooten, D. A., Campbell, R. L., Maislin, G., McCauley, C. M., & Schwartz, J. S. (2004). Transitional care of older adults hospitalized with heart failure: A randomized, controlled trial. *Journal of the American Geriatrics Society, 52,* 675–684.

Nurse practitioner entrepreneurs bring care to coastal Georgia. (2002). *Nurse Practitioner World News, 7*(5), 1–3, 10–11.

Paulus, R. A., Davis, K., & Steele, G. D. (2008). Continuous innovation in health care: Implications of the Geisinger experience. *Health Affairs, 27,* 1235–1245.

Pearson, L. J. (2002). The fourteenth annual legislative update: How each state stands on legislative issues affecting advanced nursing practice. *Nurse Practitioner, 27*(1), 10–52.

Pearson, L. J. (2009). The Pearson report. *American Journal for Nurse Practitioners, 13*(2), 8–11.

Randel, L., Pearson, S. D., Sabin, J. E., Hyams, T., & Emanuel, E. J. (2001). How managed care can be ethical. *Health Affairs, 20,* 43–56.

Sekschenski, E. S., Sansom, S., Bazell, C., Salmon, M. E., & Mullan, F. (1994). State practice environments and the supply of physician assistants, nurse practitioners, and certified nurse-midwives. *New England Journal of Medicine, 331,* 1266–1271.

Social Security Act, Sec. 1861 (aa)(4); Medicare Carrier Manual, Secs. 2158, 2160.

Sullivan-Marx, E. M., & Maislin, G. (2000). Comparison of nurse practitioner and family physician relative work values. *Journal of Nursing Scholarship, 32,* 71–76.

Tayloe, D. (2009). *Joint statement on nurse practitioners in patient-centered medical home demonstration projects.* American Academy of Pediatrics. Retrieved September 24, 2009, from http://www.txpeds.org/u/documents/tayloe_letter.pdf

Torrisi, D. L., & Hansen-Turton, T. (2005). *Community and nurse-managed health centers.* New York: Springer Publishing Company.

U.S. Department of Health and Human Services. (1992). Medicare program: Payment for federally qualified health center services. *Federal Register, 57*(11C), 24961–24985. Washington, DC: U.S. Government Printing Office.

U.S. Department of Health and Human Services, Health Care Financing Administration (1998). Part B Medicare annual data.

U.S. Department of Health and Human Services, Health Care Financing Administration (1999). Part B Medicare annual data.

U.S. Department of Health and Human Services. (1999). Medicare and Medicaid programs; Programs of all-inclusive care for the elderly (PACE). *Federal Register, 64,* 66234.

U.S. Department of Health and Human Services, Health Care Financing Administration (2001). Part B Medicare annual data.

U.S. Department of Health and Human Services, Center for Medicare and Medicaid Services. (2002). *Medicare carriers manual* (Transmittal No. 1776. Sec. 15360–15501, pp. 15-73–15-74.2).

U.S. Department of Health and Human Services, Center for Medicare and Medicaid Services. (2007). *Medicare carriers manual* (Transmittal No.1168. Sec. 120.1).

U.S. Department of Health and Human Services, Center for Medicare and Medicaid Services. (2008). *Medicare carriers manual* (Transmittal No. 1548. Sec. 30.6.12.)

Wagner, E. H., Glasgow, R. E., Davis, C., Bonomi, A. E., Provost, L., McCulloch, D., et al. (2001). Quality improvement in chronic illness: A collaborative approach. *Journal of Quality Improvement, 27,* 63–80.

21 Nurse Practitioners Navigating Managed Care

ELIZABETH MILLER

MANAGED CARE

Managed care is the system that controls the financing and delivery of health care to those who are enrolled in a specific type of health care plan. Buppert (2008) defines managed care as "the insurer is not only the payer, but also the provider of healthcare" and controls how that health care is used (p. 418). The types of plans offered by managed care organizations (MCOs) are defined by where they fall along the provider access/cost continuum. Health maintenance organizations (HMOs) and preferred provider organizations (PPOs) are two different types of programs offered by MCOs. HMOs offer enrollees controlled out-of-pocket costs, but limit their flexibility; providers serve as gate-keepers who make referrals for additional services. In theory, HMOs support coordination of care and a higher level of primary and preventive services. PPOs provide greater access to care, in that they do not require gatekeeper referrals for services like the HMO does, so the enrollee has more flexibility in determining service usage. PPO plans may cost more, with higher premiums and out-of-pocket co-pays.

According to the United States Census Bureau, the number of people with health insurance increased from 250 million in 2006 to 253 million in 2007 (DeNavis-Walt, Proctor, & Smith, 2008). Of those, 202 million were covered by private health insurance and 83 million were covered by government health insurance. Approximately 30 million individuals are covered by both government insurance and supplemental private insurance. The declining economy of 2008 and recession of 2009 have led to increasing unemployment, which effectively reduces personal income, state revenue, and overall health coverage rates. For each 1% increase in unemployment, the percentage of uninsured non-elderly adults is estimated to increase by 0.59 percentage points (Kaiser Family Foundation, 2009). For the current 2009 national unemployment rate of 9.5% (United States Department of Labor, 2009), it is estimated that we have returned to the 2006 coverage level of approximately 248 million people. The change in percentage of uninsured children was not estimated to be statistically significant (p. 8) because of corresponding increases in Medicaid/SCHIP coverage.

It is estimated that approximately 44.3 million people are enrolled in HMOs, whereas approximately 110 million people are enrolled in PPOs (Osgood, 2008). In 2008, 10.1 million enrollees, or 23% of all Medicare participants, were enrolled in a Medicare MCO plan, known as a Medicare Advantage plan (Kaiser Family Foundation, 2008). Those who are not enrolled in managed care plans remain in fee-for-service plans.

The HMO and PPO plans contract with health care providers and facilities to provide care for enrolled members at agreed-upon rates defined in a fee schedule (FS). Prior to contracting, the provider must be credentialed with the insurer. Credentialing is an essential qualification and background check to determine the legitimacy of a provider's ability to provide services. Insurers consider their credentialing to be an endorsement of the provider's ability to provide care. These credentialed, contracted providers make up the insurer's network or panel.

The FS is a listing of current procedural terminology (CPT) and healthcare common procedure and coding system (HCPCS) codes that the insurer will pay the provider for a specific visit level or procedure. Contracted providers will have a different contract and FS for each MCO. In fact, a provider may have multiple different FS addendums for each MCO contract, depending on the service lines. For example, for one MCO contract there may be a Medicaid FS appendix, a Medicare FS appendix, and a Commercial FS appendix, each offering different reimbursable codes and rates. Medicare MCO FS is typically based on the Centers for Medicare & Medicaid Services (CMS) FS. In addition, some MCO contracts include forms of capitation or pay-for-performance. Capitated arrangements give providers a per-member, per-month reimbursement to cover a range of services, whereas pay-for-performance gives a gain-sharing bonus based on success achieved in defined quality goals or cost savings. Both strategies attempt to align the incentives of the provider with those of the payer, namely, to provide high-quality, cost-effective care.

With both HMOs and PPOs, enrollees can choose to see providers outside of the contracted network, but they will have to pay higher, out-of-network co-pays. As a result, many enrollees limit themselves to the contracted providers. Consequently, if a nurse practitioner (NP) wants to see patients with coverage from a specific MCO, or, if an enrollee wants to see a specific NP, it is important that the practitioner be admitted to the MCO's panel for that particular plan and be listed in the provider directory.

THE MANAGED CARE MARKETPLACE

When considering applying to MCO panels, NPs should understand which MCOs are positioned in the market they serve. Although the national health insurance market is generally fragmented, with over 1,300 different companies, it may be concentrated in specific markets, dominated by just one or two payers. There is no national database containing enrollment figures for commercial health insurers, but the Kaiser Family Foundation does report both Medicare and Medicaid MCO enrollment information by geographic region. To further understand a payer's significance in a specific market, NPs can perform due diligence by speaking with other providers or obtaining enrollment information directly from the MCO.

Different insurance organizations have different policies to reflect their strategies for network management. Some maintain closed panels unless a need has been determined by the consumer, in an effort to control their administrative burden. Others respond more directly to providers in their requests to join plan panels, believing that more comprehensive panels are more attractive to consumers. Strategies also differ around coverage of NP services, and they may or may not independently contract and credential NPs at all.

Several states prohibit health insurers from specifically excluding qualified providers from their panels through any willing provider laws (MacEachern, 2003). Although the provision does not require that they contract with everyone, it does take steps toward ensuring due process in the contracting process. Although the provision is frequently limited to pharmacies, some states are applying the concept to all providers, including NPs. The provisions are based on the concept that by selectively contracting and excluding some providers, health plans are threatening providers' freedom to practice to the extent defined by their scope of practice, thus restricting their work and limiting patient choice. MCOs have argued against these laws, saying that they increase administration costs and impede quality monitoring (Federal Trade Commission and Department of Justice, 2003). NPs should understand their state regulations not only around their scope of practice, but also those that may impact managed care contracting.

Regulation aside, many of the large national MCOs recognize the value that NPs provide, and have policies that state they will contract with NPs in accordance with their defined scope of practice for that state. For example, Aetna, a large national health insurance provider with over 17 million medical enrollees, contracts directly with NPs for both medical and behavioral health plans (Robert J. Franzoi, personal communication, January 23, 2009). Wellpoint, with over 35 million enrollees in its Blue Cross Blue Shield plans, began credentialing NPs in 2004 (Indiana Academy of Family Physicians, 2007). Other plans such as the regional Medical Mutual of Ohio and the national UnitedHealth Group, which serves over 70 million Americans through its United, Oxford, and Pacificare health plans, have also moved to credential individual NPs, but they require evidence of collaboration with a participating physician, and only allow the physician to act as the primary care provider (Krizner, 2006; United Healthcare Oxford, 2008). Although they employ NPs directly in some plans, United does not recognize NPs for independent primary care provider contracts (Robyn King, personal communication, January 29, 2009). In addition to the MCO organizational policies around credentialing and contracting with NPs, the NPs' ability to contract independently remains subject to their State Practice Act. For example, a regional plan may require that an NP be affiliated with a network physician provider because the state practice act requires physician collaboration for NP practice (see chapter 22 in this book).

Typically, all requests for participation in MCO panels are evaluated by local network management teams, who measure those requests against the current geographical needs of the population the plan serves. So, although broad policies may be set, specific requests to admit NPs to panels are made at the regional network management level, which are subject to local market forces and influences.

MCO VALUES

Buppert (2008) identifies the numerous items that may be considered in an MCO contract, and recommends that providers seek the counsel of an attorney prior to executing this legal document. When considering the contract, the provider should understand that the contract items should be designed to protect and support the values and rights of the patient, provider, and insurer.

For practices to skillfully negotiate with MCOs, they must understand what MCOs need to operate effectively and how to present their clinical services as a value proposition in light of those needs, both individually as NPs, and collectively as a profession. Some important metrics to consider that MCOs manage their business by include: (a) the membership or number of lives covered by the plans; (b) the medical cost ratio (MCR) or benefit cost ratio (BCR), which are the percentages of every premium dollar that is paid out in medical expenses; (c) enrollee satisfaction levels; and (d) the plan performance in the Healthcare Effectiveness Data and Set (HEDIS) measures collected through the National Committee for Quality Assurance (NCQA). HEDIS is a tool used by most health plans to measure their performance on dimensions of care and service. The 70 HEDIS measures include important primary care quality indicators that are well within the scope of NPs' practice, such as "Evidence of Cholesterol Management for Patients with Cardiovascular Conditions" and "Evidence of Comprehensive Diabetes Care" (NCQA, 2009). As discussed in other chapters in this book, an established body of academic research exists that demonstrates NPs' ability to provide high-quality, cost-effective care. That said, MCOs frequently lack internal data to substantiate this fact through their own claims and medical records experience. This problem exists because these data largely identify care provided by the NP under the employing practice or physician provider numbers, making it difficult to tie outcomes to the NP (NAPNAP, 2004). Instead of direct NP billing, services may be billed under a physician or practice name and provider identification number, so that services are paid at the (higher) physician reimbursement rate or to streamline the administrative billing process. As a result, the number of enrollees who are tied to the NP (membership) and the quality outcomes (MCR, HEDIS) related to the NP provider are bundled into the physician or group practice provider number. Some insurers, such as Wellpoint/Anthem, recognize this and have begun to request that practices "refrain from billing any services provided to Anthem members under the Physicians NPI or PIN if the services are rendered by a mid-level practitioner" (Indiana Academy of Family Physicians, 2007, p. 1). This is an important step to developing a claims-based body of evidence to corroborate the research. Even if NPs are not listed as the primary provider, substantive visit quantity and outcome data can be learned by tying the claims experience directly to them. Furthermore, when NPs have and use their own provider numbers and their scope of practice permits, they are listed independently in the provider directory as being contracted and on the provider panel, which is an important marketing tool for any provider.

CREDENTIALING AND CONTRACTING

Credentialing is the process of review and verification of a health care provider's professional information. Both health care facilities and MCOs credential provider applicants as a risk management and quality assurance measure. The credentialing process involves the review and verification of professional license(s), Drug Enforcement Administration and prescriptive authority, NPI number, education, other hospital or nursing home staff privileges, levels of liability insurance, and any litigation history. Credentialing is a necessary step toward recognition as an independent and accountable provider, and is a prerequisite to MCO contracting.

As NPs are licensed as independent providers, they have several options for contracting. If the MCO policy is open to contracting NPs and the provider panel is open, meaning they are actively contracting and credentialing new providers, the NP may pursue an independent contract with that payer. Over the last 20 years, many health care markets have become consolidated, not only on the insurance side, but on the provider side, as well (Coile, 1997). On the provider side, markets have developed integrated delivery networks. These networks organize providers as groups to leverage their size when contracting with MCOs, thus negotiating more favorable contract terms. NPs can join larger provider networks, and although they will still have to independently credential with the MCO, they will be tied to the existing provider network contract. Depending on how the contract is set up, the NPs may then bill under their own provider number or through the network practice. Regardless of the contractual arrangement, NPs should be listed by name as a provider in the appropriate primary care or specialty care section of the provider directory. This is an important step in presenting oneself as a provider option to the MCO enrollees.

In addition to the traditional contract arrangements, some MCOs have used vertical integration, or the group model, to achieve their goals of cost-effective, quality care. The logic of this model is that it gives the MCO greater influence on practice patterns by aligning the goals of the provider and the insurer through an employment relationship (Casalino, 2006). The most notable model of vertical integration of NPs is the Evercare model. Here, NPs employed by the UnitedHealth Group Evercare plans maintain a caseload of enrollees, who are frail elderly patients. The result is that the intensive primary care provided by these NPs reduces the rate of costly events, such as preventable hospitalizations (Kane, Flood, Bershadsky, & Keckhafer, 2004). The model is not a production model, meaning that the NP's work is not measured by the number of visits completed. Instead, the NP provides care to a caseload of patients, adjusting the amount of time spent or number of patients seen according to acute and chronic needs. With the varying contracting models, ultimately, the type of agreement that the insurer and NP enter into depends on risk tolerance of the two parties and their motivation to achieve long-term goals for increased quality and decreased cost.

THE FUTURE OF MANAGED CARE

The Medicare Modernization Act (2003) expanded health savings accounts (HSAs) and high deductible health plans (HDHP). America's health insurance plans (AHIP) report that in 2008, greater than 6 million people were covered by HSAs coupled with HDHPs to protect them for catastrophic events. This enrollment figure has doubled since 2006. HSAs "give consumers incentives to manage their own health care costs by coupling a tax-favored savings account used to pay medical expenses with a HDHP that meets certain requirements for deductibles and out-of-pocket expense limits" (America's Health Insurance Plans, 2008, p. 3). To ensure adequate support for important preventive services such as routine medical exams, immunizations, and well-baby visits, HDHPs cover these services without requiring the enrollee to first meet the deductible, but other incidental care is paid out of the HSA. The funds in the HSA are owned by the individual and may be rolled over from year to year.

Consumers are encouraged to manage their HSA dollars as they would the rest of their budget, giving these plans the categorization of consumer-driven health plans (CDHPs). Although some evidence indicates that participants in CDHPs cut back on both evidence-based and non-evidence-based care (Dixon, Greene, & Hibbard, 2008), in an effort to save HSA funds, supporters believe that they impart a level of financial responsibility for health care use that is not existent in other health care consumer relationships. The underpinning of the CDHP is that consumers decide how and where their health care dollars are spent, within the context of price and quality transparency. They can still only choose those services or providers who are included in the payer's panel. CDHPs may be either HMOs or PPOs, but what they do is ask the consumer to consider the price of his or her incidental care. As a result, educated consumers given price and quality transparency may begin to value and request NP services more directly. Consider, for example, a patient who wants to see a primary care provider for a child's ear infection. It will cost them $60.00 HSA dollars to see a physician, and $52 HSA dollars to see an NP, and both providers have similar quality outcomes listed on the MCOs quality scorecard. This consumer will consider the value proposition and may choose the NP provider as a result. With this experience, consumers may request, or even demand, that the MCOs expand their NP provider panels to ensure adequate access.

Research by Brown (2007) indicates that greater than 90% of the consumer sample knew about NPs, that 58% of these respondents had received care provided by NPs, and that they were satisfied with that care. With increasing recognition and visibility, it is still incumbent upon NPs to continue to educate both health care payers and consumers about their preparation, scope, and outcomes. This will become increasingly important as educated consumers take greater responsibility for their health care use. To prepare for the consumer-driven demand or other managed care payment trends, NPs must also continue efforts to expand their own independent scope of practice and the direct reimbursement that goes along with it.

REFERENCES

America's Health Insurance Plans. (2008). *January 2008 census shows 6.1 million people covered by HSA/ high deductible health plans.* Washington, DC: Author.

Brown, D. J. (2007). Consumer perspectives on nurse practitioners and independent practice. *Journal of the Academy of Nurse Practitioners, 19*(10), 523–529.

Buppert, C. (2008). *Nurse practitioners business practice and legal guide.* Boston: Jones and Bartlett.

Casalino, L. (2006). The Federal Trade Commission, clinical integration, and the organization of physician practice. *Journal of Health Politics, Policy and Law, 31*(3), 569–585.

Coile, R. C. (1997). *The five stages of managed care: Strategies for providers, HMOs and suppliers.* Chicago: Health Administration Press.

DeNavis-Walt, C., Proctor, B., & Smith, J. (2008). *US Census Bureau: Income, poverty, and health insurance coverage in the United States: 2007.* Retrieved August 6, 2009, from www.census.gov

Dixon, A., Greene, J., & Hibbard, J. (2008). Do consumer-directed health plans drive change in enrollees' health care behavior? *Health Affairs, 27*(4), 1120–1131.

Federal Trade Commission and Department of Justice. (2003). *Perspectives on competition policy and the health care marketplace* (testimony of American Nurses Association). Retrieved February 4, 2010, from http://www.ftc.gov/ogc/healthcarehearings/docs/030227carsonwinifr edy.pdf

Indiana Academy of Family Physicians. (2007). *Update on Anthem Wellpoint NP and PA billing requirements.* Retrieved August 6, 2009, from http://www.in-afp.org/files/public/Update_on_Anthem_Wellpoint_NP_CredentialingI _Revised_11_27_07.pdf

Kaiser Family Foundation. (2008). *Medicare: Medicare Advantage fact sheet.* Retrieved August 6, 2009, from http://www.kff.org/medicare/upload/2052-11.pdf

Kaiser Family Foundation: Kaiser Commission on Medicaid and the Uninsured. (2009). *Rising unemployment, Medicaid & the uninsured.* Retrieved August 6, 2009, from http://www.kff.org/uninsured/upload/7850.pdf

Kane, R. L., Flood, S., Bershadsky, B., & Keckhafer, G. (2004). Effect of an innovative Medicare managed care program on the quality of care for nursing home residents. *The Gerontologist, 44,* 95–103.

Krizner, K. (2006). *Health plan networks slowly embrace nurse practitioners. Managed Healthcare executive.* Retrieved August 6, 2009, from http://managedhealthcareexecutive.modernmedicine.com

MacEachern, L. (2003). *Finance issue brief: Any willing provider: Year end report–2003.* Issue Brief Health Policy Tracking, December 31, 1–7.

NAPNAP. (2004). Position statement: Reimbursement for nurse practitioner services. *Journal of Pediatric Healthcare, 18*, 27A–28A.

NCQA. (2009). *HEDIS 2009 measures.* Retrieved August 6, 2009, from http://www.ncqa.org

Osgood, L. (2008). *National commercial managed care enrollment continues shift from HMO to PPO business lines.* Retrieved December 20, 2008, from http://www.reuters.com/article/pressRelease/idUS97330+15-Sep-2008+PRN20080915

United Healthcare Oxford. (2008). *Credentialing criteria: Nurse practitioners; nurse practitioners as empowerment coaches.* Retrieved January 23, 2009, from https://www.oxhp.com/secure/policy/credentialing_criteria_np_108. html

United States Department of Labor. (2009). *Economic news release: Employment situation summary.* Retrieved August 6, 2009, from http://www.bls.gov/news.release/empsit.nr0.htm

Community-Based Health Centers: Nurse Practitioners Contributing to Access

ANN RITTER

NURSE-MANAGED HEALTH CENTERS: A CRUCIAL PART OF THE HEALTH CARE SAFETY NET

Nurse-managed health centers are community-based health centers in which advanced-practice nurses (APNs) (usually nurse practitioners [NPs]) are the primary providers of care (Torrisi & Hansen-Turton, 2005). The vast majority of nurse-managed health centers are safety net providers, and their roots are in the public health nursing movement that first began in the 19th century. They have provided high-quality primary care to underserved and vulnerable populations throughout the United States for more than 3 decades (King, 2008, p. 14). Today, the majority of nurse-managed health center patients are uninsured, self-pay (a term that refers to patients who pay for health care with their own funds), or Medicaid beneficiaries, many of whom are living in poverty (Hansen-Turton, Ritter, & Torgan, 2008). As safety net providers, nurse-managed health centers provide care to patients regardless of their ability to pay. Although nurse-managed health centers are an essential part of the health care safety net, they face unique challenges and barriers to sustainability that physician-managed community-based health centers do not face. One such barrier is the refusal of many managed care insurers to credential and reimburse NPs as primary care providers.

The National Nursing Centers Consortium (NNCC) is an organization comprised of not-for-profit nurse-managed health centers located throughout the United States and internationally. There are approximately 250 nurse-managed health centers located in the United States, which record over 2 million patient encounters annually (National Nursing Centers Consortium, 2008). Most nurse-managed health centers are owned by academic schools of nursing and serve as important faculty and student practice sites, in addition to their role as health care providers for the underserved (Institute for Nursing Centers, 2008). The patients served by nurse-managed health centers tend to represent racial and ethnic minorities and disadvantaged populations who are more likely to experience health disparities and lack access to high-quality health care (including low-income families, the homeless, and residents of public housing) (Hansen-Turton, 2005, p. 731).

Since its creation in 1996 (originally as the Regional Nursing Centers Consortium), NNCC has worked with its health center members to pursue strategies that will improve their long-term fiscal sustainability, and ensure the continuing availability of care to vulnerable and underserved populations (Evans, Pohl, & Rothman, 2004). An important aspect of this work has been to encourage policy changes among Medicaid, Medicare, and commercial insurers to recognize NPs as primary care providers. In addition, NNCC staff and consultants provide technical assistance to nurse-managed health center staff and directors as they enter into negotiations with managed care insurers. This case study provides an overview of some of the lessons learned through NNCC's efforts.

HOW INSURER POLICIES AFFECT
HEALTH CARE ACCESS FOR THE UNDERSERVED

All primary care providers (both nurses and physicians) must go through a credentialing process and enter into a contract that sets out expectations for both parties in order to be reimbursed by health insurers for care provided to enrollees.[1] This is true regardless of whether the managed care plan provides health insurance to the commercial market or to Medicaid or Medicare beneficiaries through a contract with the government. Although each insurer has a separate credentialing and contracting process, the application process for new providers is often very similar among different managed care plans. Unless a provider is credentialed and listed in the health plan's directory as a primary care provider, the plan's enrollees will not be able to select that provider as his or her primary care provider.

NPs and other APNs in nurse-managed health centers act as primary care providers for hundreds of thousands of low-income, vulnerable, and underserved patients, despite lack of recognition for this role by many managed care insurers (National Nursing Centers Consortium, 2008). Although nursing practice laws vary in significant ways from state to state, NPs are legally authorized to prescribe controlled substances and provide comprehensive primary care in all 50 states (Ritter & Hansen-Turton, 2008). Services provided at nurse-managed health centers include treatment for acute and chronic illness, routine physical exams, immunizations for adults and children, disease screenings, prenatal care, and other services.

In recent decades, managed care organizations (MCOs) have largely only credentialed and recognized physicians as primary care providers. Insurers have rarely included NPs in provider networks as primary care providers, despite the current legal authority of NPs to perform this role. Throughout the country, MCOs have been slow to change policies to identify NPs as providers of record for a panel of patients. In 2008, NNCC published a national survey of insurer policies regarding NP primary care providers (Hansen-Turton, Ritter, & Torgan, 2008). In this study, NNCC found that only 53% of MCOs in the nation credentialed NPs as primary care providers. This was a significant increase from the results of a study conducted 2 years earlier (Hansen-Turton

---

[1]The credentialing process includes the collection and verification of a provider's licensure status, malpractice insurance, DEA certificate, and other materials. It is one of the first steps a new provider must go through in order to become part of an insurer's provider network. The CAQH Universal Provider Datasource (http://www.caqh.org/ucd.php) is used by many insurers as a central repository for information about the credentials of health care providers.

et al., 2006) that found only 33% of MCOs had a uniform policy recognizing NPs as primary care providers. Even with the progress noted in the 2008 study, however, much work remains to be done to reform health insurers' policies.

When NPs are rejected by managed care plans as primary care providers, they are often able to gain admittance to managed care provider networks in other ways. Many insurers will instead allow NPs to be credentialed in "physician extender" roles or as "specialty providers." However, both of these credentialing approaches are flawed and limiting for NP practice, because they are based on a narrow and outdated concept of the capacity of NPs to provide primary care.

The first, and perhaps most critical, flaw in these alternative credentialing options is their mislabeling of NPs. The NPs who manage and operate nurse-managed health centers are not "physician extenders." This is a term that rose to prominence in the 1970s (Fairman 2008, p. 90). It continues to be used today by the American Medical Association, which opposes the direct reimbursement of NPs by insurers on the grounds that all NPs should be supervised by physicians, and all payments for NP services should be paid to the supervising physician (American Medical Association, 2009). Thus, the concept of the NP as a "physician extender" (as opposed to an autonomous professional provider) is premised on physician supervision, even in states in which physician supervision is not required by law for NP practice. The physician-extender concept may, in part, be rooted in a time, decades ago, when NPs did not have the broad legal and social authority to provide primary care that they do today (Ritter & Hansen-Turton 2008, p. 21). It may also be based on a view that physicians have the unique authority to oversee all other primary care professionals, even though nursing is an autonomous profession. As a result, insurers' refusal to credential NPs as primary care providers does not fit the reality of day-to-day practice in a modern nurse-managed health center. As the name indicates, nurses, not physicians, direct and manage nurse-managed health centers. Although physicians provide collaborative services as needed clinically or required by law, they do not control the operation of nurse-managed health centers.

Second, "specialty provider" status does not reflect the reality of the type of care provided in nurse-managed health centers, and has important cost implications for both low-income patients and the safety net practices that serve them. Even if one sets aside the fact that NPs who provide primary care do not provide "specialty" care in any normal sense of the word, this policy also has the impact of driving primary care patients away from nurse-managed health centers because specialty co-pays tend to be significantly higher than primary care provider co-pays. This creates a major disincentive for new patients to select a nurse-managed health center for care, and creates a financial burden for patients who wish to receive care in a nurse-managed health center for reasons of convenience or preference. Furthermore, specialty providers are not listed in the same section of provider directories as primary care physicians, and they do not receive new patients through the auto-assign process that connects new enrollees with in-network primary care providers. As a result, nurse-managed primary care practices with a "specialty" designation have greater difficulty recruiting and retaining patients.

Restrictive policies such as these contribute to the financial instability of nurse-managed health centers. Nurse-managed health centers primarily focus on providing care to the uninsured (Institute for Nursing Centers 2008, p. 2). Although nurse-managed health centers use a sliding scale to collect payment from uninsured and self-pay patients, the amount collected does not approximate the actual cost of caring for the uninsured. This situation is exacerbated by managed care policies that discriminate against NPs who act as primary care providers. Because nurse-managed health centers serve a high percentage of uninsured patients, it is especially important that they are given the opportunity to attract insured patients to their practices, and are reimbursed fairly for the care that they provide to managed care enrollees.

NNCC's insurer surveys have revealed that managed care plans offer a variety of stated reasons for refusing to recognize NPs as primary care providers, all of which show a lack of understanding of NPs' capacity to provide care. Some of the reasons provided to researchers by managed care staff in the 2008 survey included:

- NPs do not meet the company's criteria for primary care providers.
- State law does not require the company to credential NPs as primary care providers.
- NPs are credentialed as primary care providers only in areas in which there is a physician shortage (Hansen-Turton, Ritter, & Torgan, 2008).

Despite NPs' proven record of high-quality care, all of these stated reasons are based either explicitly or implicitly on the understanding that NPs are primary care providers of last resort, who should be used only in situations in which physicians are unavailable. NNCC has worked for more than 10 years to encourage its health center members to develop relationships with insurer representatives to counteract this belief, and make the case for increased use of NP services (Hansen-Turton et al., 2006). Part of this process has included the creation of a credentialing tool kit for NPs, available to the public on NNCC's Web site (www.nncc.us).

THREE STEPS TO START A PRODUCTIVE DIALOGUE WITH INSURER REPRESENTATIVES

NNCC encourages its members to take a three-step approach when interacting with insurance representatives. The first step is to educate insurers about the legal authority of NPs to provide primary care in independent settings. Many insurers are unaware that the nurse-managed health center model of care has existed for decades, or that it is legal for NPs to practice in independent settings with remote physician involvement. This educational process requires that NPs understand the state laws and regulations that govern their practice, and are able to explain how their practice is in full compliance with those laws.

Second, the NP should focus on patients and explain that academic research has consistently shown that NPs provide high-quality primary care with comparable outcomes to physicians (Lenz, Mundinger, Kane, Hopkins, & Lin, 2004; Mundinger et al., 2000), and therefore, should not be considered primary care providers of last resort. Making it clear that nurse-managed health centers and NPs have a long track record of providing safe, high-quality care can make it easier for an insurer representative to justify a contract with a nurse-managed primary care practice, or the need for a plan-wide policy change, to his or her supervisors and his or her company's legal department.

Third, and most important, NPs must explain how their recognition as primary care providers will have a positive impact on the insurer's bottom line. In the case of Medicaid insurers (which often have difficulty finding physicians who are willing to accept their enrollees), this may involve explaining how nurse-managed practices can increase the number of primary care access points available to their members. For commercial and other insurers, this may include an explanation of how NPs' education makes them exceptionally well-suited to manage the care of patients with chronic illnesses, or how nurse-managed health center patients have been shown to experience fewer hospitalizations, emergency department visits, and higher generic medication prescription rates than patients of similar physician-managed practices. In some cases, NNCC may also point to the high levels of patient satisfaction and retention experienced by nurse-managed health centers. A sampling of the case studies and research findings that NNCC has cited in communications with insurers to illustrate these points is included in Table 22.1.

In addition to offering information about the quality and cost effectiveness of nurse-managed care, often the quickest way to show an insurer that contracting with NPs makes business sense is to understand the competitive nature of the insurance business and exert pressure on the insurer. Sharing information that another insurer in the region is already contracting with NPs as primary care providers can encourage other insurer representatives to consider revising their provider contracts to keep up with their competition. In addition, some NNCC members who operate academic-based health centers associated with large universities have achieved success by seeking the assistance of the health insurance purchasing department at their university. NNCC's experience has indicated that nurse-managed health centers experience better contracting outcomes when they enter into insurer negotiations with the support of a major insurance purchaser, such as a university, a state or local government, or other large employer (Hansen-Turton et al., 2006, p. 225). In addition, as nurse-managed health centers grow in size and gain community recognition, they often find it easier to successfully negotiate with insurers.

Although insurers are generally becoming more accepting of NPs in independent roles, there is still organized opposition to direct reimbursement for independent NP care (American Medical Association, 2009). For this reason, education about NP quality and outcomes alone is often not enough to convince an insurer to change its policies, especially in situations in which the insurer may fear an outcry from its physician directors or the physicians in its existing provider network. In situations such as these, earning the support of key policymakers and business leaders can help catalyze change. In Pennsylvania, for

Table 22.1

RESOURCES FOR NEGOTIATIONS WITH INSURERS

TOPIC	RESEARCH FINDINGS	SOURCE
Cost-Effectiveness	An evaluation report issued as part of a federal demonstration project found that patients of a nurse-managed health center experienced fewer hospitalizations and higher rates of generic medication fills than patients of similar providers.	(Hansen-Turton, Line, O'Connell, Rothman, & Lauby, 2004, p. 5)
Quality of Care	A randomized trial conducted at Columbia University and published in the *Journal of the American Medical Association* showed that patient outcomes among nurse practitioners and physicians are comparable.	(Mundinger et al., 2000, p. 68)
	Nurse practitioners are comparable to physicians in terms of practice patterns. A recent study found that, "NPs were comparable to the [physician sample], providing diagnostic or screening services in 99% of all encounters, and prescribing medication for primary diagnoses in 63% of these encounters."	(Deshefy-Loughi, Swartz, & Grey, 2008, p. 285)
Patient Satisfaction and Retention	A study of a school-based nurse-managed health center found very high satisfaction levels among first-time and repeat users. The highest satisfaction scores "were reported in items such as 'being treated with respect,' 'listening to you,' and 'explaining things to you.' "	(Benkert et al., 2007, p. 107)
Chronic Disease Management and Prevention	Nurse practitioners provide counseling in 84% of all patient encounters on topics such as nutrition, tobacco cessation, physical activity, family planning, child growth and development, and prenatal care. In comparison, physicians provide counseling in 61% of patient encounters.	(Deshefy-Loughi, Swartz, & Grey, 2008, p. 285)

Note: Compiled from National Nursing Centers Consortium (2009).

example, advocacy by APNs led to a decision by the Pennsylvania Department of Public Welfare to evaluate all insurers competing for its Medicaid managed care contract based on how they planned to maximize the use of APNs in their provider networks (Pennsylvania Department of Public Welfare, 2008).[2] As a result, many Medicaid managed care insurers in Pennsylvania have sought new partnerships with nursing groups, and developed a new commitment to effective use of non-physician providers. With support from policymakers and business leaders who have the power to impact insurers' revenue streams, NPs can experience credentialing and contracting breakthroughs that might otherwise be delayed.

LOOKING TO THE FUTURE

Anecdotally, NNCC is finding somewhat less resistance from insurers, or at least a better understanding of NPs' capacity to provide care, as retail clinics spread throughout the country. As insurers develop contracting models for this relatively new model of care, they are becoming increasingly familiar with the ability and authority of NPs to provide safe, high-quality, cost-effective care in independent settings (Thygeson, Van Vorst, Maciosek, & Solberg, 2008). However, many contracts with retail-based clinics are currently designed so that they are agreements between the insurer and the facility (as opposed to an agreement between the insurer and the individual NPs who provide services to patients) (Hansen-Turton et al., 2006, p. 223). This contracting model raises concerns because of its similarity to the traditional insurer contracting model in which a physician receives payment for the services of the NPs in his or her office, effectively hiding the services of the NP from the insurer. However, the growing prevalence of the retail-clinic contracting model also presents a new opportunity for nurse-managed health centers to initiate dialogues with insurers who previously would

---

[2]The RFP (request for proposals) issued in 2008 for Pennsylvania's Medicaid managed care program specifically requested the following information from all bidders: "Describe your organization's policy to ensure that all licensed health care providers—including nurses, certified registered nurse practitioners, advanced nurse practitioners, midwives, physician assistants, dental hygienists, and expanded function dental assistants—can practice to the fullest extent of their education and training. Provide the percent of your network that comprises these health care providers."

not have considered contracting with nurse-managed practices without onsite physicians.

The ongoing struggle to reform insurer policies regarding NP primary care providers is not only about ensuring equity among different types of health care providers—it is also critical to increase and sustain primary care access for the underserved in diverse communities throughout the United States. Recognizing this, NNCC staff and consultants work with health center leaders to initiate productive conversations with insurer representatives and guide negotiations to ensure fair reimbursement.

One successful example of this work has been NNCC's efforts with Project Salud, a nurse-managed health center that provides a broad scope of primary care and wellness services to more than 1,800 low-income, predominantly Latino individuals annually. It is part of La Communidad Hispaña, a nonprofit health, social services, and education organization that has served the Latino population in Chester County, PA, for more than 30 years. However, Project Salud is not part of the Federally Qualified Health Center (FQHC) program, and does not qualify for the enhanced reimbursement that is available to traditional community health centers. As a result, it is especially dependent on foundation funding and insurance reimbursement to remain sustainable.

In 2006, NNCC worked with Project Salud to successfully negotiate new provider contracts with both United Healthcare and Aetna, two of the largest commercial insurers in the country. As a result, Project Salud is now able to attract more insured patients to its practice, and has been able to expand existing partnerships with local mushroom farms in order to provide more primary care to their insured workers. In turn, these new revenue streams have allowed Project Salud to continue its important work serving uninsured patients. In addition, NNCC was able to leverage the Project Salud success to engage Aetna and United in parallel primary care provider contracting strategies for all nurse-managed health centers delivering primary care in Southeastern Pennsylvania.

CONCLUSIONS

Through its work, NNCC has learned that in order to achieve change, NPs must approach insurers as potential partners, educate insurers about the capacity of NPs to provide high-quality care, and demonstrate the value that NPs can add to insurers' provider networks. By working with insurers to make primary care credentialing policies more inclusive of NPs, we can ensure a reliable and continuing source of high-quality health care for low-income and underserved patients.

REFERENCES

American Medical Association. (2009). *Policy H-360.989: Independent nursing practice models.* Retrieved March 25, 2009, from the AMA Policy Finder, http://www.ama-assn.org/ama/no-index/legislation-advocacy/11760.shtml

Benkert, R., George, N., Tanner, C., Barkauskas, V., Pohl, J., & Marszalek, A. (2007). Satisfaction with a school-based teen health center: A report card on care. *Pediatric Nursing, 33*(2), 103–109.

Deshefy-Loughi, T., Swartz, M. K., & Grey, M. (2008). Characterizing nurse practitioner practice by sampling patient encounters. *Journal of the American Academy of Nurse Practitioners, 20*(5), 281–287.

Evans, L. K., Pohl, J. M., & Rothman, N. L. (2004). Building alliances: A survival strategy. In L. K. Evans & N. M. Lang (Eds.), *Academic nursing practice: Helping to shape the future of health care* (pp. 236–257). New York: Springer Publishing Company.

Fairman, J. (2008). *Making room in the clinic: Nurse practitioners and the evolution of modern health care.* New Brunswick, NJ: Rutgers University Press.

Hansen-Turton, T. (2005). The nurse-managed health center safety net: A policy solution to reducing health disparities. *Nursing Clinics of North America, 40,* 729–738.

Hansen-Turton, T., Line, L., O'Connell, M., Rothman, N., & Lauby, J. (2004, June). *The Nursing Center model of health care for the underserved.* Paper submitted to the U.S. Centers for Medicare and Medicaid Services (CMS). Available from the National Nursing Centers Fairness Consortium, 260 S. Broad Street, 18th floor, Philadelphia, PA 19102.

Hansen-Turton, T., Ritter, A., Begun, H., Berkowitz, S. L., Rothman, N., & Valdez, B. (2006). Insurers' contracting policies on nurse practitioners as primary care providers: The current landscape and what needs to change. *Policy, Politics, and Nursing Practice, 7*(3), 216–226.

Hansen-Turton, T., Ritter, A., & Torgan, R. (2008). Insurers' contracting policies on nurse practitioners as primary care providers: Two years later. *Policy, Politics, and Nursing Practice, 9*(4), 241–248.

Institute for Nursing Centers. (2008). *Highlight report from the Data Warehouse, October 2008.* Retrieved January 21, 2009, from http://www.nursingcenters.org/PDFs/INC%20Highlight%20Report%2010_ 6_08.pdf

King, E. S. (2008). A 10-year review of four academic nurse-managed centers: Challenges and survival strategies. *Journal of Professional Nursing, 24*(1), 14–20.

Lenz, E. R., Mundinger, M. O., Kane, R. L., Hopkins, S. C., & Lin, S. X. (2004). Primary care outcomes in patients treated by nurse practitioners or physicians: Two-year follow-up. *Medical Care Research and Review, 61*(3), 332–351.

316 **Part V** Business and Payment Structures for NPs

Mundinger, M. O., Kane, R. L., Lenz, E. R., Totten, A. M., Tsai, W., Cleary, P. D., et al. (2000). Primary care outcomes in patients treated by nurse practitioners or physicians: A randomized trial. *Journal of the American Medical Association, 283*, 59–68.

National Nursing Centers Consortium. (2008, May). *Comments regarding notice of proposed rulemaking-Designation of medically underserved populations and health professional shortage areas.* Paper submitted to United States Health Services and Resources Administration (HRSA). (Statement of Tine Hansen-Turton, Executive Director, National Nursing Centers Consortium.)Available from the National Nursing Centers Fairness Consortium, 260 S. Broad Street, 18th floor, Philadelphia, PA 19102.

Pennsylvania Department of Public Welfare. (2008). *Physical Health Southwest (PHSW)–RFP #34-08, Part II.* Retrieved March 25, 2009, from http://www.dpw.state.pa.us/omap/rfp/PHSW/PHSWrfpPart2.asp

Ritter, A., & Hansen-Turton, T. (2008). The primary care paradigm shift: An overview of the state-level legal framework governing nurse practitioner practice. *Health Lawyer, 8*(4), 21–28.

Thygeson, M., Van Vorst, K. A., Maciosek, M. V., & Solberg L. (2008). Use and costs of care in retail clinics versus traditional care sites. *Health Affairs, 27*(5), 1283–1292.

Torrisi, D., & Hansen-Turton, T. (2005). *Community and nurse-managed health centers: Getting them started and keeping them going.* New York: Springer Publishing Company.

23 Quality and Safety: Critical Components of a Nurse Practitioner Business Model

KATHRYN FIANDT AND JOANNE M. POHL

A CALL TO ACTION

Nurse practitioner (NP) care has been consistently documented as high-quality care, with very high patient satisfaction (Barkauskas, Pohl, Benkert, & Wells, 2005; Edwards, Oppewal, & Logan, 2003; Mundinger et al., 2000). In addition to the quality of their practices, NPs are well qualified to provide leadership in quality improvement (QI) initiatives based on their unique set of core competencies, which include a broad understanding of the health system, an ability to recognize the complex factors that impact health outcomes, and basic research skills (Fiandt, 2006). These competencies, and others that apply directly to QI and patient safety are identified in the core NP role competencies developed by the National Organization of Nurse Practitioner Faculties (NONPF; 2006) and, more recently, in the entry-level competencies for the Doctor of Nursing Practice (DNP) (National Panel for Nurse Practitioner Practice Doctorate Competencies, 2006). Recently, the NONPF Quality and Safety Competencies Project cross-mapped the Quality and Safety for Education of Nurses (QSEN) Graduate Competencies specific to quality and patient safety, and found that a large majority of the QSEN Graduate Competencies are reflected in the NONPF Core and DNP competencies

(Pohl, 2009). The American Association of Colleges of Nursing (AACN) Essentials for the DNP (American Association of Colleges of Nursing, 2006) role has a core essential competency, "Organizational and System Leadership for Quality Improvement and Systems Thinking" (American Association of Colleges of Nursing, 2006, p. 10). Finally, national guidelines related to NP practice include an expectation that NPs be accountable for the outcomes of their practices and maintain a formal QI program (Marian, 1996; National Nursing Centers Consortium, 2001). All this makes it increasingly clear that NPs are prepared and should be actively involved in QI and patient safety initiatives not only in their practices, but also at the larger systems level.

There is a critical need for NP leadership in QI efforts, based on extensive evidence about the crisis in quality health care in this country (Daschle, Greenberger, & Lambrew, 2008; Institute of Medicine, 2000) that will be described in detail in the next section. Based on their competencies and training, NPs must take the opportunities available now to step forward and assume a visionary and leadership role in QI and patient safety, particularly in the ambulatory/primary care and community-based practices settings in which most NPs work. NPs need to see leadership in QI and patient safety not as an "add on" or "value added" role, but as central to the services we provide in our practice settings.

Beyond the data that inform us about quality and safety concerns, there is another reason to care about and provide leadership in QI. QI, more than any other aspect of health care, is the key to successful reform of the health care system. Many experts suggest that providing high-quality health care based on best practices will go a long way toward increasing access to care *and* decreasing health care costs (Commonwealth Fund Commission on a High Performance Health System, 2008; Daschle, Greenberger, & Lambrew, 2008).

QUALITY AND SAFETY

Patient safety is generally defined by exclusion, and refers to avoiding medical errors that have the potential to result in patient injury or harm. Health care quality can be defined as ensuring that care received meets the Institute of Medicine's (IOM) aims for improvement, in other words, that patient care is "safe, effective, patient-centered, timely, efficient and equitable" (Institute of Medicine, 2001, p. 40). The recommendation for these aims was derived from the groundbreaking IOM book, *To Err is Human* (2000), which shocked the nation with the report that "preventable deaths due to adverse events" was in the top 10 causes of death in the country, and cost the health care payers anywhere from 17 to 29 billion dollars a year (p. 3).

Most data reported by the IOM were based on errors in inpatient care. There are few studies regarding errors in ambulatory settings, although a recent study on medication errors in primary care settings (Kuo, Phillips, Graham, & Hickner, 2008) suggests that medication errors, particularly prescribing errors, are not uncommon in primary settings. The emphasis in this chapter will be on the broader concept of QI, for which safe care is a necessary, but not sufficient, characteristic. The challenges of QI in the primary care setting are clearly described in ongoing reports from the Commonwealth Fund in the National Scorecard on U.S. Health System Performance (Commonwealth Fund Commission on a High Performance Health System, 2008). Commonwealth Fund data (Table 23.1) provide a comprehensive and sobering view of the poor quality of health care in the United States. These data are mirrored in other sources of health care quality evaluation (e.g., Agency for Healthcare Quality and Research, 2007a). Of particular significance to NPs in primary care settings is that all of the indicators can be positively impacted by coordinated, comprehensive, quality primary care. As the authors of the report note, "better primary care and care coordination hold potential for improved outcomes at lower costs" (p. 14).

It is easy to say that needed changes are unlikely to occur due to health care costs, however, the authors of the Commonwealth Fund report (Commonwealth Fund Commission on a High Performance Health System, 2008, p. 13) suggest that closing performance gaps would result in significant costs savings. Examples include:

- More than 100,000 fewer people would die prematurely each year.
- 37 million people would have access to a primary care provider, and 70 million adults will receive needed preventive care.
- The Medicare program could save $12 billion per year by reducing readmissions and preventable hospitalizations.
- Reducing health insurance *administrative* costs could free up $51 billion or more in avoidable health care costs.

Table 23.1

SUMMARY OF COMMONWEALTH FUND NATIONAL SCORECARD ON U.S. HEALTH SYSTEM PERFORMANCE

AREA	WHERE WE STAND
Healthy Lives	*Premature mortality*: The United States ranks the highest in 19 industrialized countries in the number of deaths that could be preventive with early and effective care. Although the United States has improved by 4% in recent years, other countries averaged a 16% improvement.
	Activity limitations: 18% of working adults report being unable to carry out work due to health problems (up from 15% in 2004).
Quality	*Patient-centered care*: Less than 50% of patients could get a rapid appointment when ill. In addition, 73% couldn't get after-hours care without going to an ER.
	Effective: Control of diabetes and HTN improved between 1999–2000 and 2003–2004; 88% of patients report at least fair control of DM, *but* there are 30–60% points difference between top- and bottom-performing health plans. Only half of all adults received 100% of recommended preventive care.
	Coordinated: Heart failure patients are more likely to receive any discharge planning (68% in 2006 compared with 50% in 2004), *but* these rates vary between 94% and 36%, depending on whether the hospital is a high or low performer.
	Safe care: There has been a recent 19% decline in reported areas, but still as many as 30% of patients report mistakes in their care. ER visits for adverse drug effects increased more than 35% between 2001 and 2004.
Access	*Insurance and access*: In 2007, 75 million (42%) working adults were uninsured or underinsured; this is up from 61 million in 2003 (35%). In 2007, 37% of people reported going without needed care due to costs.
	Affordable: The number of states in which insurance premium averaged <15% of household incomes has decreased from 58% in 2003 to 25% in 2005.

Table 23.1 *(continued)*

SUMMARY OF COMMONWEALTH FUND NATIONAL SCORECARD ON U.S. HEALTH SYSTEM PERFORMANCE

AREA	WHERE WE STAND
Efficiency	*Inappropriate, fragmented, wasteful care*: Three to four times the benchmark rate of patients report duplicated tests or that medical records or tests were not available at time of visit.
	Avoidable hospitalizations: Rates of hospitalization from preventable conditions, such as hypertension, decreased, but varied significantly across geographic regions and states.
	Variation in quality and costs: The total cost for caring for people with chronic disease varied twofold—there is good evidence to support that it is possible to lower costs and save lives with effective, efficient systems.
	Administrative costs: Costs in the United States are 30–70% higher than other countries, and are three times higher than other developed countries with the lowest rates.
	Information systems: EMR use increased from 17–28% in 2001–2006, but lags behind other developed countries in which rates are as high as 98%.
Equity	*Disparities*: The vulnerable (minorities, poor, uninsured) are more likely to wait to access care; to encounter delays and poorly coordinated care; to have dental caries, uncontrolled chronic disease, avoidable hospitalizations, and poor outcomes. They are less likely to receive preventive care or have an accessible source of primary care.

Note: Adapted from The Commonwealth Fund Commission on a High Performance Health System (2008).

The conclusion of the Commonwealth Fund is "that it is possible to prevent hospitalizations or re-hospitalizations with better primary care, planning, and follow-up care—an integrated, systems approach to care" (p. 14).

Although disparities in health care are addressed in the Commonwealth Fund report, it is important to emphasize the problem of health disparities in this country. A major quality problem in the United States is inequity of health care for populations at risk. An extensive body of literature (Agency for Healthcare Quality and Research, 2007b; Institute of Medicine, 2003) documents the disparities in health care received and clinical outcomes associated with not having insurance and/or minority status and/or low socioeconomic status. This should be of particular concern for NPs, as these are the very patients who are often seen by NPs (Fiandt, Doeschot, Lanning, & Latzke, in press; Pohl, Vonderheid, Barkauskas, & Nagelkerk, 2004). This also represents an important opportunity for NPs to impact health care quality, because their preparation and required competencies emphasize skills in quality care to diverse populations (Mundinger et al., 2000; National Organization of Nurse Practitioner Faculties, 2006).

The remainder of this chapter will provide an overview of the processes of QI and identification of national programs for QI that can serve as important resources for NPs.

THE PROCESS OF QUALITY IMPROVEMENT

There are several models for how "to do" QI. These include the Institute for Healthcare Improvement Model (www.ihi.org), Six Sigma (Barry & Smith, 2005; Barry, Murcko, & Brubaker, 2002), and Lean (Womack & Jones, 2003; 2005). Although the details of the models vary, they all involve a nonlinear process with numerous feedback loops, and are designed to address, at the most basic level, three key questions (Improving Chronic Illness Care, 2009, pp. 6–7):

1. What is the QI program trying to accomplish (e.g., improve outcomes for our patients with type 2 diabetes)?
2. How will the QI committee know whether a change is an improvement, for example, the percentage of clinic patients with type 2 diabetes who have an average A1c < 7?
3. What changes can be made in the practice that will result in this improvement? In other words, what evidence-based strategies can be implemented?

In order to successfully improve quality as measured by documented changes, the NP needs several resources. First, the NP and his/

her team need institutional support. Practice or community leadership must support the program, through both the release of time to work on the QI project and assistance in funding the work. This requires that NP leaders be able to provide a strong argument for the need for QI. One of the best tools in arguing for the need for a QI initiative is data that demonstrate patients are not meeting national benchmarks, or are not satisfied with care, or that the care processes do not meet the standards needed to receive the supplemental payment that pay-for-performance programs provide (Centers for Medicare and Medicaid Services, 2009).

Another argument in support of QI initiatives is cost effectiveness. There has been some effort to document the cost effectiveness of QI work (Kilpatrick et al., 2005). To date, the best practice for demonstrating cost effectiveness comes from the evaluation of disease management (DM) programs. DM programs are good models to use because they often involve comprehensive primary care integrated with case management, representing a strong nursing model. Health services researchers involved in evaluation of DM programs (Linden, 2006; Linden, Adams, & Roberts, 2003) recommend using the measure of "number needed to avoid" as the best marker of cost effectiveness. For example, in the case of a diabetes DM program in primary care, the key evaluation measure would be the number of preventable hospitalizations needed to support the rationale for the cost of the program in primary care (e.g., the return on investment).

Having obtained institutional support for a quality initiative, the first question to be addressed is, "What is the program trying to accomplish?" The question may have been addressed as part of the justification of the program, but the foundation of the program is data, in other words, what is the problem the initiative is working to solve. It may be poor outcomes of diabetes care, or high "no show" rates, or a low number of children with asthma who have a documented school management plan. Demonstration of the problem requires data to establish a baseline from which to start.

As health care moves to electronic health records (EHRs), it is essential that the EHR be able to provide a patient registry that includes aggregate population data, as well as individual patient-level data. However, the option of manual chart audits to document the current status of the clinical problem should not be overlooked in practices that don't have an EHR. Although it may take more resources, the inability to obtain an electronic report on populations of patients should not be an insurmountable barrier to QI.

Having determined the problem to be addressed and the measure you are using (e.g., percentage of "no show" visits), the NP and team must then address the question, "How do we know whether this is an improvement?" Establishing benchmarks is the next step. Benchmarks are the outcome standard that is established as a goal for a QI process. Benchmarks are most often evidence-based and/or recognized national standards. There is an abundance of standards available (see the resources section at the end of the chapter). Two comprehensive resources for benchmarks are the Centers for Medicare and Medicaid Services (2009) Physician Quality Reporting Initiative (PQRI) measures and the National Committee for Quality Assurance (2009) Healthcare Effectiveness Data and Information Set (HEDIS) measures. Both are well-established sets of standards. In addition to quality benchmarks, clinical practices that are believed to reflect best practices based on expert consensus can serve as benchmarks (Ellis, 2000), or national guidelines such as the U.S. Preventive Services Task Force recommendation for preventive services (U.S. Preventive Services Task Force, 2009).

Benchmarks are the goals or outcomes set for the QI project. Not all measures, however, are outcomes of practice. Some benchmarks are process measures, such as a goal that all patients with type 2 diabetes have a documented foot exam annually. A third category of outcomes are called "balancing" outcomes, related to the functioning of the system. Examples of balancing outcomes would be employee satisfaction, length of time to next open appointment slot, or "no show" rates (Fiandt, 2006).

A final component of the QI program is a planned intervention, in other words, the third question, "What changes can we make that will result in an improvement?" This is not, of course, a simple process. The intervention should be based on identified problems that have been determined to have a negative impact on the aim or goal. Many of these problems have multi-factorial causes. An example would be when a practice determines that the "no show" rate of 40% was unacceptable and leads to financial sustainability risks. The QI committee might review the practice management literature and come to the conclusion that no more than a 10% "no show" rate was reasonable, thereby establishing a benchmark of 10%. The intervention steps in this process may not be based on research, but on the judgment of experts who report on strategies they have used that had a positive impact on the "no show" rate. Multiple strategies might be identified and implemented individually in rapid improvement cycles. (A first intervention might be calling patients to remind them of appointments.) After multiple cycles of working out the "reminder call" method, the "no show" rate might be down to 30%. Because the goal is 10%, another intervention might be added to the first one, in this case, perhaps leaving open a block of afternoon appointments for urgent visits. Another series of test cycles would be used to successfully implement the urgent-visit-slots intervention. At that point, the "no show" rate might be down to 15%, and the committee will decide that is sufficient and move on to another problem.

Throughout the process, it is important to understand the difference between bad apples and bad systems. Often, the challenges to QI have to do with the systems ("bad systems") involved and policies in those systems, even though the problem is often laid incorrectly on a particular person or department ("bad apples"). A key to successful interventions is to focus on system improvements, rather than individual improvements. Recognizing quality and safety as system issues is a key cultural change that must occur to have a successful QI program.

This brief conceptual overview of the QI process demonstrates the feedback loops necessary to be successful. It also demonstrates the value of many of the skills NPs bring to QI, including research skills, evidence-based practice, and an understanding of the complex nature of the problems we encounter. The multifactorial nature of patient and system problems encountered in health care suggest the value of an organizing framework, or lens through which to look at the problems. Frameworks are discussed in the next section.

ORGANIZING FRAMEWORKS FOR IMPROVING QUALITY

Because of the complex and multifactorial nature of health care problems, organizing frameworks to evaluate practice situations are valuable tools to assist in ensuring that all aspects of care and all stakeholders' needs are addressed. There is insufficient space here to discuss any model in detail, but a brief overview of two frameworks is provided.

Michigan State University Sustained Partnership Model

One model that was designed particularly to reflect NP practice is the Michigan State University (MSU) Sustained Partnership Model (Dontje, Corser, Kreulen, & Teitelman, 2004). The model describes the unique characteristics of NP-delivered care, focusing on the process of care and the structural influences that impact the care, and then predicts potential outcomes based on the use of the processes described. The advantages of an NP-specific model as an organizing framework for a QI program is that the model emphasizes aspects that tend to be specific to NPs, in this case, the relationship between the NP and the patient.

In the MSU Sustained Partnership Model, the process of care is at the core, and focuses on the relationship that evolves between the NP and the patient. The authors suggest that the NP–patient relationship represents a special set of dynamics that include a sustained patient-centered partnership that is designed to address patient needs and preferences. The set of dynamics in the relationship are represented by four unique components of NP practice that the authors suggest often differentiate NPs from other health care providers. These dynamics include empowerment, continuity of care, shared decision making, and holistic care. The authors suggests that NPs facilitate a sense of empowerment in patients, and help them promote their own health through enhanced knowledge, skills, and attitudes that result in improved decision making and self-management. Another key component of processes of care is the importance of continuity and coordination of care as essential to an effective relationship between the NP and the patient. The NP understands patient needs in context of values, attitudes, and situation that lead to shared decision making between the NP and patient. Shared decision making leads to decisions that are consistent with patient preferences and value and, therefore, are more feasible. The fourth relationship dynamic is the ability to see each patient from a holistic, biopsychosocial-spiritual perspective, taking into account the patient's culture. Although not unique to NP practice, this focus on relationships is a significant strength of the model from the NP perspective.

In addition to the four characteristics of a sustained relationship, the model takes into account four structural factors that influence outcomes of practice. Role components include the many roles an NP has in his/her practice, in addition to the role of clinician. These include, but are not limited to, collaborator, patient advocate, leader, and change agent. The second structural factor is interdisciplinary practice relationships, the complex relationships between the NP and other members of the health care team. The third structural factors are the fiscal resources, including revenue sources, especially reimbursement, and expenses. The fourth structural factor is the environment and all the related components, including the physical environment, but also support staff, health care systems, and the community.

Unlike many models, the MSU Sustained Partnership Model identifies specific types of outcomes that are predicted based on the NP model. The authors suggest that improved outcomes are derived from the NP-specific processes of care when supported by the structural factors. Four categories of outcomes are predicted to improve, based on the relationship between the NP and patients. These outcomes include health-promoting behaviors, improved use of health care services and resources, high patient satisfaction, and improved health status.

The MSU Sustained Partnership Model provides an excellent and comprehensive framework for QI. The model is particularly designed to address all aspects of care, and is based on a holistic, system-focused perspective that acknowledges that good outcomes are the result of addressing multiple factors.

The Chronic Care Model

A commonly used model for organizing QI within primary care settings is the Chronic Care Model (CCM) (Wagner, Austin, et al., 2001; Wagner, Glasgow, et al., 2001). This model was derived from efforts to improve quality of care in patients with chronic disease. The CCM has several advantages; first, it is sufficiently descriptive to be easily applied in local practices; second, it is supported by a significant body of scientific evidence (Bodenheimer, 2003; Tsai, Morton, Mangione, & Keeler, 2005); and finally, it is holistic, accounting for system-, provider-, patient-, and community-level factors that affect health outcomes. In addition, there is evidence that the approach is effective when working with vulnerable populations (Wagner, Glasgow, et al., 2001, Wang et al., 2004). The CCM consists of six distinct concepts identified as modifiable components of health care delivery: organizational support, clinical information systems, delivery system design, decision support, community resources, and self-management support. *Organization of care* is the concept that deals with the culture of the practice. The ideal practice maintains a culture of quality as a key value, and practice leadership is committed and visibly involved, supporting change and QI. A *clinical information system*, often in the format of an EHR, is essential, and must provide timely information, in other words, data about individual patients, as well as populations of patients. The third component of the CCM is *delivery system design*, and addresses the composition and function of the practice team, the organization of visits, and the handling of follow-up care. *Decision support* includes the mechanisms for increasing provider access to evidence-based practice guidelines and specialists, and may include system prompts and reminders. A critical component of the model is *self-management support*, emphasizing the need for patient-centered interventions that include the collaboration between provider and patient to define problems, set priorities, establish goals, identify barriers, create a treatment plan, and solve problems. The final component of the CCM is *community resources*. The model acknowledges the importance of linkages with the community for peer support, care coordination, and community-based interventions.

CONCLUSIONS

The central purpose of this chapter is to describe the significance of QI in health care and the opportunities for NPs to provide leadership in QI. Not only do U.S. citizens have the most expensive health care in the world, for all the cost of the system, our citizens have poorer outcomes than any other developed country (Commonwealth Fund Commission on a High Performance Health System, 2008). If we try to solve the problems by spending more money but continue to do the same things, we are living out the sad, inane definition of insanity: we are guilty of "doing the same thing over and over and expecting different results." To get different results, we do not need to spend more money, but to do health care differently (Commonwealth Fund Commission on a High Performance Health System, 2008; Daschle, Greenberger, & Lambrew, 2008). It is clear that improving quality and implementing best practices are the keys to effective health care reform in this country.

NPs have a set of skills that puts them in an ideal position to become active participants and leaders in the move to improve health care quality in the United States. In order to participate, and more important, to lead, NPs must acknowledge and hone their skills and then make QI a central, as opposed to a "value added," component of their practice.

This chapter provides an overview of the problems with quality and the process of improving quality. There are many resources that can be used to build on this information. Some resources specific to the process of QI, and some specific to benchmarking and outcomes, are described briefly, as follows.

RESOURCES

There are multiple resources available in the area of QI. An annotated list of some resources is provided. Most are Internet-based and, therefore, the URL may change.

Guides and Tools for Implementing Quality Improvement

Improving Chronic Illness Care (ICIC): www.improvingchronic care.org

ICIC is the home site of the CCM. In addition to a great deal of information about chronic illness care, they have a downloadable practice improvement manual based on the CCM.

Institute for Healthcare Improvement: www.IHI.org

The Institute for Healthcare Improvement (IHI) is an interdisciplinary organization that has been at the core of QI since the 1990s. In addition to being involved in hospital-based QI, the IHI has provided support through their "collaboratives" model to community heath centers for over a decade. The site offers many resources and an opportunity to participate in IHI activities. The IHI "Open School" for health professions has an extensive of training resources for quality improvement.

Institute for Nursing Center: www.nursingcenters.org

The Institute for Nursing Center (INC) is a network of nursing organizations committed to the advancement of nursing center practice, particularly through the development and maintenance of databases that describe nursing center practices and their outcomes. The Web site has numerous educational resources on practice management, including QI and billing and coding. A comprehensive manual on QI (Fiandt, 2006) is available at the site in CD or hardcopy format.

Quality and Safety Education for Nurses: http://qsen.org

The primary audience for this Web site is nurse educators. Many teaching tools for education for QI are provided. In addition, competencies based on knowledge, skills, and attitudes are described.

Quality Measures

Agency for Healthcare Quality and Research: www.AHRQ.gov

The Agency for Healthcare Quality and Research (AHRQ) is charged with describing the state of health care in the United States, and provides support for health care research focused on quality. The Web site leads to the quality measures used by AHRQ, their current reports, and the health disparities data sets (Hughes, 2008).

Centers for Medicare and Medicaid Services: www.cms.hhs.gov/pqri

In 2006, a law was passed requiring the establishment of a physician QI reporting system to be tied with incentive payment. This is the foundation of pay for performance. The Web site describes the program in detail, including information on how to code bills for incentive payments. The comprehensive list of benchmarks is available at the Web site.

National Committee for Quality Assurance: www.ncqa.org

The National Committee for Quality Assurance (NCQA) is a nonprofit organization founded almost 20 years ago to "improve health care quality through measurement, transparency, and accountability" (National Committee for Quality Assurance, 2009). Many large health care plans seek accreditation through the NCQA. An NCQA benchmark, the Healthcare Effectiveness Data and Information Set (HEDIS), is used by the majority of managed health care plans and serves as an important benchmark for quality.

REFERENCES

Agency for Healthcare Quality and Research. (2007a). *2007 national healthcare quality report*. Retrieved February 2, 2009, from www.ahrq.gov/qual/nhqr07

Agency for Healthcare Quality and Research. (2007b). *2007 national healthcare disparities report*. Retrieved February 2, 2009, from www.ahrq.gov/qual/nhdr07

American Association of Colleges of Nursing. (2006). *The essentials of doctoral education in advanced nursing practice*. Retrieved August 6, 2009, from www.aacn.nche.edu/DNP/pdf/Essentials.pdf

Barkauskas, V. H., Pohl, J. M., Benkert, R., & Wells, M. A. (2005). Measuring quality in nurse-managed centers using HEDIS measures. *Journal for Healthcare Quality*, 27(1), 4–14.

Barry, R. D., Murcko, A., & Brubaker, C. (2002). *The Six Sigma book for healthcare: Improving outcomes by reducing errors*. Chicago: Health Administration Press.

Barry, R. D., & Smith, A. C. (2005). *The manager's guide to Six Sigma in healthcare: Practical tips and tools for improvement*. Milwaukee, WI: ASQ Quality Press.

Bodenheimer, T. (2003). Interventions to improve chronic illness care: Evaluating their effectiveness. *Disease Management*, 6(2), 63–71.

Centers for Medicare and Medicaid Services. (2009). *Physician quality reporting initiative*. Retrieved August 6, 2009, from www.cms.hhs.gov/pqri/

Commonwealth Fund Commission on a High Performance Health System. (2008). *Why not the best? Results for the national scorecard on US health system performance*. New York: Commonwealth Fund.

Daschle, T., Greenberger, S. S., & Lambrew, J. M. (2008). *Critical: What we can do about the health-care crisis*. New York: Thomas Dunne Books, St. Martin's Press.

Dontje, K., Corser, W., Kreulen, G., & Teitelman, A. (2004). A unique set of interactions: The MSU Sustained Partnership Model for nurse practitioner primary care. *Journal of the American Academy of Nurse Practitioners*, 16(2), 63–69.

Edwards, J., Oppewal, S., & Logan, C. L. (2003). Nurse-managed primary care: Outcomes of a faculty practice network. *Journal of the American Academy of Nurse Practitioners*, 15(12), 563–569.

Ellis, J. (2000). Sharing the evidence: Clinical practice benchmarking to improve continuously the quality of care. *Journal of Advanced Nursing*, 32(1), 215–225.

Fiandt, K. (2006) *Quality improvement manual for nurse practitioners*. Okemos, MI: The Institute for Nursing Centers.

Fiandt, K., Doeschot, C., Lanning, J., & Latzke, L. (In press). Characteristics of risk in patients of nurse practitioner safety net practices.*Journal of the American Academy of Nurse Practitioners*.

Hughes, R. (Ed.). (2008). *Patient safety and quality: An evidence-based handbook for nurses* (Prepared with support from the Robert Wood Johnson Foundation). AHRQ publication No. 08-0043. Rockville, MD: Agency for Healthcare Research and Quality.

Improving Chronic Illness Care. (2009). *Improving your practice manual.* Retrieved January 30, 2009, from www.improvingchroniccare.org

Institute of Medicine. (2000). *To err is human: Building a safer health system.* Washington, DC: National Academy Press.

Institute of Medicine. (2001). *Crossing the quality chasm: A new health system for the 21st century.* Washington, DC: National Academy Press.

Institute of Medicine. (2003). *Unequal treatment: Confronting racial and ethnic disparities in healthcare.* Washington, DC: National Academy Press.

Kilpatrick, K. E., Lohr, K. N., Leatherman, S., Pink, G., Buckel, J. M., Legarde, C., et al. (2005). The insufficiency of evidence to establish a business case for quality. *International Journal for Quality in Health Care, 17*(4), 347–355.

Kuo, G. M., Phillips, R. L., Graham, D., & Hickner, J. M. (2008). Medication errors reported by US family physicians and their office staff. *Quality and Safety in Health Care, 17,* 286–290.

Linden, A. (2006). What will it take for disease management to demonstrate a return on investment? New perspectives on an old theme. *American Journal of Managed Care, 12*(4), 217–222.

Linden, A., Adams, J. L., & Roberts, N. (2003). Evaluating disease management programs effectiveness: An introduction to time-series analysis. *Disease Management, 6*(4), 243–255.

Marian, L. (Ed.). (1996). National Organization of Nurse Practitioner Faculties (NONPF) guidelines for evaluation of faculty practice. *Faculty practice: Applying the models.* Washington, DC: NONPF.

Mundinger, M., Kane, R., Lenz, E., Totten, A., Tsai, W., Cleary, P., et al. (2000). Primary care outcomes in patients treated by nurse practitioners of physicians. *Journal of the American Medical Association, 283*(1), 59–68.

National Committee for Quality Assurance. (2009). *HEDIS and quality improvement.* Retrieved February 1, 2009, from www.ncqa.org

National Nursing Centers Consortium. (2001). *Guidelines for quality management for nursing centers.* Washington, DC: Author.

National Organization of Nurse Practitioner Faculties. (2006). *Domains and core competencies of nurse practitioner practice.* Washington, DC: Author

National Panel for Nurse Practitioner Practice Doctorate Competencies. (2006). *Practice doctorate nurse practitioner entry-level competencies.* Retrieved January 29, 2009, from www.nonpf.org

Pohl, J. (2009, January). *Quality and safety in doctoral education: Crossmapping QSEN advanced practice competencies with NONPF NP and DNP competencies.* Paper presented at the American Association of Colleges of Nursing Doctoral Conference, San Diego, CA.

Pohl, J. M., Vonderheid, S. C., Barkauskas, V. H., & Nagelkerk, J. (2004). The safety net: Academic nurse managed centers' role. *Policy, Politics, & Nursing Practice, 5*(2), 84–94.

Tsai, A. C., Morton, S. C., Mangione, C. M., & Keeler, E. B. (2005). A meta-analysis of intervention to improve care for chronic illnesses. *American Journal of Managed Care, 11*(8), 478–488.

U.S. Preventive Services Task Force. (2009). *Guide to clinical preventive services.* Retrieved February 2, 2009, from www.ahrq.gov/clinic/pocketgd.htm

Wagner, E. H., Austin, B., Davis, C., Hindmarsh, M., Schaefer, J., & Bonomi, A. (2001). Improving chronic illness care: Translating evidence into action. *Health Affairs, 20*(6), 64–78.

Wagner, E. H., Glasgow, R. E., Davis, C., Bonomi, A. E., Provost, L., McCulloch, D., et al. (2001). Quality improvement in chronic illness care: A collaborative approach. *Joint Commission Journal on Quality and Safety, 27*(2), 63–80.

Wang, A., Wolf, M., Carlyle, R., Wilkerson, D., Porterfield, D., & Reaves, J. (2004). The North Carolina experience with the diabetes health disparities collaboratives. *Joint Commission Journal on Quality and Safety, 30*(7), 396–404.

Womack, J. P., & Jones, D. T. (2003). *Lean thinking.* New York: Free Press.

Womack, J. P., & Jones, D. T. (2005). *Lean solutions.* New York: Free Press.

Global Health and Future Challenges

The nurse practitioner (NP) role in the United States is being examined by nurses and policymakers, business leaders, and others around the world to determine the adaptability of the NP role to local models of care, gaps and needs, professional and regulatory structure, acceptance, and the capability of education programs to produce graduates equipped for a different type of practice. As helpful as examining the U.S. model is for other countries, practitioners in the United States should also value international lessons learned, as those countries that develop the role do so in a context that is fresh and potentially more flexible.

Ward describes the global impact of the NP role and the adaptability of the model to different cultural and system requirements around the world. Citing Canada, Botswana, the United Kingdom, Australia, New Zealand, and other Asian and European countries, Ward makes the case that the NP role is being developed multi-nationally for three common reasons: need for cost containment, improved access, and better services to the underserved.

Hansen-Turton and Hughes sharpen Ward's global view by providing details of the development of the NP role in New Zealand, and some of the political and policy considerations that have influenced the role evolution. Although countries may differ in their health care system requirements, some factors seem pandemic, including opposition from other professions and political and regulatory complexity.

NP service is basic to the country's strategy to provide all citizens access to culturally competent primary, secondary, and tertiary care that is locally determined.

Access to health care in Ireland is universal, as a result of the Health Act of 2004. New developments, including raising the preregistration level of education, expanding nurses' scope of practice, new clinical positions, and prescriptive authority have occurred over a relatively short period of time. MacLellan describes how advanced-practice nursing roles are now imbedded in Ireland's health care system and regulations. Health and nursing policies have been crafted to avoid some of the role, title, scope, and education issues that potentially are barriers for nursing professionals.

McGivern, Sullivan-Marx, and Fairman outline the challenges and opportunities that lie ahead for advanced practice generally, and NPs in particular. Their analysis serves as a jumping-off point for readers whose experiences, aspirations, and investment in individual and organizational activism will more precisely define the future.

Finally, Greenberg has compiled a summary of the Web sites most likely to fully inform readers about the topics discussed in these chapters. These sites, fully vetted and described, provide the most current and authoritative data from organizations responsible for representing, advocating, credentialing, and informing NP practice.

24

Global Health and Future Challenges

HELEN WARD

Chapter 1 discusses the historical emergence of the nurse practitioner (NP) role in the 1960s as a solution to meeting the community health needs of Americans in rural and poor urban areas. Following the establishment of the role of the NP in the United States, other countries have adapted the role to meet health challenges in their own countries. This chapter will discuss the global impact that the role of the NP is having, and will explore how different countries have introduced the role. The term "nurse practitioner" is not one that has been globally adopted, and tends to be used synonymously with the term "advanced-practice nurse" (APN). For the purposes of this chapter, the term *nurse practitioner* will be used unless otherwise stated.

The role of the NP is evolving in response to rapidly changing health policies seeking to meet the challenges of aging populations, the increased complexity of chronic disease, and underserved populations in both the developed and developing countries. Different countries have responded to health care challenges by introducing the NP as a provider of direct patient care within his or her individual health care system. Each nation has its own reason for supporting the development of the NP role.

WHY IS IT IMPORTANT TO LOOK AT THE GLOBAL ROLE OF NURSE PRACTITIONERS?

Global health policy faces disparate challenges and focuses on meeting an array of complex health needs within the context of environmental factors. The concept of the NP role and standards for education and practice vary from country to country, and sometimes even within countries. Challenging issues include lack of role clarification, proliferation of titles, differing educational requirements, scope of practice conflicts, and variability in standards of educational programs (Schober & Affara, 2006). The work of the International Council of Nurses (ICN) has been pivotal in evaluating the role of the NP (Sheer & Wong, 2008) and influencing regulation. Indeed, recognizing the global trend in the development of advanced nursing was the impetus for members of the ICN to launch an International Nurse Practitioner/Advanced-Practice Network (INP/APNN) in 2000. The aim of this network is to facilitate communication among nurses throughout the world who share the same interest. In 2002, a definition of an NP/APN was published by the ICN, with the aim of providing a framework for different countries to develop their own model, but at the same time adhering to a global conceptualization:

> The APN is a registered nurse who has acquired the expert knowledge base, complex decision-making skills and clinical competencies for expanded practice, the characteristics of which are shaped by the context and/or country in which s/he is credentialed to practice. A master's degree is recommended for entry level. (International Council of Nurses [ICN], 2002, cited in ICN, 2008, p. 7)

The ICN has also developed a *Scope of Practice, Standards and Competencies for the Advanced Practice Nurse* (International Council of Nurses, 2008). Under the three main headings of professional, ethical, and legal practice; care provision; and management and professional, personal, and quality development, a range of domains with an expectation of the competencies are documented. This framework is designed to be generic, and aims to provide individual countries with a model from which they can work when developing practice competencies for the role of the NP. Ideally, standardized global competencies would provide international benchmarks for the NP. However, this is not realistic, due to the diversity of global health care systems.

The role of the NP was relatively slow to emerge in countries apart from the United States until the mid-1980s. Canada attempted to adopt the role in the 1960s due to a perceived physician shortage, but lack of legitimization resulted in its disappearance until the 1990s (International Council of Nurses, 2008). Recently, the Canadian Nurse Practitioner Initiative (CNPI), led by the Canadian Nurses Association (CNA), developed a pan-Canadian framework for the promotion and the sustained integration of the role of NPs across Canada (Canada Nurse Practitioner Initiative, (2006). The CNA has published a national framework for advanced nursing practice to provide a common understanding of the roles (Canadian Nurses Association, 2008). This document supports the *Canadian Nurse Practitioner Core Competency Framework* (Canadian Nurses Association, 2005).

Botswana was amongst the first countries outside the United States to implement an education program for NPs (International Council of Nurses, 2008). This initiative was developed in response to a physician shortage, and the subsequent expectation that nurses with a generalist education were expected to not only provide nursing care, but also to make medical decisions. The NP role is now well established in Botswana, where the Institute of Health Sciences in Gaborone is educating nurses at the master's level (Sheer & Wong, 2008).

The United Kingdom (U.K.) saw the first NP emerge in general practice in 1986. Barbara Stilwell completed an NP educational program in the United States, and returned to the United Kingdom to implement a service providing for the health care needs of Muslim women in an inner city area, whose needs were not met by a single male physician (Bowling & Stilwell, 1988). Stilwell then established the first educational program for NPs in the United Kingdom supported by the Royal College of Nursing (RCN). The NP movement in the United Kingdom was relatively slow to evolve, and did so within the primary care setting. Lack of regulation and protection of the title NP has led to confusion among employers and a proliferation of titles and roles. Regulation of the title continues to threaten the role, and has become embroiled in a new argument for the regulation of all health professionals (Department of Health, 2008). In 1998, the RCN developed a set of competencies and educational standards for NPs adapted from the NONPF competencies; these were updated in 2008 (Royal College of Nursing, 2008). Despite lack of regulation, the role of the NP is now well established in the United Kingdom, with over 3,500 nurses working with the title "nurse practitioner." The majority are working in the primary care setting, but more recently, the role has been developing into specialty areas, such as cancer care and pediatrics.

Learning from the experiences of other countries, Australia and New Zealand developed educational programs and protected the title NP before establishing the role. Access to cost-effective health care in remote and rural areas was one stimulus for the development of the NP in Australia, where the role was first established in New South Wales (Offredy, 1999). By 2008, there were more than 320 authorized NPs in Australia. In New Zealand, the role of the NP is just becoming established, following a joint project by the Australian Nursing and Midwifery Council (ANMC) and Nursing Council of New Zealand to develop competency standards for the NP. These competency standards are used to assess the license renewal process, assess NPs educated overseas, and are used by universities to assess standards when developing the curriculum (Australian Nursing and Midwifery Council, 2006; Hughes, Clarke, Sampson, Fairman, & Sullivan-Marx, 2003).

Not all countries have followed the competency framework for NPs, although many are building on existing postregistration pathways to enable clinical nurses to progress through a structured career pathway to become an NP. A good example of this is Singapore, where in 2001, the Singapore Ministry of Health provided the opportunity for clinicians to become APNs after completing an accredited master's program in nursing. The APNs were perceived as being at the same level as Assistant Directors of Nursing and Principal Nurse Educators. Previously, good nurse clinicians were promoted into management or education. In 2005, the Nurses and Midwifery Act was amended to provide for an ANP register, and in 2006, the Singapore Nursing Board registered the first two APNs (A. B. Choo, personal communication, 2008).

In Asia, the role of the NP is developing in a variety of ways, mainly linked to socioeconomic and political backgrounds. Taiwan and Hong Kong led the way in developing the role of the clinical nurse specialist (CNS) in the mid-1990s, and in 2004, Taiwan issued the regulation for an NP program accreditation. In Hong Kong, nurses can now see patients independently in nurse-led clinics, and are in the process of developing an Academy of Nursing to establish regulation and accreditation of APNs in the future (Sheer & Wong, 2008). In mainland China, there is a need to develop the role of the NP, and it appears on the nursing development agenda for the future. However, it is deterred by the fact that nursing education is still at a basic level, and the number of physicians is higher than the number of nurses. However, some hospitals are introducing the CNS in areas such as diabetes and stoma care, and educational courses are available in collaboration with Hong Kong (Sheer & Wong, 2008).

In some developing areas of the world, education is not a barrier to the autonomy experienced by some nurses. For example, in remote areas of sub-Saharan Africa, nurses working with the highest degree of autonomy are often those with the least educational preparation, as these positions are not regarded as attractive and are poorly supported and remunerated. Gaining further education is often the route to the towns and into hospitals in which a nurse's ranking is linked to professional hierarchy. In most African countries, any further education following initial registration would be considered "advanced."

In Europe, the role of the advanced nurse is accepted and commonplace, although variable, and comes in a variety of guises (CNS, nurse anesthetist, advanced nurse, nurse consultant). In the Netherlands, the role of the NP is well established, with approximately 2,000 nurses working in advanced roles, mostly in the hospital setting as CNSs. Nurses in this country are in the process of establishing a register for the Nurse Specialist (Sheer & Wong, 2008). In Belgium, Switzerland, and Germany, it is the role of the CNS that is being developed, rather than that of the NP. France launched the NP role in February 2009, and already has an established nurse anesthetist role. The Nordic countries of Denmark, Finland, and Norway are all hoping to establish the role of the NP. In particular, Denmark is looking to the United Kingdom, Netherlands, and the United States for models of health care to meet the demand for effective management of chronic diseases, which are challenging the current health care system (Danish Nurses Organisation, 2008).

Experiences in different countries show that NPs are developing as a result of the challenges that center on current health care systems. There is a need to contain cost, improve access to patient care, reduce waiting times, serve the underprivileged populations, and maintain the health of patients. The 21st century will see the establishment of the NP across the globe, particularly in areas such as chronic disease management, in which nurse-led services will complement those provided by our medical colleagues. In countries where there is a physician shortage, the role is expanding rapidly to reduce the medical/nursing gap in health care services. Educational programs will provide nursing with an advanced career option, which may encourage nurses to stay in their countries and provide a respected contribution to health care. The evolution of the NP role is clearly linked to the political agenda, and its autonomy is linked to educational preparation, and in many cases, prescriptive authority. Although prescribing by NPs is well established in the United States, this is generally not the case worldwide, with many countries having to provide evidence that NPs can make a difference before legislative changes are made to allow nurses to prescribe.

REFERENCES

Australian Nursing and Midwifery Council. (2006). *National competency standards for the nurse practitioner*. Retrieved February 2009, from http://www.anmc.org.au/docs/Publications/Competency%20Standards%20for%20the%20Nurse%20Practitioner.pdf

Bowling, A., & Stilwell B. (Eds.). (1988). *The nurse in family practice*. London: Scutari Press.

Canadian Nurse Practitioner Initiative. (2006). *Canadian Nurse Practitioner Initiative technical report: Legislative and regulatory framework*. Ottawa, ON, Canada: Canadian Nurses Association.

Canadian Nurses Association. (2005). *Canadian Nurse Practitioner core competency framework*. Ottawa, ON, Canada: Author.

Canadian Nurses Association. (2008). *Advanced nursing practice: A national framework* (revised). Ottawa, ON, Canada: Author.

Danish Nurses Organisation. (2008). *Advanced nurse practitioners: Improved health care to the chronically ill*. Copenhagen, Denmark: Author.

Department of Health. (2008). *Implementing the white paper Trust, Assurance and Safety: Enhancing confidence in healthcare professional regulators. Final report*. AB, Canada: London, Ontario: Crown Publications

Hughes, F., Clarke, S., Sampson, D. A., Fairman, J., & Sullivan-Marx, E. (2003). Research in support of nurse practitioners. In M. D. Mezey, D. O. McGivern, & E. M. Sullivan-Marx (Eds.), & S. A. Greenberg (Managing Ed.), *Nurse practitioners: Evolution of advanced practice* (4th ed., pp. 84–107). New York: Springer Publishing Company.

International Council of Nurses. (2008). *The scope of practice, standards and competencies of the advanced practice nurse*. Geneva, Switzerland: Author.

Offredy, M. (1999). The nurse practitioner role in New South Wales: Development and policy. *Nursing Standard, 13*(43), 38–41.

Royal College of Nursing. (2008). *Advanced nurse practitioners. An RCN guide to the advanced nurse practitioner role, competencies and programme accreditation*. London: Author.

Schober, M., & Affara, F. (2006). *Advanced nursing practice.* Oxford, U.K.: Blackwell Publishing.

Sheer, B., & Wong, F. (2008). The development of advanced nursing practice globally. *Journal of Nursing Scholarship, 40,* 204–211.

25

The Evolution and Future of Nurse Practitioners in New Zealand

TINE HANSEN-TURTON AND FRANCES HUGHES

FOREWORD

In June 2005, one of the authors of this chapter, who currently directs the National Nursing Centers Consortium in the United States, a non-profit association of 250 nurse-managed health centers, spent 5 weeks in New Zealand on an Eisenhower Fellowship to study the overall health care infrastructure and the new role of nurse practitioners (NPs) in the country. As part of the fellowship, the author worked with the Ministry of Health and Nursing Council of New Zealand, its regulatory agency for nursing, to implement their 2002 Strategic Plan to deploy NPs in primary care and community care in New Zealand. She also explored the feasibility of establishing nurse-managed health centers in partnership with the Ministry of Health and local nursing schools.

The chapter is based on the author's first-hand experience during 2005, working with health care leaders in New Zealand, interviewing key nursing, physician, and health care leaders, along with traditional researchers. Because the information for this chapter was initially gathered in 2005, some updated material has been provided as an addendum to the report. However, many of the issues in this report remain current, particularly the need for NPs to become better recognized as leaders within the primary health system.

INTRODUCTION

NPs in New Zealand are educated and licensed to be independent primary care providers with authority to treat, diagnose, and prescribe medications. They integrate public health nursing practice to promote health and prevent disease, using nursing frameworks for behavior change at the individual and population levels of contact. However, it was not always so. Prior to 2001, New Zealand primarily followed common practices in most countries of the world, in which nurses, for the most part, finish their training at the bachelor's degree or lower educational levels. In 2001, the New Zealand government recognized that, "using nurse practitioners would be an important part of delivering the Government's priorities for health, as outlined in the New Zealand Primary Health Care Strategy" (New Zealand Ministry of Health, 2002, pp. 1–2). Thus, New Zealand universities are currently graduating master's-prepared NPs to be deployed throughout the country. These NPs work in nurse-led practices in primary care, specialty care, and chronic disease management throughout the country's health care institutions.

PART I: BACKGROUND

Overview of the New Zealand Health Care System

The Minister of Health has the overall responsibility for the health care system in New Zealand. The Minister works through the Ministry of Health, which employs civil servants to enter into management agreements with District Health Boards (DHBs), determines the health strategy for the country, and decides with government colleagues how much public funding will be spent on the public delivery of health service (New Zealand Ministry of Health, 2003b). The Ministry of Health provides policy advice on improving health outcomes and reducing health disparities, acts as the Minister's agent, monitors the performance of DHBs and other health entities, implements, administers, and enforces legislation and regulations, provides health information, facilitates collaboration across sectors, and plans and funds public health, disability support services, and other services (New Zealand Ministry of Health, 2003b).

Although the New Zealand belief is that health care is a right for all its citizens, over the last decade, the health care sector in New Zealand has undergone four major structural changes that have had an impact on access to care for many New Zealand residents. The changes have ranged from a purchaser/provider market-oriented model in 1994, to a more community-oriented model that is currently in place to promote access (World Health Organization, 2005a). In December 2000, New Zealand launched a new health care strategy to ensure that all citizens have access to health care services, including primary, secondary, and tertiary care. The goal of the plan is for New Zealand to have healthy and thriving communities by 2010. Up until 2000, the health care system had focused on a more traditional medical model, emphasizing treatment of illnesses, and not prevention. Care was provided under a fee-for-service arrangement under the direction of a physician, with little acknowledgment of the role of nursing, and services that were provided in a Western manner, without recognition of cultural competence or local ethnicities, like the Maori and Pacific Island populations (King, 2001). To change the direction of the medical model, the first major policy step was to create a strategy to build a strong primary health care system (King, 2001). Accordingly, the New Zealand Ministry of Health, under the leadership of the then-Minister of Health, Annette King, decentralized the delivery of health care in the country through the establishment of 21 local DHBs, giving them the full responsibility of providing health care in a designated service area (World Health Organization, 2005a).

DHBs report and are responsible to the Minister of Health. Each DHB Board of Directors has up to 11 members, 7 of whom are elected by the community. The Minister of Health appoints four members. In recognition of the unique status of Maori in New Zealand, each DHB must have at least two Maori members. DHBs function as a cross between a state health department and a large county or city health department in the United States, and are primarily responsible for planning, funding, and guaranteeing the provision of health and disability services to a geographically defined population in 21 regions. The Ministry of Health provides broad guidelines on what services the DHBs must provide, and national priorities have been set in the New Zealand Primary Health Care strategy. Health care services, such as assessment, treatment, rehabilitation, and some public health services, come directly under the arm of DHBs, whereas primary care provided by general practitioners

(GPs), primary health care organizations (PHOs), nursing homes, and independent midwifery services are independent, and are contracted by DHBs to supply services. Currently, there are 80 public hospitals in New Zealand (New Zealand Ministry of Health, 2003b). DHBs control all the funding, and are responsible for managing their budgets, which are created on a fairly complicated population health formula. The non-governmental organizations (NGOs), which the DHBs fund, often serve the indigent populations, and those who for cultural or other reasons are not comfortable using mainstream health services.

Health Disparities in New Zealand

Maori and South Pacific Island populations suffer the most health disparities in New Zealand. Maori have a higher rate of smoking, especially among younger women, than non-Maori. The cancer mortality and diabetes rates are higher, oral health is poor, vaccine-preventable diseases among children are higher, and obesity is higher, particularly among men (World Health Organization, 2005b). The Maori mortality rate in the 35–64-year-old age group is 3.4 times as high as that of non-Maori and non-Pacific Islanders. For the 65–74-year-old Maori male, the mortality rate was twice that of non-Maori. For female Maori in the 35–64-year-old age group, the mortality rate was 5.6 times as high as that of non-Maori, and in the age group of 65–74, the mortality rate was 3.3 times the non-Maori rate (National Health Committee, 2005). To address health disparities in the Maori population, the principles of the New Zealand Primary Health Care Health Strategy include acknowledging the special relationship between Maori and the English Crown under the Treaty of Waitangi. In the Treaty, the New Zealand government committed to work with Maori communities to develop strategies for Maori health gains and appropriate services. The government involved Maori at all levels of health care decision making, planning, development, and delivery of health services. The treaty ensured the safeguarding of Maori cultural concepts, values, and practices (King & Turia, 2002). Maori and Pacific communities have also demonstrated considerable leadership in developing and pursuing their own health initiatives.

Although the New Zealand government publicly acknowledged that the current health disparities among ethnic groups are not acceptable, it has a long way to go to actually address them (I. Ernura, personal communication, October 10, 2005).[1] The Ministry of Health has also emphasized in its publication on *Investing in Health* a framework for activating primary health care nursing in New Zealand, including an enhanced role for nursing and NPs (New Zealand Ministry of Health, 2003a).

A Ten-Year Primary Health Care Strategy

In February 2001, the Ministry of Health launched a new 10-year primary health care strategy. The vision of the strategy involved a new direction for primary health care with greater emphasis on population-based health care, and the integration of the community, health promotion, and preventive care with primary care (King, 2001; World Health Organization, 2005a). The Ministry of Health laid out six goals for the primary care strategy vision: (a) work with local communities; (b) identify and remove health inequalities; (c) offer access to comprehensive services to improve, maintain, and restore people's health; (d) coordinate care across service areas; (e) develop a primary health care workforce; and (e) continuously improve quality using good information (King, 2001). In line with the World Health Organization's Alma Ata Declaration, New Zealand has defined quality primary health care as, "essential health care based on practical, scientifically sound, culturally appropriate and socially acceptable methods that is universally accessible to people in their communities, involves community participation, integral to...New Zealand's health system and the first level of contact...with the health system" (King, 2001, p. 5).

Although the strategy is impressive, in interviews with many providers, the author found that practitioners and leaders of the DHBs were hesitant to put their energy behind it. According to Eldred Gilbert, (then) Director of Nursing at the Capital and Coast DHB, "our health care system has undergone four major policy changes in the past decade, with an upcoming September 2005 election, where it is not sure Labor will prevail, a new leadership could get in office and change the system

---

[1]Inia Ernura, formerly of New Zealand's Northland District Health Board.

yet another time" (E. Gilbert, personal communication, June 20, 2005).[2]
Incidentally, elections took place in September 2005, and Labor retained
its control, and thus the primary care strategy is still in effect as the
government's main health care policy strategy.

The New Zealand system from the primary, secondary, and tertiary
levels remains very segregated. For example, the secondary sector,
which provides public health nursing care such as immunizations,
disease management, and hospitalization, is not integrated with the
primary care sector. Consumers access these services independently
from the GPs, "although the idea of the primary health care strategy
was to provide these services as extensions of primary care," according
to Dr. Frances Hughes (personal communication, June 21, 2005).[3]
Furthermore, unlike the American system, GPs cannot follow their
patients in the hospital. The high levels of specialization have created
an "isolation mentality among providers, which will be hard to break
as it has been part of the New Zealand health care culture for so long,"
according to Jenny Carryer (personal communication, June 20, 2005).[4]

Discussion of the Primary Health Care Strategy Impact on District Health Boards, General Practitioners, and Primary Health Care Organizations

The establishment of DHBs had four objectives: (a) Health improvement: maintaining, improving and promoting the health of the population; (b) Responsiveness: meeting the legitimate expectations of
communities for quality health services (person-centered, timely, appropriate, accessible, effective, safe); (c) Equity: ensuring equal distribution
of health through strategic planning and funding to address population
need; and (d) Efficiency: technical efficiency, including value for money
through minimizing costs and maximizing outcomes, and efficiency
allocations by maximizing overall health from resources provided (New

---

[2]Eldred Gilbert is the Director of Nursing at the Capital and Coast District Health Board in Wellington, New Zealand.
[3]Dr. Frances Hughes was Professor and Director of the Centre for Mental Health Research, Policy and Service Development at the University of Auckland in Wellington, N.Z.
[4]Jenny Carryer is a Professor of Nursing at Massey University in Palmerston North, N.Z.

Zealand Health and Development Act of 2000, 2002). The mechanisms to reach the health improvement, responsiveness, equity, and efficiency objectives include collaboration at all levels, using health needs assessments to strategically plan and fund services, targeting areas of need, particularly the Maori population, and use evidence-based governance, policy, planning, funding, and service delivery.

The purpose of establishing DHBs was to move from a centralized health care delivery system to a local community-access strategy, with a focus on improving population health status in New Zealand (World Health Organization, 2005c). This has been a hard cultural change for all providers, especially the physician community, and health care systems, which traditionally looked at health care from an individual standpoint and not a population focus. The DHB system was designed to be open to new ideas, and break the cycle of specialization and silo-mentality. These new ideas include the introduction of NPs and the establishment of NP-led clinics and nurse-managed health centers to further the development of the primary care workforce, and especially to address gaps in service among the Maori and Pacific Island populations.

Unlike the United States, where family physicians have to navigate the myriad of private insurance company policies, Medicaid, and managed care to get reimbursement for primary care services, GPs in New Zealand are funded through the DHBs. Traditionally, GP practices have been run like small businesses. Since 2002, DHBs have changed the funding formula of GPs to a capitation fee formula, similar to the U.S. model. The difference is that primary care and preventive services in the DHB government model are funded as part of an overall payment for the individual's care, rather than privately funded through insurance companies on a fee-for-service basis. According to Pauline Cook, the then-Acting Chief Nurse Policy Advisor to the Minister of Health, the care provided by GPs is partially sponsored under capitation by the DHBs to the tune of $10 per patient or patient visit per month; however, users are still responsible for co-payment for services, which averages $40–$50 New Zealand dollars per GP visit (P. Cook, personal communication, June 21, 2005).[5] Hence, capitation has not necessarily reduced the GP fees; they have just offset some of the costs to the New Zealand

---

[5]Pauline Cook is Former Acting Chief Advisor of Nursing, Clinical Services Improvement, Clinical Services Directorate, at the Ministry of Health in Wellington, N.Z.

population. The co-payment has provided some obstacles for low-income residents, thus, the Ministry of Health has subsidized some of the co-payments for low-income residents and for children under the age of 6. In these incidences, New Zealand residents are only required to pay $20 at certain income levels. However, the co-pay has still proven to be an obstacle for a lot of people seeking care.

There are some concerns in the health care community that payment of physicians for primary care on a capitation model is a disincentive to provide regular primary care to the capitated patients. For example, in Aranui, a low-income area in the South Island city of Christchurch, local physicians are struggling to keep their practices going, "serving the underserved" (D. Deering, personal communication, July 4, 2005).[6] The nonprofit PHOs described in the following do not provide any bonus or other incentive payments for good patient outcomes. In addition to subsidies for underserved populations, the Ministry of Health has started the Access Plus program, in which residents can enroll directly within their GP office, and that entitles them to management of certain chronic diseases (P. Cook, personal communication, June 21, 2005).

Although the Ministry of Health has given DHBs overall responsibility for assessing the health needs of communities in their regions, and managing the resources and services to meet the needs under the direction of the Ministry, it also established local nonprofit PHOs to carry out the new vision and direction at the local level (King, 2001). DHBs fund the local PHOs. In turn, PHOs can contract with a range of providers from individual physicians, NPs, and nurse-managed clinics. These providers are required to offer services directed to improving and maintaining the health of the population. PHOs are expected, but not required (unlike the DHBs), to involve local communities in their governing process. All providers, including nurses, must be involved in the PHO organization's decision making, rather than one dominant group, which traditionally had been physicians (GPs) (King, 2001). Membership in the PHOs is voluntary. GPs are not required to join a local PHO, although it is strongly encouraged by the government.

---

[6]Daryle Deering is the Director of Nursing Practice at the Christchurch District Health Board in Christchurch, N.Z.

PART II: A COMPARISON OF NURSE PRACTITIONERS IN THE UNITED STATES AND NEW ZEALAND

In 2001, the Ministry of Health and the Nursing Council of New Zealand unveiled their decision to educate and graduate NPs to address a growing problem of primary health care access for all populations in New Zealand. The NP degree was envisioned and marketed as a way to change primary health care in New Zealand. In December 2003, the New Zealand General Assembly passed the Health Practitioners Competence Assurance Act, which established a new scope of practice for NPs in the country (New Zealand Health and Development Act of 2000, 2002). Following the adoption of the Act, the Nursing Council of New Zealand, which functions as the country's regulatory nursing oversight Board, developed the regulations to accompany the act. These regulations were adopted on September 18, 2004 (New Zealand Health and Development Act of 2000, 2002).[7] The establishment of NPs is seen as a strong policy component of the country's new Primary Health Care Strategy to close gaps in health care, especially for New Zealand's indigent populations, such as the Maoris and Pacific Islanders. Since 2001, there has been considerable investment from both the Ministry of Health and various professional nursing organizations in developing the NP role (Dr. F. Hughes, personal communication, June 21, 2005). To date, several hundred NPs have graduated, and 50 are recognized as registered NPs in New Zealand.

In New Zealand, to receive a NP degree, registered nurses (RNs) spend 3–4 years in postgraduate studies, and 1 additional year in practi-

---

[7]Health Practitioners Competence Assurance Act, Title 12 (2): Scope of practice —Nurse Practitioners: Nurse Practitioners are expert nurses who work within a specific area of practice incorporating advanced knowledge and skills. They practice both independently and in collaboration with other health care professionals to promote health, prevent disease, and to diagnose, assess, and manage people's health needs. They provide a wide range of assessment and treatment interventions, including differential diagnoses, ordering, conducting, and interpreting diagnostic and laboratory tests and administering therapies for the management of potential or actual health needs. They work in partnership with individuals, families, whanau, and communities across a range of settings. NPs may choose to prescribe medicines within their specific area of practice. NPs also demonstrate leadership as consultants, educators, managers, and researchers, and actively participate in professional activities, and in local and national policy development.

cum and licensing formalities to become an NP (New Zealand Health and Development Act of 2000, 2002). In general, the scope and competencies of NPs in New Zealand are similar to that of U.S.-educated NPs. Revised requirements for education and continuing competence for NP prescribing authority came into force in December 2005. These requirements replaced those made in 2002 and in 2005. In addition, approved training programs that include nurse prescribing at the master's level are in place at the following institutions:

- Auckland University of Technology—Master of Health Science in Advanced Nursing Practice
- Eastern Institute of Technology—Master of Nursing
- Massey University—Master of Nursing
- Otago Polytechnic—Master of Nursing
- The University of Auckland—Master of Nursing
- University of Otago—Christchurch School of Medicine
- Victoria University of Wellington—Master of Nursing (Clinical)
- Waikato Institute of Technology—Master of Nursing (Clinical)

Specifically, the Nursing Council of New Zealand requirements for NP competencies include: registration with the Nursing Council in the Registered Nurse Scope of Practice, a minimum of 4 years of experience in a specific area of practice, successful completion of a clinically focused master's degree program approved by the Council, passing a Nursing Council assessment of NP competencies, and successful completion of an approved prescribing class of a clinically focused master's degree program (Nursing Council of New Zealand, 2005a). Although U.S. schools of nursing must be accredited by national organizations to administer an approved NP degree program, the schools of nursing in New Zealand are not accredited (Nursing Council of New Zealand, 2005a). Instead, the Council of Nursing accredits the individual NP candidate through a 2-day intense exam following the student's completion of the educational and clinical course work (Nursing Council of New Zealand, 2005a). The Nursing Council recently evaluated its process for registering NPs in October 2007 and concluded that process is credible for applicants and reviewers.

In New Zealand, nurses who have entered into NP education have gravitated to their current areas of expertise, and not moved into primary care. Thus, in order for the New Zealand's nursing community to become an active and visible player in the country's new primary health care strategy, it must be able to meet the demand and fulfill the identified needs, which are in primary care.

Policies, Regulations, and Reimbursement for Nurse Practitioners in the United States and New Zealand

Similar to American NPs, New Zealand NPs have also met some opposition from organized medicine (Mackay, 2003). The criticism particularly has had to do with the debate on whether NPs in New Zealand should be able to prescribe (Moller, 2005). Physicians have made claims that nurse prescribing will lead to adverse patient outcomes (New Zealand Nurses Organization, 2005). Associations like the New Zealand Society of Anesthetists have supported the development of NP roles in some areas, but have been particularly concerned about the safety of NP autonomous prescribing when it comes to anesthesia types of drugs (New Zealand Society of Anesthetists, 2005).

Managed-care company credentialing and reimbursement policies are the biggest barrier to nurse-managed health center practice in the United States today. Although New Zealand has only a small private health insurance market, establishing a reimbursement mechanism for NPs will be critical to their success as a new provider type in the country (F. Hughes, personal communication, June 21, 2005). Although the NP role in New Zealand has been identified in several government policies and strategies as a key vehicle to deliver health goals, the development to date has been around individuals, not services or environments for NPs to deliver their practice once they are registered as an NP. To date, there have been no incentives for the current DHBs or PHOs to create NP jobs or training sites for them. Although the DHBs are responsible for providing health care through a population-based approach, a focus in which NPs traditionally have proven effective, there has been no integrated workforce approach at the local levels to include NPs in care delivery. Thus, one strategy for the Health Ministry to consider is to institute a financial incentive for these funders to encourage them to develop NP positions to allow for the role to become established and validated.

Since July 2005, the Ministry of Health has moved forward with providing some pilot funding to hire NPs to provide primary care services to the Maori population in Northland. Subsequently, the National Nursing Centers Consortium, the newly established New Zealand Consortium, and schools of nursing in New Zealand began to plan a global health care conference. On January 15–17, 2008, close to 200 health professionals, representing 11 countries, gathered in Auckland, New Zealand, at the first Global Healthcare Solutions to Vulnerable Populations Conference, sponsored by the National Nursing Centers Consortium, along with Auckland University of Technology Fulbright New Zealand and Eisenhower Fellowships. The Conference was a direct outcome of the author's work in New Zealand, and provided an exciting opportunity for health care professionals from around the world to share innovative health care models and services, and to discuss best practices for vulnerable populations. Since 2005, more than 30 New Zealand health care professionals attended conferences and visited the United States on sabbaticals to learn more about integrating NPs into primary care.

PART III: THE CHALLENGES AND OPPORTUNITIES FOR ESTABLISHING NURSE PRACTITIONER PRACTICES IN NEW ZEALAND

The New Zealand Primary Health Care Strategy supports development and funding of both NPs and nurse-managed health centers. A strengths–weakness–opportunity–threats (SWOT) analysis done in 2005 indicates that the strengths and opportunities of developing NP-run health centers include better provision of holistic care that is community-based and more likely to address health disparities among the Maori and Pacific Island populations, yet, the weaknesses and threats are considerable and need to be addressed (World Health Organization, 2005c).

One major weakness for NPs to overcome is achieving prescriptive authority to fully function as primary care providers. NP prescriptive authority was under intense debate with major opposition from the medical community in New Zealand when the author visited the country (New Zealand Nurses Organization, 2005; New Zealand Society of Anesthetists, 2005). The author was interviewed by both nursing and medical journals about prescriptive authority for NPs in the United States. The medical journals and physician providers expressed unqualified concerns about NP competencies in prescribing; however, they found it hard to argue against U.S. NP prescribing trends. They also found it hard to argue with studies conducted in New Zealand, supporting that nurse practitioners performed quality of care and good health outcomes (Laurant et al., 2004). In a meeting with the [former] Minister of Health, Annette King, the author stressed the importance of ensuring that NPs get prescriptive authority prior to the election in September, 2005. Despite significant GP opposition, 3 days prior to the election, the Minister of Health signed prescriptive authority into law, and thus a major political barrier for NPs in New Zealand has now been overcome (Fox, 2005; Hodgson, 2005). The prescribing regulations took effect on November 1, 2005 (Nursing Council of New Zealand, 2005b).

In terms of threats, physicians currently receive capitated payments from the PHOs for their primary care patients. Further, as discussed earlier, the health care sector has undergone four major restructures under the last four administrations, which have changed every 3 years. The Labor party was re-elected in September, 2005, which gave the administration 3 more years to implement the primary care health care strategy. The reelection of the government may have removed some of the provider fears that a new government administration could make another health care system overhaul, and thus give health care funders, such as the DHBs and PHOs, a new incentive to support the primary health care strategy.

More recently, New Zealand underwent a further general election, and a national government has been elected (November, 2008). The new government has not indicated any significant changes to the provision of primary health care, and its policies retain a strong focus on enhancing and improving the delivery of primary health services, including clinical leadership.

Finally, the GP community in New Zealand has control over the provision of primary care. Unlike the United States, where the specialist physician community traditionally has had broader political powers, the GPs have a lot of political power and control in New Zealand (F. Hughes, personal communication, June 21, 2005). Both NP and nurse-managed health centers pose severe threats to the current GP-centered medical model of care, and ultimately, their funding for primary care. However, despite these political challenges, with the reelection of the administration, the strengths and opportunities for NPs in New Zealand seem stronger than the weaknesses and threats from other providers (D. Oliff, personal communication, June 15, 2005).[8] Nevertheless, to successfully integrate NPs into the health care infrastructure in New Zealand, the new NP development in New Zealand must become more integrated with current government policies and strategies of the government, and be seen as an integrated solution to the country's health care access challenges.

Interestingly, in 2006, the Ministry of Health released its implementation work program for 2006–2010. One of the goals of the work program is "shared ownership and responsibility for the primary health care system and outcomes." The role of NPs is crucial in ensuring that this and other goals are met.

Finally, in September 2007, the Ministry of Health published an Evaluation of the Eleven Primary Health Care Nursing Innovation Projects: A Report to the Ministry of Health by the Primary Health Care Nurse Innovation Evaluation Team. The evaluation was focused on nursing innovations that supported the development of new models of primary care nursing practice and fostering nurse leadership, including innovations based on the role of the NP.

CONCLUSIONS

Although New Zealand can learn a lot from the U.S. NP and nurse-managed health center movement in addressing access issues and health disparities, the U.S. health care system and other countries have a great deal to learn from New Zealand, as well. Health care in New Zealand is considered a right and not a privilege, as many would describe the U.S. health care system. New Zealand's socialized health care system provides primary, secondary, and tertiary health services to all citizens. In the United States, we continue to struggle with increasing health care costs. The U.S. GDP per capita for health care is higher than any other country, twice as high as that of New Zealand, and yet, the U.S. government neglects to provide care to 47 million people. New Zealand, on the other hand, has recognized its primary health care problem in

---

[8]Dale Oliff is Director of Nursing, Middlemore Hospital, Auckland, N.Z.

underserved communities, and is systemically doing something about it by the introduction of a new provider who can fill the gap in service.

In summary, to ensure the proper integration of NPs and nurse-managed health centers in New Zealand as part of the Primary Health Care Strategy, the following areas should be addressed by the Ministry of Health and Council of Nursing to ensure success of their primary health care strategy: (a) NPs must be integrated with PHOs. Similarly, pilot programs should also be developed to integrate NP service delivery in conjunction with both PHOs and NGOs, with a focus on vulnerable populations, such as the Maori, through a funding mechanism from the DHBs; (b) New Zealand should consider the development of the family NP, with a general scope of primary care for all age groups, to fill the gaps of GP service; (c) to ensure the success of the NP program, the Ministry of Health should put pressure on the DHBs to provide set-aside funding for PHOs to try alternative NP models in primary care, such as nurse-managed health centers, to provide care for indigent populations, in which DHBs have a shortage of GPs, and there is a lack of access to primary care; and (d) The Nursing Council should enter into a dialogue with universities and consider the possibility of credentialing Schools of Nursing to award the NP degree, and then administer a national test for all graduates. This would assure fairness and equity in the process.

In March 2006, the Ministry of Health released its implementation work programs for 2006–2010. One of the goals of the work programs is "shared ownership and responsibility for the primary health care system and outcomes." The role of NPs is crucial in ensuring that this and other goals are met. In September 2007, the Ministry of Health published an *Evaluation of the Eleven Primary Health Care Nursing Innovation Projects: A Report to the Ministry of Health* by the Primary Health Care Nurse Innovation Evaluation Team. The evaluation was focused on nursing innovations that supported the development of new models of primary care nursing practice and fostering nurse leadership, including innovations based on the role of the NP. The evaluation report noted that fundamental to the progress made in establishing and facilitating the innovations was nursing leadership, demonstrated at either a clinical or organizational level (New Zealand Ministry of Health, 2008).

In conclusion, the nursing community in New Zealand is a passionate group who stands firmly behind the evolution of the NPs and the next step, the establishment of nurse-managed health centers. They understand the obstacles they face, but are united in making the implementation of NPs and nurse-managed health centers a success. The exchange of information about nurse-managed health centers and the autonomy of NPs as fully recognized primary care providers in the United States, provided by the author's fellowship, provided the nursing leadership and nurses fuel for their passion that nursing can become a real player and change agent in GP-dominated New Zealand.

REFERENCES

Fox, J. (2005, September 13). *New prescribing role will add power to primary care team.* The Royal New Zealand College of General Practitioners. Retrieved August 22, 2009, from http://www.rnzcgp.org.nz/new-prescribing-role-will-add-power-to-primary-care-team/

Hodgson, P. (2005). *Nurse practitioner prescribing rights take effect.* Retrieved July 14, 2009, from http://www.beehive.govt.nz/node/24539

King, A. (2001). *The primary health care strategy.* Wellington, NZ: New Zealand Health Ministry.

King, A., & Turia, T. (2002). *He korowai oranga: Maori health strategy.* Wellington, NZ: New Zealand Ministry of Health.

Laurant, M., Reeves, D., Hermens, R., Braspenning, J., Grol, R., & Sibbald, B. (2004). Substitution of doctors by nurses in primary care. *Cochrane Database of Systematic Reviews,* Issue 4. Art. No.: CD001271. DOI: 10.1002/14651858.CD001271.pub2.

Mackay, B. (2003). General practitioners perceptions of the nurse practitioner role. *New Zealand Medical Journal, 116,* 1170.

Moller, P. (2005). Independent nurse prescribing in New Zealand. *New Zealand Medical Journal, 118,* 1225.

National Health Committee. (2005). *Decision-making about new health interventions. A report to the New Zealand Ministry of Health.* Wellington, NZ: New Zealand Health Ministry.

National Nursing Centers Consortium. (2005a). *Managed care credentialing and reimbursement policies: Barriers to healthcare access and consumer choice.* Philadelphia: Author.

National Nursing Centers Consortium. (2005b). *Congressional briefing* (March 18, 2005). Philadelphia: Author.

New Zealand Health and Development Act of 2000. (2002). Wellington, NZ: New Zealand Health Ministry.

New Zealand Ministry of Health. (2002). *Nurse practitioners in New Zealand.* Retrieved on March 4, 2010, from http://ww.moh.govt.nz/moh.nsf/01e65F72c8749e74c25696-220000b7ce?OpenDowment.

New Zealand Ministry of Health. (2003a). *Investing in health, a framework for activating primary health care nursing in New Zealand.* Wellington, NZ: Author.

New Zealand Ministry of Health. (2003b). *New Zealand health and disability sector overview.* Wellington, NZ: Author.

New Zealand Ministry of Health. (2008). *The evaluation of the eleven primary health care nursing innovation projects: A report to the Ministry of Health by the primary health care nurse innovation evaluation team.* Wellington, NZ: Author.

New Zealand Nurses Organization. (2005, November 5). *Medical fears regarding nurse prescribing groundless.*

New Zealand Society of Anesthetists. (2005). *Submission from the New Zealand Society of Anesthetists, implementing nurse practitioner prescribing.* New Zealand Society of Anesthetists.

Nursing Council of New Zealand. (2005a). *Notice of scope of practice and related qualifications prescribed by the Nursing Council of New Zealand.*

Nursing Council of New Zealand. (2005b). *Designated prescriber: Nurse practitioners regulations 2005.*

World Health Organization. (2005a). *Case study: New Zealand.* Geneva, Switzerland: Author.

World Health Organization. (2005b). *New Zealand nutrition overview.* Geneva, Switzerland: Author.

World Health Organization. (2005c). *New Zealand national health plan and priorities.* Geneva, Switzerland: Author.

26 Advanced-Practice Nursing in Ireland

KATHLEEN MacLELLAN

INTRODUCTION

Ireland operates a public health care system funded through general taxation and governed by the Health Act (Government of Ireland, 2004). Irish citizens are generally entitled to public inpatient and outpatient services. However, some may have to pay partial charges. Approximately one third of the population is entitled to a medical card, which allows free health care at all points of access, and a further segment is eligible for a doctor visit card for general practice services (Organisation for Economic Co-operation and Development, 2008). Ireland also has a growing private health care market, and over half the population has private health insurance.

The government, the Minister for Health and Children, and the Department of Health and Children are at the head of health service provision in Ireland. The Department's primary role is to support the Minister in formulating and evaluating policies for the health services. The Department also has a role in the strategic planning of health services, and has introduced a modern health service reform program to meet the changing health care needs of Irish society. Delivery of the public health and personal social services in Ireland is the responsibility of the Health Service Executive (HSE). The HSE was established by the Health Act (Government of Ireland, 2004), and came into being in January 2005. In essence, the Department of Health and Children are responsible for policy direction for health, and the HSE is responsible for policy implementation through health service delivery.

Ireland's population of 4.4 million continues to grow, with increases of over 11% since 2003. There have been unexpected significant population increases at both ends of the lifespan. Such demographics present challenges to the delivery of appropriate health services. For example, an older population means an increasing incidence of chronic illnesses, such as diabetes, heart failure, and kidney disease. Changes in health technology and clinical practice will continue to drive health service delivery.

Ireland is currently facing a prolonged period of economic challenge, with rising unemployment levels in tandem with a global recession. Such socioeconomic issues will challenge both funding and provision of a quality health service.

NURSING IN IRELAND

Ireland has more than 80,000 registered nurses (RNs) and midwives, of whom an estimated 44,000 currently work in the health care system. This makes nurses the largest group of health service professionals in Ireland. Nursing has seen unprecedented education and clinical practice developments. Specifically, new initiatives, such as developing the clinical career pathway, expanding scope of practice, nurse-led services, and medication prescribing to retain clinical nursing and midwifery expertise at the interface with patients or clients have been introduced. These developments have been supported and driven by a number of government reports (such as the Report of the Commission on Nursing in Ireland [Government of Ireland, 1998]), the setting up of the National Council for the Professional Development of Nursing and Midwifery (NCNM) in 1999, modern legislation to permit nurse prescribing of medication and ionizing radiation, and education developments. Since 2002, preregistration nursing education is a 4-year honors-degree program. Five programs lead to registration with the Irish Nursing Board: Children's and General Nursing, General Nursing, Intellectual Disability Nursing, Midwifery, and Psychiatric Nursing. This education is augmented by a significant growth in postregistration education at higher levels and postgraduate diploma, bachelor's, and master's degree levels. In 2006, there were 285 postregistration courses run by 14 higher education institutes in Ireland (Health Services Executive, 2008). In providing for more highly qualified nurses, the status of the profession as a whole is elevated.

Ireland has built nursing research capacity through the implementation of a *Research Strategy for Nursing and Midwifery in Ireland*, published in 2003 (Department of Health and Children, 2003). The strategic approach has been to identify research fellowships for nurses, expand expertise in research at the service level, and increase the number of PhD programs available.

The European Union Directive 2005/36/EC was transposed into Irish law in 2008, and repeals previous directives. It has implications for recognition of the qualifications of nurses who were educated and trained in other member states who wish to travel and work as RNs in Ireland. It will take time to assess the impact of this directive in relation to assessing and providing reciprocity of qualifications of nurses at the registration level, and those wishing to practice at specialist and advanced-practice levels.

NURSE PRESCRIBING OF MEDICATIONS AND IONIZING RADIATION

In March 2006, the Minister for Health and Children introduced primary legislation to allow medication prescriptive authority for nurses. This followed 7 years' collaborative working between NCNM and the Irish Nursing Board, An Bord Altranais (An Bord Altranais & National Council for the Professional Development of Nursing and Midwifery, 2005, 2008). This collaboration tested an education program and appropriate governance processes, making several recommendations that have resulted in the implementation of nurse medication prescribing. To date, almost 250 nurses and midwives are undergoing or have completed the 6-month education program, with broad representation from 61 different clinical areas, and there are 58 registered nurse practitioners.

The swift advancement of the implementation of prescriptive authority and, indeed, expanded medication management practice in Ireland is a significant accomplishment when realizing the resources and planning required, and when making comparisons with other countries' experiences. It is anticipated that across the health care service, patients and service users will also be the beneficiaries of this expansion of practice. Benefits (as reported internationally) such as convenience and increased accessibility for patients, greater emphasis on non-pharmacological interventions, improved medication compliance, and patient self-management may be realized with commencement of this initiative (An Bord Altranais & National Council for the Professional Development of Nursing and Midwifery, 2008).

The Statutory Instrument (SI) No. 303 of 2007 incorporated an amendment to the previous definition of prescriber of ionizing radiation to include nurses as prescribers. Requirements and standards for nurse education programs giving nurses authority to prescribe ionizing radiation were developed in 2008, and the education program is under development. The introduction of this initiative will support the streamlining of patient journeys, prevent duplication of resources, and maximize the capacity of nursing skills.

CLINICAL CAREER PATHWAY

Expanded, enhanced, and advanced-practice nursing roles are part of the strategic development of the overall Irish health service. There are more than 120 advanced nurse practitioner (ANP) and 2,050 clinical nurse specialist (CNS) posts. Exhibits 26.1 and 26.2 provide examples of the titles/areas of practice of these posts.

Ireland adopted a strategic approach to clinical career pathway development closely aligned with health service requirements, in order to avoid issues that caused considerable confusion, and even international resistance, among the nursing profession, the multidisciplinary team, and the general public. Such issues regarding new nursing roles relate to lack of role definition, lack of clarity of nomenclature, integration, disparate scope of practice, and inconsistent educational preparation. Figure 26.1 outlines the levels of nursing practice and corresponding educational preparation in Ireland.

NCNM sets the criteria for CNS and ANP posts and personnel, and monitors the clinical career pathway for nurses (National Council for the Professional Development of Nursing and Midwifery, 2008a, 2008b, 2008c). Irish nurses continue to be regulated through the Nurses Act

Exhibit 26.1

EXAMPLES: TITLES/AREAS OF PRACTICE, CNS POSTS IN IRELAND

CNS (Behavior Therapy)

CNS (Breast Care)

CNS (Cardiology)

CNS (Child & Adolescent Mental Health)

CNS (Community Mental Health)

CNS (Dementia)

CNS (Diabetes)

CNS (Dyspnoea)

CNS (Epilepsy)

CNS (Gastroenterology)

CNS (Haematology)

CNS (Heart Failure)

CNS (Infection Control)

CNS (Liver Liaison)

CNS (Liaison Psychiatry)

CNS (Multiple Sclerosis)

CNS (Neurology)

CNS (Occupational Health)

CNS (Older Person)

CNS (Oncology)

CNS (Osteoporosis)

CNS (Pain Management)

CNS (Palliative Care)

CNS (Primary Care)

CNS (Respiratory)

CNS (Rheumatology)

CNS (Stroke Care)

CNS (Tissue Viability)

CNS (Urology)

Exhibit 26.2

TITLES/AREAS OF PRACTICE, ANP POSTS IN IRELAND

ANP (Addiction & Mental Health)
ANP (Breast Care)
ANP (Cardiology)
ANP (Cardiothoracic)
ANP (Care of the Older Person)
ANP (Child & Adolescent Mental Health & Psychotherapy)
ANP (Child Health & Parenting)
ANP (Children's Emergency)
ANP (Children's Renal)
ANP (Cognitive Behavior Therapy)
ANP (Cognitive Behavioral Psychotherapy)
ANP (Colorectal)
ANP (Community Older Adults)
ANP (Diabetes)
ANP (Eating Disorders)
ANP (Emergency)
ANP (Emergency Cardiology)
ANP (Epilepsy)
ANP (Gastroenterology)
ANP (Haematology)
ANP (Haematology Oncology)
ANP (Heart Failure)
ANP (Liaison Psychiatry)
ANP (Neonatology)
ANP (Occupational Health)
ANP (Older Person with Dementia)
ANP (Oncology)
ANP (Pain Management)
ANP (Palliative Care)
ANP (Positive Behavior Support)
ANP (Primary Care)
ANP (Rheumatology)
ANP (Sexual Health)
ANP (Specialist Palliative Care)
ANP (Stroke Care)
ANP (Tissue Viability)
ANP (Urology)
ANP (Women's Health)

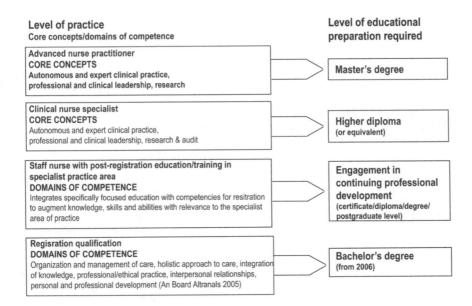

Figure 26.1 Clinical career pathway: Levels of practice and corresponding educational preparation.
Reprinted from National Council for the Professional Development of Nursing and Midwifery. (2006). *Position Paper 2: Clinical Nurse Specialist and Advanced Nurse Practitioner Roles in Intellectual Disability Nursing* by permission of the National Council for the Professional Development of Nursing and Midwifery, Ireland.

of 1985, and the Irish nursing board ensures that nurses are registered, fit to practice, and sets education program standards. Employment as a CNS or ANP is contingent on the nurse and the post meeting NCNM criteria. The Statutory Instrument (SI) No. 3 of 2010 provides for accreditation of ANP posts and registration of ANPs by the Irish nursing board in accordance with NCNM criteria.

NCNM maintains a national database of CNSs and ANPs. Figures 26.2 and 26.3 outline growth in CNS and ANP posts over the past number of years.

SCOPE OF PRACTICE:
AN EMERGENCY DEPARTMENT EXEMPLAR

To ensure safe and effective care, nurses require development and maintenance of specific competencies. These competencies should be

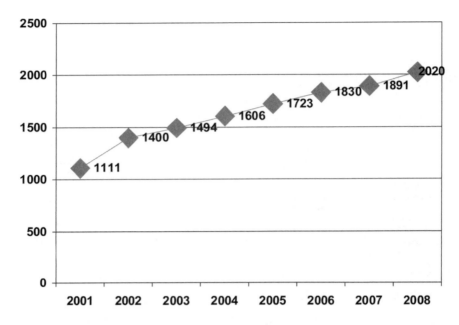

Figure 26.2 Growth of clinical nurse/midwife specialist posts, 2001–2008.

required by the health service, in line with service needs analysis and evidence-based practice. Competencies are developed in a number of ways, such as formal education programs, continuing professional development, clinical exposure, clinical supervision, and experience.

To ensure a coherent and meaningful clinical career pathway, the level of clinical decision making and scope of practice expected of nurses working at different levels within the Irish system should be explicit. A recent Irish paper outlining current and future enhanced clinical nursing roles in an emergency department (ED) describes the levels of care provided by nurses in the ED (National Council for the Professional Development of Nursing and Midwifery, 2008d). Generally, the clinical lead in the ED will be an emergency physician/consultant or an ANP, depending on the specific caseload. On-going clinical support, clinical supervision, and peer review is provided for all nurses based on their level of experience, education, and competency development.

The ED staff nurse is assigned to a designated patient group or area within the unit. The nurse will engage in nursing assessment and carry

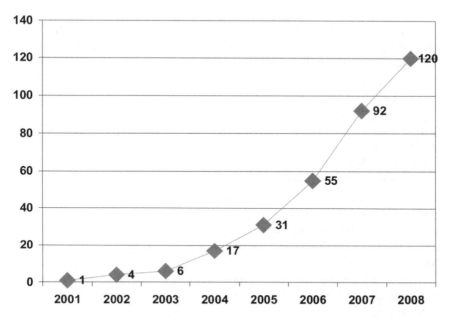

Figure 26.3 Growth of advanced nurse/midwife practitioner posts, 2001–2008.

out interventions using enhanced clinical skills, as per the level of competence along agreed guidelines. Examples of enhanced skills used by the staff nurse range from venepuncture, cannulation, male catheterization, application of plaster of Paris, management of patient medication through medication management protocols, and prescribing. The staff nurse is engaged in monitoring and evaluating the patient's response to intervention and treatment, and reports to the clinical lead at appropriate stages throughout the patient journey. The decision regarding interventions and to conclude an episode of care rests solely with the clinical lead. The clinical lead will either be the ANP or the Emergency Consultant.

Following formal triage, the CNS may select a patient from an agreed caseload. The caseload may include patients with uncomplicated minor injury, surgical, respiratory, cardiac, mental health conditions, or other. The CNS performs a focused assessment relevant to the clinical condition. The CNS will initiate investigations and holistic care based on his/her findings, and initiate continuous monitoring of the patient's response to interventions, while liaising with the staff nurse assigned to the patient care area and an identified clinical lead. Decision making regarding the definitive management and further care of the patient is shared by the CNS and clinical lead. The ultimate decision to conclude an episode of care will rest with the clinical lead. The clinical lead will either be the ANP or the Emergency Consultant.

The ANP also selects a patient from an agreed caseload following formal triage. In this instance, the caseload includes more complex conditions, illnesses, and injuries than those managed by the CNS. The ANP will accept referred patients who fall within the agreed scope of ANP practice from CNS, medical staff, and professions allied to medicine, or patients who self-refer. The ANP will elicit a full history and carry out a comprehensive physical examination. The ANP will formulate a working diagnosis, initiate investigations, and carry out specific interventions/treatments based on patient history and physical assessment. The ANP will initiate continuous monitoring of patient response to interventions and treatment. Staff nurses assigned to the patient care area or the CNS may provide support in the continuous monitoring of the patient, and report to the ANP on the patient response to interventions.

Interpretation of investigation results will assist the ANP to formulate a definitive diagnosis and plan of management for each patient episode. The decision to refer the patient for further immediate specialist care (for advice or admission), to outpatient clinics, or discharge home, thus concluding a complete episode of care, rests with the ANP. Clinical judgment and decision making carried out by the ANP are based on expert knowledge, specific education, and vast clinical experience grounded in the art and science of nursing.

The ANP provides a comprehensive holistic service to the ED attendee. For example, an older woman who attends the ED for management of an ankle injury following a fall will have the following assessment and care provided: The ankle injury will be assessed, and appropriate diagnostics ordered as the history and physical examination dictate. Interventions following radiological investigation may require application of a lower limb cast if the investigation reveals a fracture. In the course of the history taking, the psychosocial history and activities of daily living are also assessed, and this allows discharge planning to commence, usually in conjunction with family or a specific carer at a very early stage. The ANP will liaise with allied professionals in the hospital, such as the falls clinic, occupational therapists, and physiotherapists to arrange for acute assessment of the older woman from a safety and mobility point of view. At the same time, arrangements are put in place with community agencies, such as a community intervention team, to plan for an ongoing safe and seamless transition for the patient from the ED back to the community. As a result of the ANP coordinating the activities of multiple professionals and agencies, she/he provides a "one-stop shop" approach to managing the patient who attends the ED with an injury, particularly those patients who have additional needs that are related to age, social circumstances, mobility, and safety.

CONCLUSIONS

This chapter provides an update on developments in Irish nursing. An evidence-based strategic approach has been taken to develop nursing to its current level. This has ensured a transparent, high-quality process that has produced significant deliverables that have an impact on patient outcomes. Ireland needs to consolidate and expand the current initiatives, maintaining best-practice standards going into the future. The goal has been to improve the patient journey in a safe, accountable, and effective manner through the provision of quality evidence-based nursing.

A focused evaluation of the clinical services provided by CNSs and ANPs in Ireland is underway through research with teams from Trinity College, Dublin, and University College, Galway. This research will involve undertaking original data collection to evaluate the clinical outcomes, service delivery, and economic implications. Evaluation of the introduction of nurse medication prescribing is underway. These independent evaluations will further contribute to refining and developing the strategic direction of nursing in Ireland.

REFERENCES

An Bord Altranais and the National Council for the Professional Development of Nursing and Midwifery. (2005). *The review of nurses and midwives in the prescribing and administration of medicinal products.* Dublin, Ireland: Authors.

An Bord Altranais and the National Council for the Professional Development of Nursing and Midwifery. (2008). *Final Report: The implementation of the review of nurses and midwives in the prescribing and administration of medicinal products.* Dublin, Ireland: Authors.

Department of Health and Children. (2003). *Research strategy for nursing and midwifery in Ireland.* Dublin, Ireland: Stationery Office.

Government of Ireland. (1998). *Report of the Commission on Nursing: A blueprint for the future.* Dublin, Ireland: Stationery Office.

Government of Ireland. (2004). *Health act.* Dublin, Ireland: Stationery Office.

Health Services Executive. (2008). *Report of the post-registration nursing and midwifery education review group.* Dublin, Ireland: Author.

National Council for the Professional Development of Nursing and Midwifery. (2008a). *Framework for the establishment of clinical nurse/midwife specialist posts intermediate pathway* (4th ed.). Dublin, Ireland: Author.

National Council for the Professional Development of Nursing and Midwifery. (2008b). *Framework for establishment of advanced nurse practitioner and advanced midwife practitioner posts* (4th ed.). Dublin, Ireland: Author.

National Council for the Professional Development of Nursing and Midwifery. (2008c). *Accreditation of advanced nurse practitioner and advanced midwife practitioner posts* (2nd ed.). Dublin, Ireland: Author.

National Council for the Professional Development of Nursing and Midwifery. (2008d). *Position paper 4: Enhanced nursing practice in emergency practice.* Dublin, Ireland: Author.

Organisation for Economic Co-operation and Development. (2008). *Ireland toward an integrated public service.* Paris: Author.

27 One Look at the Future

DIANE O. McGIVERN, EILEEN M. SULLIVAN-MARX, AND
JULIE A. FAIRMAN

Commenting on the dynamics of power and change, Frederick Douglass said that, "Every day our numbers grow, and they will speak for us." As numbers of nurse practitioners (NPs) grow in the United States and take hold around the world, their presence is influencing health outcomes and providing greater access to services. Because the number of NPs is greatest and their history the longest in the United States, their footholds in health care have become standard in many areas of practice, such as in nurse-managed centers and gerontological care. To speculate on the future of NPs, we can see further growth, particularly with respect to improving access to care and achieving quality and offering a cost-effective approach.

As this book is published in 2010, we must recognize that the United States is again grappling with health care reform. Whether it is achieved through legislation or, if legislation fails, is driven by the momentum unleashed by the years of debate, NPs are well positioned to capitalize on the moment. Capitalizing on the moment means gaining recognition of and payment for services, legislative and regulatory support for more autonomous practice, and providing a broader array of service choices that will allow patients to tailor care to their requirements.

375

Nurses highly invested in the profession may be suspect, particularly if their view of the future of advanced-practice nursing is too optimistic, too rosy. So predictions are subject to skepticism and, we hope, reader comment. But here is the important question that arises from the narratives found in all of our chapters: What is positive about this moment in the 45-year history of practice? Several historic factors are operating. The demand for NPs services is as related to demographics as to other drivers, including insurance regulations and practices. So, too, should the sheer weight of numbers of elderly, chronically ill, and worried well move NP services to the front and center of the system.

Organized nursing's political profile has never been higher, and to the extent that the profession's organizational support of politicians and social movements is mutually beneficial, the dividends to nursing may accrue over the next decade. Articulate voices for nursing and advanced practice emanating from the Center to Champion Nursing, the Raise the Voice Campaign, and the Robert Wood Johnson Commission on the Future of Nursing at the Institute of Medicine are positive and effective, reaching out to consumers and patients, media, and nurses practicing across the spectrum. The incrementally positive changes in reimbursement and practitioners' understanding of payment structures and requirements are also a positive force at this juncture. Informed providers more conversant with the current system, and future possibilities bode well for more autonomous practice and patient access.

The current promise of federal funding for education aid and institutional support could, if realized, support a major boost in enrollments, graduations, and practice placements that will be most meaningful in meeting social and health care needs. However, the opportunities are balanced by several significant challenges, namely, incentives to continue prelicensure education programs producing a skewed and underskilled workforce, and the highly segmented and uncertain consumer population unsure about the intended and unintended consequences of proposed reform. The economic stimulus package, which supports community colleges and their vocational and technical programs as a way to stimulate the economy and job preparation, may also expand the associate-degree registered nurse population. More associate-degree nurses may further constrict the pipeline to graduate degree programs preparatory to advanced practice and functional roles, including teaching, administration, and informatics. Although we recognize the importance of associate-degree programs as a viable entry point for many with limited access to higher education, support should be targeted to helping these groups enter baccalaureate programs.

The current environment is highly politicized, creating a more polarized dialogue about everything from health care to education reform, to professional collaboration. Nursing throughout the globe, but particularly in the United States, is also becoming more fragmented, with new levels of preparation, degrees, specialties, and titles. Yet, at the same time, NPs achieved historically significant progress through the development of the consensus on models of advanced practice. Europe and Taiwan have agreed on standards of preparation for advanced practice, and the United States has promulgated revised recommendations for standardizing NP regulation throughout the country.

What factors will create the tipping point, the events that will promote and accelerate NPs' control of their role and destiny in health care delivery? Three efforts will move the agenda forward: creative collaborative efforts to attract, educate, and graduate baccalaureate and higher degree nurses; strong united voices in the policy arena; and support for funding and developing clear messages to consumers and payers about the desirability, cost effectiveness, and efficaciousness of NP services. As the editors and authors of the chapters in this book have shown, these efforts are not impossible, nor simply applied. NPs' success in moving these efforts forward will rest on relationships with patients and the historical notions of context and contingency. History tells us that the place and time of political opportunities, as well as the politics and power of consensus, economics, race, class, and gender will shape the future of NPs. Understanding the complexities that confront us today, gaining and nurturing the tools of flexibility and strategic thinking, and being prepared to expect and embrace those that we will encounter in the future will be the key to maintaining NPs' position as central and normative providers in the health care system.

28 Online Resources

SHERRY A. GREENBERG

WEB SITES

Many of the chapters in this book include online resources as they pertain to the specific topic. This is a compilation of national and international nurse practitioner (NP) organizations, with a brief description of each and their Web sites. Included are those NP organizations focused on education, clinical practice, credentialing, and policy.

Nurse Practitioner Organizations

American Academy of Nurse Practitioners (AANP): http:// www.aanp.org/

AANP, established in 1985, was the first national organization created for NPs of all specialties. AANP provides networking opportunities and represents the interests of NPs currently practicing in the United States. AANP advocates at local, state, and federal levels for the recognition of NPs as providers of high-quality, cost-effective health care. There are currently over 26,000 individual members, and 139 NP group members. AANP offers a national certification examination for adult, family, and gerontological NPs.

American College of Nurse Practitioners (ACNP): http://www.acnp
web.org/

ACNP, established in 1993, is a national, nonprofit membership organization that ensures a strong policy and regulatory foundation that enables NPs to continue to provide accessible, high-quality health care to those residing in the United States. Membership includes both individual NPs as well as national and state NP organizations.

Gerontological Advanced Practice Nurses Association (GAPNA):
https://www.gapna.org/

GAPNA, formerly NCGNP and founded in 1981, represents nearly 10,000 certified advanced-practice nurses (APNs) who work with older adults in a various clinical practice settings. GAPNA provides continuing education in gerontological nursing care and provides peer support from experienced clinicians.

National Association of Nurse Practitioners in Women's Health
(NPWH): http://www.npwh.org/

NPWH, founded in 1980, assures the provision of quality health care by NPs to women of all ages, in terms of their physical, emotional, spiritual, and cultural needs. Continuing education is available.

National Association of Pediatric Nurse Practitioners (NAPNAP):
http://www.napnap.org/

NAPNAP, established in 1973, aims to improve child health for infants, children, and adolescents through leadership, clinical practice, advocacy, education, and research. There are currently over 7,000 members, as well as 48 chapters, nationally.

Nurse Practitioner Credentialing Organizations

American Academy of Nurse Practitioners: http://www.aanp.org/

See Nurse Practitioner Organizations section in the preceding text.

American Nurses Credentialing Center (ANCC): http://www.nurse
credentialing.org/

ANCC, a subsidiary of the American Nurses Association and established in 1990, is the largest credentialing organization in the United States.

There are currently over 75,000 APNs certified. These include NPs and clinical nurse specialists in all specialty arenas, as well as other advanced-practice specialists with expertise in nursing areas such as diabetes management and public health nursing. ANCC also provides certifications to those registered nurses who have demonstrated expertise in a nursing specialty area, such as in cardiac rehabilitation, college health, informatics, or pain management, to name just a few. Aside from individual certification, those health care organizations that demonstrate excellence in nursing care may seek Magnet recognition through ANCC's Magnet Recognition Program. Additionally, ANCC provides accreditation for continuing nursing education programs throughout the country.

National Council of State Boards of Nursing (NCSBN): https://www.ncsbn.org/

NCSBN, founded in 1978, is a not-for-profit organization comprised of Member Boards. NCSBN develops licensing examinations in nursing, monitors trends in public policy, clinical practice, and education, conducts research on nursing practice issues, and provides a forum for collaboration amongst members and other health care organizations.

National Council of State Boards of Nursing: Advanced-Practice Registered Nurses (APRN): https://www.ncsbn.org/170.htm/

This is a nursing initiative of NCSBN. The APRN committee worked with the APRN Consensus Work Group to develop the *Consensus Model for APRN Regulation: Licensure, Accreditation, Certification, & Education.* For more information, refer to chapter 9.

Nurse Practitioner Data Bank (NPDB): Healthcare Integrity and Protection Data Bank (HIPDB): http://npdb-hipdb.hrsa.gov/

Managed by the U.S. Department of Health and Human Services (HHS), Health Resources and Services Administration (HRSA), Bureau of Health Professions (BHPr), Division of Practitioner Data Banks (DPDB). The NPDB is primarily an alert system intended to provide supplemental information to facilitate a comprehensive review of health care practitioners' professional credentials. The HIPDB was developed to combat fraud and abuse in health insurance and health care delivery. It alerts users when a comprehensive review of a practitioner's, provider's, or supplier's past actions may be needed.

U.S. Department of Health and Human Services: Health Resources and Services Administration (HRSA): Nursing Workforce Reports & Data: http://bhpr.hrsa.gov/healthworkforce/nursing.htm/

Under the Bureau of Health Professions, this Web site provides nursing workforce reports and data, including NP data.

Educational/Practice Organizations

American Association of Colleges of Nursing (AACN): http://www.aacn.nche.edu/

AACN establishes quality standards for bachelor's and graduate degree nursing education, assists deans and directors to implement those standards, influences nursing to improve health care, and promotes public support for the education, research, and practice of nursing. Faculty development and resources for nurse educators are available, including the *Essentials* series, competency guidelines in various specialty areas, and guidelines for designing curricula. Student scholarship programs are available, as well.

American Nurses Association (ANA): http://www.nursingworld.org/

ANA promotes excellence in nursing care, promotes rights for nurses in the work environment, and lobbies on health care issues affecting nurses and the public. Continuing education modules are available for members. ANA has 51 constituent member nursing associations and 24 specialty nursing and workforce advocacy affiliate nursing organizations.

ANA Constituent Member Associations: http://www.nursingworld.org/FunctionalMenuCategories/AboutANA/WhoWeAre/CMA.aspx/

This Web site provides links to ANA's constituent member nursing associations.

ANA Specialty Nursing Practice: http://www.nursingworld.org/EspeciallyForYou/Links/SpecialtyNursi ng.aspx/

This Web site provides links to ANA's specialty nursing organizations.

American Organization of Nurse Executives (AONE): http:// www.aone.org/

AONE, a subsidiary of the American Hospital Association and founded in 1967, is comprised of over 6,400 nurse leaders. AONE provides professional development, advocacy, and research in order to advance nursing practice, improve patient care, promote nursing leadership excellence, and shape health care public policy.

National Organization of Nurse Practitioner Faculties (NONPF): http://www.nonpf.com/

NONPF, which began in 1974 as a group of educators developing the first set of NP curriculum guidelines, has become a much larger organization, representing over 1,200 educators. NONPF provides resources and enhances the promotion and tenure of NP faculty.

National League for Nursing (NLN): http://www.nln.org/

NLN, founded in 1893 as the American Society of Superintendents of Training Schools for Nurses, was the first nursing organization in the United States. Its members include nurse educators, educational institutions, and health care agencies. NLN provides a Certified Nurse Educator (CNE) examination accredited by the National Commission for Certifying Agencies (NCCA). The Web site provides links to *Excellence Initiatives* in nursing education. Various nursing education research grants are available.

Policy Organizations

American Academy of Nursing (AAN): http://www.aannet.org/

AAN, established in 1973, advances health policy and practice through the generation, synthesis, and dissemination of nursing knowledge. The current 1,500 Fellows of the AAN are nursing leaders in education, practice, management, and research. Current initiatives include the Building Academic Geriatric Nursing Capacity Program (BAGNC), Disparities in Health Care Initiative, Geropsychiatric Nursing Collaborative (GPNC), and the Quality of Care Initiative.

American Association of Retired Persons (AARP): http://www.aarp.org/

AARP, founded in 1958, is a nonprofit, nonpartisan membership organization for adults over 50. With over 40 million members, AARP advocates for social change on important issues such as health care, social security, and community issues. Products and publications are available.

Center to Champion Nursing in America: http://championnursing.org/

The Center to Champion Nursing in America, a joint initiative between AARP, the AARP Foundation, and the Robert Wood Johnson Foundation, is developing initiatives to increase and retain skilled nurses, and seek funding sources to expand nursing education programs in a national effort to address the nursing shortage. For more information, refer to chapter 4.

The Commonwealth Fund: http://www.commonwealthfund.org/

The Commonwealth Fund, a private foundation, promotes a health care system that achieves better access, improved quality, and greater efficiency, particularly for those most vulnerable, including low-income people, the uninsured, minority Americans, young children, and older adults. The Fund supports independent research on health care issues, and provides grants to improve health care practice and policy. An international program in health policy is designed to stimulate innovative policies and practices in the United States and other industrialized countries.

All topics: http://www.commonwealthfund.org/Topics.aspx State health policy information: http://www.commonwealthfund.org/Topics/State-Health-Policy.aspx/

Updates on state health care improvements and reform initiatives are provided.

Institute of Medicine of the National Academies (IOM): http://www.iom.edu/

The IOM, established in 1970, provides evidence-based health care information and guidance to Congress and all policymakers, health care professionals, the private sector, and the public on health, biomedical science, and medical issues. The IOM publishes reports on U.S. health care issues, such as aging, mental health, minority health, nutrition, public health, and others, through their *National Academies Press* series.

Kaiser Permanente: http://www.kaiserpermanente.org/

Kaiser Permanente, opened to public enrollment as a health care organization in 1945, consists of the Kaiser Foundation Health Plan, Inc. and Hospitals and the Permanente Medical Groups. Kaiser Permanente is the largest not-for-profit health plan in the United States, with approximately 8.6 million members. Kaiser Permanente also provides community resources.

National Academy for State Health Policy: http://www.nashp.org/

The National Academy for State Health Policy conducts policy analysis, provides training and technical assistance to states, produces informational resources, and convenes state, regional, and national forums.

**National Nursing Centers Consortium (NNCC):
http://www.nncc.us/**

NNCC advocates for NPs as primary health care providers and represents nurse-managed health centers throughout the United States. For more information, refer to chapter 13.

Robert Wood Johnson Foundation: http://www.rwjf.org/

The Robert Wood Johnson Foundation provides private grant funding for current areas of focus such as childhood obesity, health coverage, public health, and vulnerable populations, as well as building human capital by encouraging health careers and training providers and leaders to conduct research.

**Robert Wood Johnson Foundation Initiative on the Future of
Nursing, at the Institute of Medicine:
http://www.iom.edu/CMS/28312/64233.aspx/**

The IOM committee is working to address the nursing and nursing faculty shortage, and ensure that nurses receive the skill competencies to provide safe, innovative, and quality health care in a variety of clinical settings. System changes and institutional policies will be implemented at national, state, and local levels.

**The U.S. Department of Health and Human Services Centers for
Medicare & Medicaid Services (CMS): http://www.cms.hhs.gov/**

CMS is the federal agency responsible for administering the Medicare, Medicaid, Children's Health Insurance Program (CHIP), Health Insurance Portability and Accountability Act (HIPPA), and Clinical Laboratory Improvement Amendments (CLIA). Contact information is available for questions and/or program issues.

The U.S. Department of Health and Human Services (HHS), Health Resources and Services Administration (HRSA): http://www.hrsa.gov/

HRSA, established in 1982, is the primary federal agency for improving access to culturally competent, quality health care services for those who are uninsured, underserved, or medically vulnerable. HRSA focuses on these populations in its goals and program activities. HRSA provides leadership and financial support to health care providers in every state and U.S. territory.

The White House, Washington, DC: http://www.whitehouse.gov/

This is the official Web site of the White House and U.S. government.

International Organizations

International Council of Nursing: http://www.icn.ch/

The ICN, founded in 1899, represents nurses in more than 128 countries. ICN position statements on topics such as nursing roles in health care services, the nursing profession, the socioeconomic welfare of nurses, health care systems, and social issues are available online at http://www.icn.ch/policy.htm. The ICN revised its *Code of Ethics for Nurses* in 2006. Fact sheets in the *"Nursing Matters"* series provide information and international perspectives on current global health and social issues.

International Council of Nursing: Nurse Practitioner Advanced Practice Network: http://www.icn-apnetwork.org/

This organization developed a definition and characteristics of an NP/APN. The definition and characteristics reflect ICN's official position and represent current and potential roles globally. Additionally, the *Scope of Practice, Standards, and Competencies of the Advanced Practice Nurse* document is available from this Web site.

Sigma Theta Tau International Honor Society of Nursing: http://www.nursingsociety.org/

Sigma Theta Tau supports the learning, knowledge, and professional development of nurses globally. Leadership programs are available through the International Leadership Institute. Research grants and continuing education are also available.

World Health Organization (WHO): http://www.who.int/en/

WHO provides leadership on global health issues, shapes the health research agenda, sets standards, and monitors and assesses global health trends. Countries from the United Nations may become members. Other countries may apply to join.

**World Health Organization Collaborating Centres:
http://www.who.int/collaboratingcentres/en/**

The WHO Collaborating Centres are institutions such as research institutes, parts of universities or academies, which are designated by the Director General to carry out activities in support of the Organization's programs. Currently, there are over 800 WHO Collaborating Centres in 90 Member States working with WHO on interdisciplinary areas such as nursing, occupational health, communicable diseases, nutrition, mental health, chronic diseases, and health technologies.

Index

A

ACNP. *See* American College of Nurse Practitioners

An Act Providing Access to Affordable, Quality, Accountable Health Care, 114–115

An Act to Promote Cost Containment, Transparency and Efficiency in the Delivery of Quality Health Care, 118

Adult Health Nurse Practitioner, 205

Advanced-practice registered nurses, 34, 125

African countries, health care in, 341

Agency for Healthcare Quality and Research, 330

AHNP. *See* Adult Health Nurse Practitioner

AIDS, 213–221

American Academy of HIV Medicine, 217

Association of Nurses in AIDS Care, 216
cancers, 213
cardiovascular disease, 220
comorbidities, 220
expectations of HIV specialist, 218–219
first special care unit for people with HIV, 214–215
future of HIV advanced practice, 220
hepatitis C, 220

highly active antiretroviral therapies, 215–216
infectious diseases, 214
liver disease, 220
Morrison, Cliff, 214–215
New York State Department of Health AIDS Institute, 215
opportunistic infections, 213
quality of NP care, 217–220
renal disease, 220
specialists, 214
substance use, 220

Alternative medicine, 227–228

AMA. *See* American Medical Association

American Academy of HIV Medicine, 217

American Academy of Nurse Practitioners, 128, 379–380

American Academy of Nurse Practitioners Certification Program, 130

American Academy of Nursing, 383

American Association of College of Nursing, 126–127, 130, 191, 382

American Association of Nurse Anesthetists, 130

American Association of Retired Persons, 383–384

American Board of Comprehensive Care, 135

American College of Nurse-Midwives, 130, 133
American College of Nurse Practitioners, 24, 380
   establishment of, 22
American Council of Graduate Medical Education, 171
American Diabetes Association, guidelines of, 201
American Medical Association, CPT coding system, 277
American Nurses Association, 130, 382
   Congress of Nursing Practice, 18–19
   Social Policy Statement, 22–23
American Nurses Credentialing Center, 128, 134, 380–381
American Organization of Nurse Executives, 130, 382–383
American Recovery and Reinvestment Act, 174
ANA. *See* American Nurses Association
ANA Constituent Member Associations, 382
ANA Specialty Nursing Practice, 382
ANAC. *See* Association of Nurses in AIDS Care
ANCC. *See* American Nurses Credentialing Center
ANMC. *See* Australian Nursing and Midwifery Council
AONE. *See* American Organization of Nurse Executives
Applicants to nursing schools, 37
APRN. *See* Advanced-Practice Registered Nurses
Asia, health care in, 340
Association of Academic Health Centers, 21
Association of Nurse Anesthetists, 133
Association of Nurses in AIDS Care, 216
Association of Physical Therapists, 177
Auckland University of Technology, 354
Audiences, reaching, 56–58

Facebook, 56
Gallup poll, 57
Internet as news source, 57
local news, 57
Twitter, 56
Australia, health care in, 340
Australian Nursing and Midwifery Council, 340
Autonomy to care for patients, 32

B
Balanced Budget Act, 257, 271
Bartol, Tom, 59
Bates, Barbara, 7
Becoming Influential, A Guide for Nurses, 59
Behavioral change, 50–51
Belgium, health care in, 341
Beneficence, 240–241, 244
Billing coding systems, 277–278
BON, Texas. *See* Texas Board of Nursing
Botswana, health care in, 339
Breckinridge, Mary, 5, 185
Brown Report, 4
Bureau of Health Professions, Division of Nursing, 185–187
Business, 257–269
Balanced Budget Act of 1997, 257
   business policy, 260–261
   Center for Nurse Entrepreneurship, 264–265
   Chiverton, Patricia, 264
   Collins, J., 257–268
      framework of, 258
   convenience care clinics, 265
   culture of discipline, 264–265
   discipline, culture of, 264–265
   economic drivers, 262
   electronic health record systems, 265–266
   factors moving practice toward greatness, 258–268
   Family Practice & Counseling Network, 259

Federally Qualified Health Center, 261
focus of practice, 262–264
Good to Great, 258, 262
greatness, factors moving practice toward, 258–268
Health Annex, 260–261
Health Resources and Services Administration, 260
hedgehog concept (simplification), 261–264
home monitoring devices, 265–266
interpersonal skills, 260
Living Independently For Elders Program, 263
McDonald, Cheryl, 266
Medicaid plans, 261
Minute Clinics, 265
momentum in organizations, 266–268
transformations in organizations, 266
online claims billing, 265–266
policy, 260–261
political contexts, 260–261
Program of All-Inclusive Care for Elders model of care, 263
recruitment, 259
reimbursement, 257
retail care clinics, 265
School of Nursing Penn Nursing Network, University of Pennsylvania, 260
simplification, 261–264
status quo, 260
technical skills, 260
technology accelerators, 265–266
telehealth communication, 265–266
Torrisi, Donna, 259
University of Pennsylvania School of Nursing, 262–263

C
CACC. *See* Council for Advancement of Comprehensive Care
Callahan, Jennifer, 117

Canadian Nurse Practitioner Initiative, 339
Capitation, 173
Catheter-related infections, 231
CCM. *See* Chronic Care Model
CCNE. *See* Commission on Collegiate Nursing Education
Center for Health Professions, 166–167, 177
Center for Nurse Entrepreneurship, 264–265
Center to Champion Nursing in America, 43–48, 384
Centers for Medicare and Medicaid Services, 168, 330–331
Certification, 133–136
    historic perspective, 133–135
Certified nurse anesthetists, 33–34
Certified nurse midwives, 33–34, 273
Chiverton, Patricia, 264
Cholesterol levels, 97
Chronic care management, payment, 290–291
Chronic Care Model, 327–328
Chronic disease management, 96–98
Chronically ill mental health, 234
Cleary, Brenda, 43–48
Clinical Nurse Leader, 174
Clinical Nurse Scholars, 7
Clinical nurse specialists, 33–34
CMHCs. *See* Community Migrant Health Centers
CNAP. *See* Coalition for Nurses in Advanced Practice; Texas Coalition for Nurses in Advanced Practice
CNL. *See* Clinical Nurse Leader
CNMs. *See* Certified nurse midwives
CNPI. *See* Canadian Nurse Practitioner Initiative
CNSs. *See* Clinical nurse specialists
Coalition for Nurses in Advanced Practice, 145

Cognitive neuroscience, 241
Collegiate Commission for Nursing
    Education, 128
Collins, J., 257–268
    framework of, 258
Commission on Collegiate Nursing
    Education, 136–137
Committee to Study Credentialing in
    Nursing, 126
Commonwealth Foundation, 7
Commonwealth Fund, 385
Commonwealth Fund Commission on
    High Performance Health
    System, 319–322
Commonwealth Fund report, 319–322
Communities, partnering with, 36
Community-based health centers,
    305–316
    alternative credentialing options, 308
    chronic disease management,
        prevention, 312
    cost-effectiveness, 312
    dialogue with insurer representatives,
        310–313
    Federally Qualified Health Center
        program, 314
    future developments, 313–314
    health care safety net, 305–306
    insurer policies, 306–310
    patient satisfaction, retention, 312
    quality of care, 312
    resources for negotiating with
        insurers, 312
    restrictive policies, 309
    specialty provider status, 308–309
    underserved, access for, 306–310
Community Migrant Health Centers,
    193
Comorbidities of diabetes, 201–202
Compact Administrators, 130
Competition, 68–70, 73–74
Conflicts of interest, 241, 245

Congress of Nursing Practice, American
    Nurses Association, 18–19
Consensus model, 125–142
    accreditation, 136–139
        historic perspective, 136–137
    certification, 133–136
        historic perspective, 133–135
    clinical career pathway, 127
    education programs, 139–140
    licensure, 138–139
    new regulatory model, 129–133
Consolidated Health Center Plan, 194
Consumer-driven health plans, 30
Consumer organizations, partnerships
    with, 43–48
Convenience care clinics, 265
Cooper, Richard, 31
Council for Advancement of
    Comprehensive Care, 135
CPT coding system. *See* Current
    procedural terminology coding
    system
Credentialing, 38–39
    Web sites, 380–382
Critical care, 32
Crossing the Quality Chasm, 10, 87
CSCN. *See* Committee to Study
    Credentialing in Nursing
Culture of discipline, 264–265
Current procedural terminology coding
    system, 75–76
Curtis, Val, 51

D
DCCT. *See* Diabetes Complications and
    Control Trial
Deep vein thrombosis, 94
Denmark, health care in, 341
Department of Health and Children,
    Ireland, 363–364
Department of Health and Human
    Services, 31, 186, 385–386

Centers for Medicare Medicaid Services, 385–386
Health Resources and Services Administration, 382, 386
Registered Nurse Sample Survey, 31
Developing countries, 32
Development model, 33–34, 38
DHBs. *See* District Health Boards
Diabetes
  adolescent, 202
  American Diabetes Association, guidelines of, 201
  comorbidities of diabetes, 201–202
  counseling, 200–203
  developmental issues, 201–202
  Diabetes Complications and Control Trial, 200–201
  financial costs, 202
  goal of diabetes management, 200
  mortality, 202
  multidisciplinary management, 202–203
  pediatric, 199–204
  prescribing medications, 200–203
  problem-solving skills, 200–203
  psychosocial issues, 201–202
  racial disparities, 202
  risk of death, 202
  screening for complications, 201–202
  self-management training, 200–203
  social costs, 202
Diabetes Complications and Control Trial, 200–201
Discipline, culture of, 264–265
Distributive justice issues, 244
District Health Boards, New Zealand, 346–347, 350–352
Division of Nursing, Bureau of Health Professions, 185–187
Doctorate degree in nursing practice, 37, 135, 174, 317
Douglass, Frederick, 375

Drug Enforcement Agency, 169
DVT. *See* Deep vein thrombosis

E
Eastern Colorado Health Care System Home-Based Primary Care Program, 229–230
Eastern Institute of Technology, 354
Educational organization Web sites, 382–383
Electronic health record systems, 105, 265–266, 323–324
End-of-life care, 241
Entrepreneurial nurses, 35–36
Equity within health care system, 240–241
Essentials for Doctoral Education for Advanced Practice Nurse Practitioners, 137
Essentials of Master's Education for Advanced Practice Nursing, 126–127
Ethical issues, 239–253
  acute care, 243–247
  beneficence, 240–241, 244
  boundary blurring, 246
  child/parent/practitioner relationship, 245
  chronic care, 243–247
  cognitive neuroscience, 241
  collaborative practice, 247–249
  conflicts of interest, 241, 245
  decision making, strategies to improve, 249–250
  distributive justice issues, 244
  end-of-life care, 241
  equity within health care system, 240–241
  ethics education, 249
  genetic markers, 241
  human subjects, recruitment, retention of, 241
  impaired physician, 245

informed consent, 244
integrity, 245
justice, 244
medication refilling, 245
misrepresentation, 245
models of ethical decision making,
    250–251
moral concerns, 244
moral dilemma, 241
moral distress, 242
moral uncertainty, 241
patient advocacy goals, 240–241
patient–provider relationships, 244
personal values, 245
physician collaboration, 245
pressure to prescribe, 245
primary care, 243
reimbursement in collaborative
    practice, 248
resource allocation, 241
respect for persons, 240–241, 244
supportive practice concerns, 244
Ethics education, 249
Ethnicity of NP workforce, 31–32
Europe
    health care in, 341
    regulatory policy, 39
Evolution of nurse practitioners
    practice, 31–32

F
Facebook, 56
Factors moving practice toward
    greatness, 258–268
Fairman, Julie A., 85–87
Family Practice & Counseling Network,
    259
Faso, Burkina, 51
Federal Employee Health Benefit Plan,
    284–285
Federal funding guidelines, 39
Federally Qualified Health Centers, 188,
    193–195, 261, 283–384

Fee schedule, Medicare, 276–277
Feedback loops, 325
FEHBP. See Federal Employee Health
    Benefit Plan
Finance. See Business
Finland, health care in, 341
First special care unit for people with
    HIV, 214–215
Flexner Report, 1
Food and Drug Administration, 169
Ford, Loretta, 7, 17, 162, 186
FPCN. See Family Practice &
    Counseling Network
FQHCs. See Federally qualified health
    centers
France, health care in, 341
Frontier Nursing, midwifery service,
    school, 5
Funding for scholarships, 173
Future developments, 375–377

G
Gallup poll, 57
GAPNA. See Gerontological Advanced
    Practice Nurses Association
Genetic markers, 241
Germany, health care in, 341
Gerontological Advanced Practice
    Nurses Association, 380
Gerontology, 205–211
    Adult Health Nurse Practitioner, 205
    eating, 209
    extended care centers, 228–229
Gerontology Nurse Practitioner, 205
    hip fracture, 208
    home physical therapy, 209
    National Council of State Boards of
        Nursing, 205–206
    participating in therapies, 209
    serotonin reuptake inhibitors, 209
    zoster lesions, 208
Gerontology Nurse Practitioner, 205
Global health, 33–35, 337–343

Africa, sub-Saharan, 341
African countries, 341
Asia, 340
Australia, 340
Australian Nursing and Midwifery
    Council, 340
Belgium, 341
Botswana, 339
Canadian Nurse Practitioner Initiative,
    339
Denmark, 341
Europe, 341
Finland, 341
France, 341
Germany, 341
Hong Kong, 340
International Council of Nurses, 338
International Nurse Practitioner/
    Advanced-Practice Network, 338
New South Wales, 340
New Zealand, 340
Norway, 341
nurse practitioner global role,
    338–342
Nursing Council of New Zealand, 340
Royal College of Nursing, 339
Singapore Ministry of Health, 340
sub-Saharan Africa, 341
Switzerland, 341
Taiwan, 340
United Kingdom, 339
usage of terms, 337
Global Public-Private Partnership for
    Handwashing with Soap, Ghana,
    51
GMENAC. *See* Graduate Medical
    Education, Nursing, and Allied
    Professions Commission
GNP. *See* Gerontology Nurse
    Practitioner
Goal of diabetes management, 200
Goal of standardization, 23–36

Goffman, Erving, 53
Goldmark Report, 4
Good to Great, 258, 262
Gordon, Suzanne, 53
Graduate level, 37
Graduate Medical Education, Nursing,
    and Allied Professions
    Commission, 72
Great Society initiatives, 149–150
Greatness, factors moving practice
    toward, 258–268
Growth in NP workforce, 31

H
HAART. *See* Highly active antiretroviral
    therapies
Hastings, Marguerite, 151–152
HDHP. *See* High deductible health plans
Health Act, Ireland, 363–364
Health Annex, 260–261
Health care finance, 257–269
    Balanced Budget Act of 1997, 257
    business policy, 260–261
    Center for Nurse Entrepreneurship,
        264–265
    Chiverton, Patricia, 264
    Collins, J., 257–268
        framework of, 258
    convenience care clinics, 265
    culture of discipline, 264–265
    discipline, culture of, 264–265
    economic drivers, 262
    electronic health record systems,
        265–266
    factors moving practice toward
        greatness, 258–268
    Family Practice & Counseling
        Network, 259
    Federally Qualified Health Center,
        261
    focus of practice, 262–264
    Good to Great, 258, 262

greatness, factors moving practice toward, 258–268
Health Annex, 260–261
Health Resources and Services Administration, 260
hedgehog concept (simplification), 261–264
home monitoring devices, 265–266
interpersonal skills, 260
Living Independently For Elders Program, 263
McDonald, Cheryl, 266
Medicaid plans, 261
Minute Clinics, 265
momentum in organizations, 266–268
transformations in organizations, 266
online claims billing, 265–266
political contexts, 260–261
Program of All-Inclusive Care for Elders model of care, 263
recruitment, 259
reimbursement, 257
retail care clinics, 265
School of Nursing Penn Nursing Network, University of Pennsylvania, 260
simplification, 261–264
status quo, 260
technical skills, 260
technology accelerators, 265–266
telehealth communication, 265–266
Torrisi, Donna, 259
University of Pennsylvania, School of Nursing Penn Nursing Network, 260
University of Pennsylvania School of Nursing, 262–263
Health Care for Homeless Programs, 193
Health care reform, 3–13, 113–123, 162–165
An Act Providing Access to Affordable, Quality, Accountable Health Care, 114–115
An Act to Promote Cost Containment, Transparency and Efficiency in the Delivery of Quality Health Care, 118
Callahan, Jennifer, 117
grassroots efforts, 121–123
legal consultants, 121–123
legislative efforts, 117–119
lobbying efforts, 121–123
Massachusetts Coalition of Nurse Practitioners, 115–116
Minute Clinics, 117
Murray, Therese, 118
political action committee efforts, 121–123
Rourke, Nancy, 116
transformative effect on health care, 115–117
Health Plan Employer Data and Information Set, 188–189
Health Resources and Services Administration, 260
U.S. Department of Health and Human Services, 186
Health savings accounts, 301–302
Health Service Executive, 364
Health services needs, 35
access, 35
developing countries, 35
nutrition, 35
World Health Organization, 35
Hedgehog concept (simplification), 261–264
HEDIS. See Health Plan Employer Data and Information Set
Henry Street Settlement, 185
Hepatitis C, 220
HHS. See U.S. Department of Health and Human Services
High deductible health plans, 301–302
Highly active antiretroviral therapies, 215–216
Hip fracture, 208

HIV. *See* Human immunodeficiency
   virus
Home monitoring devices, 265–266
Home physical therapy, 209
Hong Kong, health care in, 340
Hospital services, payment, 280–281
HRSA. *See* Health Resources and
   Services Administration
HSAs. *See* Health savings accounts
HSE. *See* Health Service Executive
Human immunodeficiency virus,
   213–221
   American Academy of HIV Medicine,
      217
   Association of Nurses in AIDS Care,
      216
   cancers, 213
   cardiovascular disease, 220
   comorbidities, 220
   expectations of HIV specialist,
      218–219
   first special care unit for people with
      HIV, 214–215
   future of HIV advanced practice, 220
   hepatitis C, 220
   highly active antiretroviral therapies,
      215–216
   infectious diseases, 214
   liver disease, 220
   Morrison, Cliff, 214–215
   New York State Department of Health
      AIDS Institute, 215
   opportunistic infections, 213
   quality of NP care, 217–220
   renal disease, 220
   specialists, 214
   substance use, 220
Human subjects, recruitment, retention
   of, 241
Hypertension, 35

I
ICIC. *See* Improving Chronic Illness
   Care

Impaired physician, 245
Improving Chronic Illness Care, 329
Indemnity plan reimbursement, 285
Independence Foundation, 187
Independent practice association, 273
Infection, 35
Informed consent, 244
Initiative on Future of Nursing
   Committee, 4
Institute for Healthcare Improvement,
   329
Institute for Nursing Center, 330
Institute of Medicine, 4
Institute of Medicine of National
   Academies, 384
Insurers, negotiating with, resources for,
   312
Integrity, 245
Interdisciplinary outcomes research, 107
International Council of Nursing, 32,
   338, 386
   Nurse Practitioner Advanced Practice
      Network, 386
International Nurse Practitioner/
   Advanced Practice Nursing
   Network, 34, 338
International organization Web sites,
   386–387
Internet as news source, 57
IOM. *See* Institute of Medicine of
   National Academies
IPA. *See* Independent practice
   association
Ireland, 363–374
   areas of practice, 367–368
   career pathway, 366–369
   Department of Health and Children,
      363–364
   economic challenges, 364
   educational preparation, 369
   emergency department exemplar,
      369–373
   funding of public health care, 363

Health Act, 363–364
Health Service Executive, 364
ionizing radiation, 365–366
levels of practice, 369
medication prescriptive authority,
    365–366
midwives, 364
National Council for Professional
    Development of Nursing and
    Midwifery, 364
prescribing of medications, 365–366
registered nurses, 364
regulatory policy, 39
research, 365
socioeconomic issues, 364
unemployment, 364
Ivins, Molly, 155

J
Johnson, Lyndon B., 149–150
Joint dialogue groups, 130
Justice, 244

K
Kaiser Family Foundation, 190
Kaiser Permanente, 384
Kissick, William, 70
Kitzman, Harriet, 7

L
LDL-C. *See* Low density lipoprotein-
    cholesterol
Legal consultants, 121–123
Lewis, Charles, 7
Licensure, 38–39, 138–139
    levels of, 138
LIFE Program. *See* Living Independently
    For Elders Program
Living Independently For Elders
    Program, 263
Loan forgiveness, 173
Lobbying efforts, 121–123
Long-term outcomes research, 93–110

acute care/transitional care, 94–96
    activities of daily living, 96
    acute care nurse practitioners, 94
    deep vein thrombosis, 94
    randomized controlled trial, 95
chronic disease management, 96–98
    low density lipoprotein-cholesterol,
        97
    total cholesterol levels, 97
conceptual/methodological challenges,
    99–104
    design, 99–101
    intervention effectiveness, 103–104
    long-term outcomes, 101–103
    methods, 99–101
    obtaining clarity in theoretical
        framework, 99
electronic medical record, 105
emerging health information, 105–106
interdisciplinary outcomes research,
    107
practice preparation, 107–108
social determinants of health equity,
    106
studies of long-term outcomes, 94–98
Low density lipoprotein-cholesterol, 97
Lynaugh, Joan, 7, 86

M
Made to Stick, 55
Making Room in the Clinic, 6
Managed care, 168–169, 183–198,
        273–275, 295–304
    bonus payment plans, 275
    clinical privileges, 274
    consumer-driven health plans, 30
    consumers, 273–274
    contract, 274
    contracting, 300–301
    credentialing, 300–301
    financial arrangements, 274–275
    future of, 301–303
    health savings accounts, 301–302

high deductible health plans, 301–302
malpractice insurance, 274
Medicare Modernization Act, 301
percentage of payment to physician, 275
risk sharing, 274
role of advanced-practice nurses, 274
values, 299–300
MANP. *See* Massachusetts Association of Nurse Practitioners
Maori population, health care for, 348–349
Massachusetts Association of Nurse Practitioners, 164
Massachusetts Coalition of Nurse Practitioners, 115–116
Massachusetts health care reform, 113–123
  An Act Providing Access to Affordable, Quality, Accountable Health Care, 114–115
  An Act to Promote Cost Containment, Transparency and Efficiency in the Delivery of Quality Health Care, 118
  Callahan, Jennifer, 117
  grassroots efforts, 121–123
  legal consultants, 121–123
  legislative efforts, 117–119
  lobbying efforts, 121–123
  Massachusetts Coalition of Nurse Practitioners, 115–116
  Minute Clinics, 117
  Murray, Therese, 118
  political action committee efforts, 121–123
  Rourke, Nancy, 116
  transformative effect on health care, 115–117
Massey University, 354
Master's program, 33, 173
Maternity Center Association, New York City, 5

McDonald, Cheryl, 266
McLane, Susan, 152
Medicaid, 146, 168–170, 261, 282
  policy changes in, 33
Medicare, 168–169, 271–272, 275–277, 285–289
  Advantage program, 282–283
  AMA Relative Value Update Committee, 276
  current procedural terminology coding system, 276
  fee schedule, 276–277
Medicare Payment Advisory Committee, 275
  Modernization Act, 301
  policy changes in, 33
Medicare part B, 279–280
  "incident to" billing under, 281
  payment structure, 273
Medicine's Dilemmas: Infinite Needs vs. Finite Resources, 70
Medoff-Cooper, Barbara, 85
Messaging, 54–56
  Made to Stick, 55
Michigan State University Sustained Partnership Model, 326–327
Military health insurance, 284
Ministry of Health and Nursing Council of New Zealand, 345
Minute Clinics, 117, 265
MNP. *See* Massachusetts Coalition of Nurse Practitioners
Model for Differentiated Nursing Practice, 23
Models of ethical decision-making, 250–251
Momentum in organizations, 266–268
  transformations in organizations, 266
Moral dilemma, 241
Moral distress, 242
Moral uncertainty, 241
Morrison, Cliff, 214–215

Murray, Therese, 118
Myers, Maynard, 151–152

N
NANCS. *See* National Association of
    Clinical Nurse Specialists
NAPNAP. *See* National Association of
    Pediatric Nurse Practitioners
National Association of Clinical Nurse
    Specialists, 130, 137
National Association of Nurse
    Practitioners in Women's
    Health, 380
National Association of Pediatric Nurse
    Practitioners, 380
National Center for Complementary and
    Alternative Medicine, 227
National Certification Corporation, 128
National Certification Corporation for
    Obstetric, Gynecological, and
    Neonatal Nursing Specialties,
    134
National Commission for Study of
    Nursing and Nursing Education,
    4
National Committee for Quality
    Assurance, 331
National Council for Professional
    Development of Nursing and
    Midwifery, 364
National Council of State Boards of
    Nursing, 22, 128, 130, 205–206,
    381
  Advanced-Practice Registered Nurses,
    381
National League for Nursing, 383
National League for Nursing Accrediting
    Commission, 128, 130, 136–137
National League of Nursing, 136
National Nursing Centers Consortium,
    188–189, 384
National Organization of Nurse
    Practitioner Faculties, 23, 32,
    137, 150, 317, 383

NCC. *See* National Certification
    Corporation for Obstetric,
    Gynecological, and Neonatal
    Nursing Specialties
NCCAM. *See* National Center for
    Complementary and Alternative
    Medicine
NCNM. *See* National Council for
    Professional Development of
    Nursing and Midwifery
NCSBN. *See* National Council of State
    Boards of Nursing
NCSBN APRN Advisory Committee
    Representatives, 130
Negotiating with insurers, resources for,
    312
New Hampshire, 151–152
New regulatory model, 129–133
New South Wales, health care in, 340
New York State Department of Health
    AIDS Institute, 215
New Zealand, 345–361
  Auckland University of Technology,
    354
  District Health Boards, 346–352
  Eastern Institute of Technology, 354
  establishing practices in, 356–358
  general practitioners, 347–348,
    350–352
  health care in, 340
  health care system, 346–348
  health disparities in, 348–349
    South Pacific Island populations,
    348–349
    Treaty of Waitangi, 348
  Maori, 348–349
  Massey University, 354
  Ministry of Health and Nursing
    Council of New Zealand, 345
  nurse practitioners in U.S., New
    Zealand, comparison, 353–355
  Otago Polytechnic, 354
  policies, 355–356

primary health care strategy, 349–350
primary healthcare organizations, 348, 350–352
regulations, 355–356
regulatory policy, 39
reimbursement, 355–356
South Pacific Island population, 348–349
training programs, 354
University of Auckland, 354
University of Otago, 354
Victoria University of Wellington, 354
Waikato Institute of Technology, 354
NLN. *See* National League for Nursing; National League of Nursing
NLNAC. *See* National League for Nursing Accrediting Commission
NMHCs. *See* Nurse-managed health centers
NNCC. *See* National Nursing Centers Consortium
NONPF. *See* National Organization of Nurse Practitioner Faculties
Norway, health care in, 341
Norwood, Susan, 52
NPDB. *See* Nurse Practitioner Data Bank
NPWH. *See* National Association of Nurse Practitioners in Women's Health
Number of NPs in United States, 31
Nurse-managed health centers, 183–198
    American Association of Colleges of Nursing, 191
    Breckinridge, Mary, 185
    challenges, 187–188
    Community Migrant Health Centers, 193
    Consolidated Health Center Plan, 194
    designation by FQHC, 194–195
    disparities in health care, 190–191
    Division of Nursing, Bureau of Health Professions, 185–187
    Federally Qualified Health Center, 188, 193–195
    financial sustainability, 192–193
    Ford, Loretta, 186
    future developments, 195–196
    Health Care for Homeless Programs, 193
    Health Plan Employer Data and Information Set, 188–189
    Health Resources and Services Administration, U.S. Department of Health and Human Services, 186
    Henry Street Settlement, 185
    Independence Foundation, 187
    Kaiser Family Foundation, 190
    medically underserved area/ populations, 193
    National Nursing Centers Consortium, 188–189
    nurse-managed primary health center, 184–185
    patients served, 189–190
    policy recommendations, 195–196
    Regional Nursing Centers Consortium, 187
    role in nursing education, 191
    safety net providers, role as, 189
    Silver, Henry, 186
    staffing, 191
    Wald, Lillian, 185
    workplace gap, filling, 191–192
Nurse midwifery, 34
Nurse Practitioner Data Bank, Healthcare Integrity and Protection Data Bank, 381
Nurse practitioner development model, 34
"Nurse Practitioners, Physician Assistants, and Certified Nurse-Midwives," 72–73
Nurse Training Acts, 7
Nursing Against the Odds, 53

Nursing career advancement, 36–38
Nursing Council of New Zealand, 340
Nursing homes, 32
Nursing regulatory bodies, 38–39

O
Occupational Health and Safety
  Administration, 169
OEF. *See* Operation Enduring Freedom
Office of Technology Assessment, 72–73
OIF. *See* Operation Iraqi Freedom
Olds, David, 7
Online claims billing, 265–266
Online resources, 379–387
Operation Enduring Freedom, veterans
  returning from, 235–237
Operation Iraqi Freedom, veterans
  returning from, 235–237
Organ transplant services, 32
Organizing frameworks, 325–328
OTA. *See* Office of Technology
  Assessment; U.S. Office of
  Technology Assessment
Otago Polytechnic, 354
Outcomes research, 78–81

P
PAC. *See* Political Action Committee
Participating in therapies, 209
Partnering with communities, 36
Partnerships with consumer
  organizations, 43–48
Pathogen-borne illnesses, 35
Patient advocacy goals, 240–241
Patient safety, 317–333
  Agency for Healthcare Quality and
    Research, 330
  benchmarks, 324
  Centers for Medicare and Medicaid
    Services, 330–331
  Chronic Care Model, 327–328
  Commonwealth Fund Commission on
    High Performance Health
    System, 319–322

  Doctor of Nursing Practice, 317
  electronic health records, 323–324
  To Err is Human, 319
  feedback loops, 325
  Improving Chronic Illness Care, 329
  Institute for Healthcare Improvement,
    329
  Institute for Nursing Center, 330
  institutional support, 323
  Michigan State University Sustained
    Partnership Model, 326–327
  National Committee for Quality
    Assurance, 331
  National Organization of Nurse
    Practitioner Faculties, 317
  organizing frameworks, 325–328
  planned intervention, 324–325
  Quality and Safety Education for
    Nurses, 330
  quality measures, 330–331
  resources, 329
Payment systems, 271–294
  American Medical Association, 277
  Balanced Budget Act, 271
  billing coding systems, 277–278
  certified nurse midwives, 273
  chronic care management, 290–291
  direct Medicare reimbursement,
    271–272
  Federal Employee Health Benefit Plan,
    284–285
  federally qualified health centers,
    283–384
  hospital services, 280–281
  indemnity plan reimbursement, 285
  independent practice association, 273
  managed care, 273–275
    bonus payment plans, 275
    clinical privileges, 274
    consumers, 273–274
    contract, 274
    financial arrangements, 274–275
    malpractice insurance, 274

percentage of payment to physician, 275
risk sharing, 274
role of advanced-practice nurses, 274
Medicaid, 282
Medicare, 275–277, 285–289
AMA Relative Value Update Committee, 276
current procedural terminology coding system, 276
fee schedule, 276–277
Medicare Payment Advisory Committee, 275
Medicare Advantage program, 282–283
Medicare part B, 279–280
"incident to" billing under, 281
payment structure, 273
military health insurance, 284
payment issues, 285–289
payment mechanisms, 272–273
potential payment, 289–291
Program for All-Inclusive Care for Elderly model, 283
provider payment incentives, 289–290
readjustment of fee for service, 289
resource-based relative value scale process, 278–279
Social Security Act, 279
transitional care model, 291
TRICARE, 284
Pearson Report, 167
Pearson Report, 138
Pediatric diabetes, 199–204. *See also* Diabetes
Pediatric Nursing Certification Board, 128
Pension examination program, 226–227
Perceptional change, 50–51
Physician supply, 31, 161–162
PICC catheter-related infections, 231
Planned intervention, 324–325

Pluralistic workforce, 31
Policy organization websites, 383–386
Political action committee efforts, 121–123
Political contexts, 260–261
Postoperative surgical patients, 32
Posttraumatic stress disorder, 234
symptom levels, 234
Practice organization websites, 382–383
Prescriptive authority, 144–145, 149–158
Great Society initiatives, 149–150
Hastings, Marguerite, 151–152
Ivins, Molly, 155
Johnson, Lyndon B., 149–150
McLane, Susan, 152
Myers, Maynard, 151–152
New Hampshire, 151–152
Richards, Ann, 153
Texas, 152–155
Texas Coalition for Nurses in Advanced Practice, 154
TMA Political Action Committee, 155
Press release, writing, 58–59
Becoming Influential, A Guide for Nurses, 59
case study, 59–60
Pressure to prescribe, 245
Primary care, 5–6, 170–171
Procedural terminology coding system, 75–76
Program diversity, 174–175
Program of All-Inclusive Care for Elders model of care, 8–9, 263, 283
PTSD. *See* Posttraumatic stress disorder
Public relations, 49–61
Bartol, Tom, 59
Curtis, Val, 51
Faso, Burkina, 51
Global Public-Private Partnership for Handwashing with Soap, Ghana, 51
Goffman, Erving, 53

Gordon, Suzanne, 53
messaging, 54–56
  Made to Stick, 55
Norwood, Susan, 52
Nursing Against the Odds, 53
perceptional change, 50–51
reaching audience, 56–58
  Facebook, 56
  Gallup poll, 57
  Internet as news source, 57
  local news, 57
  Twitter, 56
Sigma Theta Tau International, 52
Waters, David, 54
writing press release, 58–59
  Becoming Influential, A Guide for Nurses, 59
  case study, 59–60

Q
Quality and Safety Education for Nurses, 330
Quality of care, 35, 317–333
  Agency for Healthcare Quality and Research, 330
  benchmarks, 324
  Centers for Medicare and Medicaid Services, 330–331
  Chronic Care Model, 327–328
  Commonwealth Fund Commission on High Performance Health System, 319–322
  Doctor of Nursing Practice, 317
  electronic health records, 323–324
  To Err is Human, 319
  feedback loops, 325
  Improving Chronic Illness Care, 329
  Institute for Healthcare Improvement, 329
  Institute for Nursing Center, 330
  institutional support, 323
  Michigan State University Sustained Partnership Model, 326–327
  National Committee for Quality Assurance, 331
  National Organization of Nurse Practitioner Faculties, 317
  organizing frameworks, 325–328
  planned intervention, 324–325
  Quality and Safety Education for Nurses, 330
  quality measures, 330–331
  resources, 329

R
Randomized controlled trial, 95
RCN. *See* Royal College of Nursing
RCT. *See* Randomized controlled trial
Reaching audience, 56–58
  Facebook, 56
  Gallup poll, 57
  Internet as news source, 57
  local news, 57
  Twitter, 56
Readjustment of fee for service, 289
Realtime ultrasound, 231
Regional Nursing Centers Consortium, 187
Registered Nurse Sample Survey, 31
Regulation, 38–39
Reimbursement, 39, 165–169
Reinhard, Susan, 43–48
Report of Surgeon General Consultant Group on Nursing, 4
Research, 65–92
  competition, 68–70, 73–74
  context, 66–67
  cost, 71–73
  Crossing the Quality Chasm, 87
  current procedural terminology coding system, 75–76
  exemplars, 67–68

Fairman, Julie A., 85–87
future developments, 82–83
Graduate Medical Education, Nursing, and Allied Professions Commission, 72
innovations, 70–76
innovative models, 75–76
international agenda, 83–84
Kissick, William, 70
Lynaugh, Joan, 86
Medicine's Dilemmas: Infinite Needs vs. Finite Resources, 70
Medoff-Cooper, Barbara, 85
"Nurse Practitioners, Physician Assistants, and Certified Nurse-Midwives," 72–73
Office of Technology Assessment, 72–73
   "Nurse Practitioners, Physician Assistants, and Certified Nurse-Midwives," 72–73
outcomes research, 78–81
procedural terminology coding system, 75–76
proving worth, 66–70
quality, 71–73
social context, 66
Sullivan-Marx, Eileen M., 85–87
Thomas F. Gailor Out-Patient Clinics, 68
Resnick, Barbara, 7
Resource-based relative value scale process, 278–279
Resources for negotiating with insurers, 312
Respect for patient, 240–241, 244
Retail care clinics, 265
Retail convenience clinics, 36
Richards, Ann, 153
RNCC. *See* Regional Nursing Centers Consortium

Robert Wood Johnson Foundation, 4–5, 7, 43–48, 385
   Initiative on Future of Nursing, 385
Rourke, Nancy, 116
Royal College of Nursing, 339

S
Safety issues. *See* Patient safety
School of Nursing Penn Nursing Network, University of Pennsylvania, 260
Serotonin reuptake inhibitors, 209
Sigma Theta Tau International, 52, 386–387
Silver, Henry, 17, 186
Simplification, 261–264
Singapore Ministry of Health, 340
Social costs of diabetes, 202
Social determinants, health equity, 106
Social Security Act, 279
South Pacific Island population, New Zealand health care for, 348–349
Spheres of interaction, 33–34
Standardization, 175–176
   goal of, 23–36
Standards of Clinical Practice, and Scope of Practice for Acute Care Nurse Practitioner, 22
State borders, standardized practice, 39
State environment, 165–168
Statement on Clinical Nurse Specialist Practice and Education, 137
Sub-Saharan Africa, health care in, 341
Sullivan-Marx, Eileen M., 32, 43, 85–87
Switzerland, health care in, 341

T
Taiwan
   health care in, 340
   regulatory policy, 39
Technology accelerators, 265–266
Telehealth communication, 265–266

TEX-PAC. *See* TMA Political Action
  Committee
Texas, 152–155
  nurse practitioner regulation, 143–148
  Coalition for Nurses in Advanced
    Practice, 145
  education, 146–147
  Medicaid, 146
  prescriptive authority, 144–145
  professional organization
    development, 145
  Texas Board of Nursing, 143–144
  Texas Higher Education Coordinating
    Board, 146–147
  Texas Nursing Practice Act, 145
Texas Board of Nursing, 143–144
Texas Coalition for Nurses in Advanced
  Practice, 154
Texas Higher Education Coordinating
  Board, 146–147
Texas Nursing Practice Act, 145
Thailand, regulatory policy, 39
THECB. *See* Texas Higher Education
  Coordinating Board
Thomas F. Gailor Out-Patient Clinics,
  68
Tipping point, factors creating, 377
TMA Political Action Committee, 155
To Err is Human, 319
Torrisi, Donna, 259
Total cholesterol levels, 97
Transformations in organizations, 266
Transitional care model, 291
Treaty of Waitangi, 348
TRICARE, 284
Twitter, 56

U
Underseved, access for, 306–310
United Kingdom
  health care in, 339
  regulatory policy, 39

United States Medical Licensing
  Examination, 135–136
University of Auckland, 354
University of Otago, 354
University of Pennsylvania, School of
  Nursing Penn Nursing Network,
  260
University of Pennsylvania School of
  Nursing, 262–263
U.S. Department of Health and Human
  Services, 186, 385–386
  Centers for Medicare Medicaid
    Services, 385–386
  Health Resources and Services
    Administration, 382, 386
U.S. Office of Technology Assessment,
  72–73
USMLE. *See* United States Medical
  Licensing Examination

V
Veterans Affairs, 223–238
  alternative medicine, 227–228
  ambulatory care, 224
  chronically ill mental health, 234
  compensation, 226–227
  complementary medicine, 227–228
  data, 224
  Eastern Colorado Health Care System
    Home-Based Primary Care
    Program, 229–230
  employees, 224
  future developments, 235–238
  gerontology, extended care centers,
    228–229
  home-based primary care, 229–230
  home care programs, 224
  informatics, 230–231
  interventional radiology, 231
  National Center for Complementary
    and Alternative Medicine, 227
  nurse managers, 231–232
  nurse practitioners, 224

nurse practitioners' roles, 226
nursing homes, 224
Operation Enduring Freedom,
    veterans returning from,
    235–237
Operation Iraqi Freedom, veterans
    returning from, 235–237
outpatient clinics, 224
pension examination program,
    226–227
PICC catheter-related infections, 231
posttraumatic stress disorder, 234
    symptom levels, 234
primary care, 232–234
programs, 224
projected U.S. veterans population,
    224
psychiatric care, 234–235
realtime ultrasound, 231

registered nurses, 224
residential rehabilitation treatment,
    224
Victoria University of Wellington, 354

W
Waikato Institute of Technology, 354
Wald, Lillian, 185
Waters, David, 54
Web sites of nurse practitioner
    organizations, 379–380
WHO. *See* World Health Organization
World Health Organization, 35, 387
Writing press release, 58–59
    *Becoming Influential, A Guide for
    Nurses,* 59
    case study, 59–60

Z
Zoster lesions, 208